New Trends in Sport and Exercise Medicine

New Trends in Sport and Exercise Medicine

Editor

Daniela Galli

MDPI • Basel • Beijing • Wuhan • Barcelona • Belgrade • Manchester • Tokyo • Cluj • Tianjin

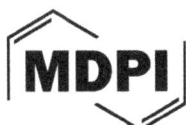

Editor
Daniela Galli
University of Parma
Italy

Editorial Office
MDPI
St. Alban-Anlage 66
4052 Basel, Switzerland

This is a reprint of articles from the Special Issue published online in the open access journal *Applied Sciences* (ISSN 2076-3417) (available at: https://www.mdpi.com/journal/applsci/special_issues/trends_in_sport_exercise_medicine).

For citation purposes, cite each article independently as indicated on the article page online and as indicated below:

LastName, A.A.; LastName, B.B.; LastName, C.C. Article Title. *Journal Name* **Year**, *Volume Number*, Page Range.

ISBN 978-3-0365-2502-0 (Hbk)
ISBN 978-3-0365-2503-7 (PDF)

© 2021 by the authors. Articles in this book are Open Access and distributed under the Creative Commons Attribution (CC BY) license, which allows users to download, copy and build upon published articles, as long as the author and publisher are properly credited, which ensures maximum dissemination and a wider impact of our publications.

The book as a whole is distributed by MDPI under the terms and conditions of the Creative Commons license CC BY-NC-ND.

Contents

About the Editor vii

Daniela Galli
Special Issue "New Trends in Sport and Exercise Medicine"
Reprinted from: *Appl. Sci.* **2021**, *11*, 8353, doi:10.3390/app11188353 1

Tanaka Kungwengwe and Richard Evans
Sana: A Gamified Rehabilitation Management System for Anterior Cruciate Ligament Reconstruction Recovery
Reprinted from: *Appl. Sci.* **2020**, *10*, 4868, doi:10.3390/app10144868 7

Andrea Di Credico, Pascal Izzicupo, Giulia Gaggi, Angela Di Baldassarre and Barbara Ghinassi
Effect of Physical Exercise on the Release of Microparticles with Angiogenic Potential
Reprinted from: *Appl. Sci.* **2020**, *10*, 4871, doi:10.3390/app10144871 27

Hyun Chul Jung, Nan Hee Lee, Young Chan Kim and Sukho Lee
The Effects of Wild Ginseng Extract on Psychomotor and Neuromuscular Performance Recovery Following Acute Eccentric Exercise: A Preliminary Study
Reprinted from: *Appl. Sci.* **2020**, *10*, 5839, doi:10.3390/app10175839 47

Vittoria Carnevale Pellino, Matteo Giuriato, Gabriele Ceccarelli, Roberto Codella, Matteo Vandoni, Nicola Lovecchio and Alan M. Nevill
Explosive Strength Modeling in Children: Trends According to Growth and Prediction Equation
Reprinted from: *Appl. Sci.* **2020**, *10*, 6430, doi:10.3390/app11186430 61

Sergio Sebastia-Amat, Alfonso Penichet-Tomas, Jose M. Jimenez-Olmedo and Basilio Pueo
Contributions of Anthropometric and Strength Determinants to Estimate 2000 m Ergometer Performance in Traditional Rowing
Reprinted from: *Appl. Sci.* **2020**, *10*, 6562, doi:10.3390/app10186562 71

Takuma Miyamoto, Yasushi Shinohara, Tomohiro Matsui, Hiroaki Kurokawa, Akira Taniguchi, Tsukasa Kumai and Yasuhito Tanaka
Effects of Achilles Tendon Moment Arm Length on Insertional Achilles Tendinopathy
Reprinted from: *Appl. Sci.* **2020**, *10*, 6631, doi:10.3390/app10196631 81

Moo Sung Kim and Jihong Park
Immediate Effects of an Inverted Body Position on Energy Expenditure and Blood Lactate Removal after Intense Running
Reprinted from: *Appl. Sci.* **2020**, *10*, 6645, doi:10.3390/app10196645 93

Fermín Valera-Garrido, Sergio Jiménez-Rubio, Francisco Minaya-Muñoz, José Luis Estévez-Rodríguez and Archit Navandar
Ultrasound-Guided Percutaneous Needle Electrolysis and Rehab and Reconditioning Program for Rectus Femoris Muscle Injuries: A Cohort Study with Professional Soccer Players and a 20-Week Follow-Up
Reprinted from: *Appl. Sci.* **2020**, *10*, 7912, doi:10.3390/app10217912 105

Juan Pablo Medellín Ruiz, Jacobo Ángel Rubio-Arias, Vicente Javier Clemente-Suarez and Domingo Jesús Ramos-Campo
Effectiveness of Training Prescription Guided by Heart Rate Variability Versus Predefined Training for Physiological and Aerobic Performance Improvements: A Systematic Review and Meta-Analysis
Reprinted from: *Appl. Sci.* **2020**, *10*, 8532, doi:10.3390/app10238532 123

Abdelaziz Ghanemi, Aicha Melouane, Mayumi Yoshioka and Jonny St-Amand
Exercise Training of Secreted Protein Acidic and Rich in Cysteine *(Sparc)* KO Mice Suggests That Exercise-Induced Muscle Phenotype Changes Are SPARC-Dependent
Reprinted from: *Appl. Sci.* **2020**, *10*, 9108, doi:10.3390/app10249108 139

Sung-Woo Kim, Myong-Won Seo, Hyun-Chul Jung and Jong-Kook Song
Effects of High-Impact Weight-Bearing Exercise on Bone Mineral Density and Bone Metabolism in Middle-Aged Premenopausal Women: A Randomized Controlled Trial
Reprinted from: *Appl. Sci.* **2021**, *11*, 846, doi:10.3390/app11020846 163

Daniela Galli, Cecilia Carubbi, Elena Masselli, Mauro Vaccarezza, Valentina Presta, Giulia Pozzi, Luca Ambrosini, Giuliana Gobbi, Marco Vitale and Prisco Mirandola
Physical Activity and Redox Balance in the Elderly: Signal Transduction Mechanisms
Reprinted from: *Appl. Sci.* **2021**, *11*, 2228, doi:10.3390/app11052228 175

Oscar F. Araneda, Franz Kosche-Cárcamo, Humberto Verdugo-Marchese and Marcelo Tuesta
Pulmonary Effects Due to Physical Exercise in Polluted Air: Evidence from Studies Conducted on Healthy Humans
Reprinted from: *Appl. Sci.* **2021**, *11*, 2890, doi:10.3390/app11072890 193

Dongmin Lee, Kyengho Byun, Moon-Hyon Hwang and Sewon Lee
Augmentation Index Is Inversely Associated with Skeletal Muscle Mass, Muscle Strength, and Anaerobic Power in Young Male Adults: A Preliminary Study
Reprinted from: *Appl. Sci.* **2021**, *11*, 3146, doi:10.3390/app11073146 205

José Raúl Hoyos-Flores, Blanca R. Rangel-Colmenero, Zeltzin N. Alonso-Ramos, Myriam Z. García-Dávila, Rosa M. Cruz-Castruita, José Naranjo-Orellana and Germán Hernández-Cruz
The Role of Cholinesterases in Post-Exercise HRV Recovery in University Volleyball Players
Reprinted from: *Appl. Sci.* **2021**, *11*, 4188, doi:10.3390/app11094188 215

Melania Gaggini, Cristina Vassalle, Fabrizia Carli, Maristella Maltinti, Laura Sabatino, Emma Buzzigoli, Francesca Mastorci, Francesco Sbrana, Amalia Gastaldelli and Alessandro Pingitore
Changes in Plasma Bioactive Lipids and Inflammatory Markers during a Half-Marathon in Trained Athletes
Reprinted from: *Appl. Sci.* **2021**, *11*, 4622, doi:10.3390/app11104622 225

About the Editor

Daniela Galli In 1997, she obtained a single-cycle master's degree in Biological Sciences cum laude from "La Sapienza" University (Rome, IT). In December 2000, she obtained a diploma of specialization in Applied Genetics, and in 2004, she obtained a PhD in Morphogenetic and Cytological Sciences from "La Sapienza" University. From 2005 to 2007, she was awarded a post-doc fellow at Pasteur Institute (Paris, France). From 2007 to 2013, she spent time in Pavia and Parma as a post-doc fellow. From 2013–2017, she worked as a researcher at the University of Parma (Parma, IT). Since 2018, she has been an Associate Professor at the University of Parma. Her research themes cover subjects including stem cell application studies for the prevention and treatment of heart attacks, mechanisms of cardiogenesis, and tissue engineering studies for bone regeneration. Her most recent publications also concern anthropometric evaluations of children in relation to diet and sport and postural and metabolic studies in elite athletes.

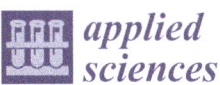

Editorial

Special Issue "New Trends in Sport and Exercise Medicine"

Daniela Galli

Department of Medicine and Surgery, University of Parma, 43125 Parma, Italy; daniela.galli@unipr.it

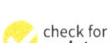

Citation: Galli, D. Special Issue "New Trends in Sport and Exercise Medicine". *Appl. Sci.* **2021**, *11*, 8353. https://doi.org/10.3390/app11188353

Received: 30 August 2021
Accepted: 6 September 2021
Published: 9 September 2021

Publisher's Note: MDPI stays neutral with regard to jurisdictional claims in published maps and institutional affiliations.

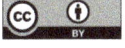

Copyright: © 2021 by the author. Licensee MDPI, Basel, Switzerland. This article is an open access article distributed under the terms and conditions of the Creative Commons Attribution (CC BY) license (https://creativecommons.org/licenses/by/4.0/).

1. Introduction

The practice of regular physical activity has been proposed as a determinant in many disciplines, from wellness to physiotherapy; in fact, it reduces the risks of cardiovascular diseases and diabetes. Moreover, physical exercise decreases the incidence of some types of cancer, such as breast and colon cancer. Finally, rehabilitation protocols need correct exercise training to reach the complete "return to play" of the patients. Unfortunately, the mechanisms associated with the beneficial effects of physical activity are still under study. Therefore, advances in all aspects of sport and exercise medicine will be relevant for physicians, recreational sport practitioners and elite athletes.

This was the aim of this Special Issue "New trends in sport and exercise medicine", that achieved great success. Sixteen papers have been published, which are briefly described below. They range from mobile applications in physiotherapy to changes in bioactive lipids in half-marathoners [1–16].

However, sport and exercise medicine are wide subjects and require more papers to clarify their different aspects. Therefore, we proposed a new Special Issue (https://www.mdpi.com/journal/applsci/special_issues/Sport_Exercise_Medicine_II, accessed on 8 September 2021) to continue on this path and receive new insights in sport and exercise medicine.

2. Sana: A Gamified Rehabilitation Management System for Anterior Cruciate Ligament Reconstruction Recovery

The Anterior Cruciate Ligament (ACL) surgery reconstruction is necessary in approximately 76.6% of ACL ruptures. The rehabilitation following ACL reconstruction includes long-term programs that are often performed at home by patients, without supervision. The failure of rehabilitation programs increases the onset of secondary pathologies in the years after surgery. In this paper, Kungwengwe and Evans [1] studied a mobile application, called Sana, based on gamification theory, to improve the results of post-operative physiotherapy after ACL reconstruction. The program content is based on the Royal National Orthopedic Hospital guidelines for ACL rupture reconstruction. The data show that the patients are satisfied with the application, find it convenient, engaging and user-friendly, and that physiotherapists state that the system improves therapy administration and interactions with the patients, suggesting that the Sana system can make a positive contribution to ACL rupture post-surgery rehabilitation.

3. Effect of Physical Exercise on the Release of Microparticles with Angiogenic Potential

Microparticles (MP) are extracellular vesicles involved in cell-to-cell communications. They are present in physiological conditions, but their levels change in response to oxidative stress, inflammation, hypoxia and shear stress. Interestingly, these situations are also caused by physical activity. Notably, microparticles induced by physical activity are involved in angiogenesis. Di Credico et al. [2] reviewed the effects of different types of exercise on microparticle release in correlation with new vessel formation. Although training status, drugs and disease can affect microparticle formation, future studies will be necessary to clarify the effect of acute and chronic exercise on vascular adaptations.

4. The Effects of Wild Ginseng Extract on Psychomotor and Neuromuscular Performance Recovery Following Acute Eccentric Exercise: A Preliminary Study

Ginseng is a widely diffused anti-inflammatory agent with positive actions on the nervous system and cognitive function. Thus, it is a reasonable alternative to decrease exercise-induced inflammation. Jung et al. [3] studied the effect of ginseng extract (700 mg/day) on psychomotor and muscular performance after acute eccentric exercise. Although they only found a significant decrease in exercise-induced inflammatory markers such as Interleukin-6 (IL-6), this preliminary study opens new issues, which a future project, with a large sample, will elucidate.

5. Explosive Strength Modeling in Children: Trends According to Growth and Prediction Equation

Strength training is usually only performed in adults. Recently, the relevance of muscular strength in youth and adolescents has been shown to prevent cardiovascular diseases, metabolic disorders and obesity. However, it is very important to monitor developmental aspects in parallel with training and increases in performance. Looking at this scenario, Carnevale Pellino et al. [4] elaborated a model of predictive equations to correlate anthropometric parameters, fitness levels and the maturation of children.

This will provide practical suggestions for coaches who should consider age, body shape and body mass for strength training and, in particular, lower limb performance.

6. Contributions of Anthropometric and Strength Determinants to Estimate 2000 m Ergometer Performance in Traditional Rowing

Traditional rowing is a widely diffused sport, and many scientists are studying the importance of physiological characteristics to optimize the rowers' performance. Although, to date, the papers were focused on Olympic rowing, the paper by Sebastia-Amat et al. [5] analyzes the contribution of physical determinants such as height, body mass and strength of the lower/upper body on row ergometer performance in traditional rowing. The authors found that higher anthropometric determinants were positively correlated with higher performance, but upper body strength factors (determined by bench pull training) showed the best correlation with positive performance, evidencing the role of upper body strength in rowing execution.

7. Effects of Achilles Tendon Moment Arm Length on Insertional Achilles Tendinopathy

The Achilles tendon is the largest tendon in the body, and it is very important in the gait cycle because it links the ankle joint to the triceps surae. The insertional Achilles tendinopathy (IAT) is a painful chronic disorder that requires suture bridge surgical therapy. This technique is still under investigation and its level of effectiveness is unclear. Miyamoto et al. [6] performed a retrospective study to analyze the moment arm length in both healthy subjects and in post-operative patients. They observed a significant increase in the force of the IAT group after surgery, suggesting that a long moment arm is one of the causes of IAT and that suture bridge surgery is an effective technique that reduces the Achilles tendon moment arm.

8. Immediate Effects of an Inverted Body Position on Energy Expenditure and Blood Lactate Removal after Intense Running

Overtraining and overreaching are challenges for all athletes. Thus, physiological and psychological recoveries after training are important for health and optimal performance.

Kim and Park [7] studied the effect of a cool-down strategy with an inverted body position (IBP) on fatigue perception, blood lactate concentration and heart rate in 22 athletes. While the fatigue perception was not significantly modified by this recovery technique, blood lactate level and energy expenditure were significantly lower than in controls, suggesting that this technique could be useful in many disciplines that have short breaks during matches, such as martial arts and wrestling.

9. Ultrasound-Guided Percutaneous Needle Electrolysis and Rehab and Reconditioning Program for Rectus Femoris Muscle Injuries: A Cohort Study with Professional Soccer Players and a 20-Week Follow-Up

One of the most common sports injuries is rectus femoris muscle strain. Therefore, it is very important to elaborate rehabilitation programs that can induce a fast "return to play" in the athletes. Valera-Garrido et al. [8] studied the effects of a combination of percutaneous needle electrolysis and a specific rehabilitation program in professional soccer players with Rectus femoris muscle strain. The authors demonstrated that the combination of the two techniques permitted a safe "return to play", with no re-injuries seen in a long-term check.

10. Effectiveness of Training Prescription Guided by Heart Rate Variability Versus Predefined Training for Physiological and Aerobic Performance Improvements: A Systematic Review and Meta-Analysis

During physical activity, the balance between the training load and the physiological responses to training, including neuromuscular and cardiovascular activity, is very important. Mendellin Ruiz et al. [9] conducted a systematic review comparing the effects of heart-rate variability-guided training versus a predefined training designed to optimize the aerobic performance of athletes.

Although they did not find significant differences between the two training methods, this review evidences the potential of the heart-rate variability methodology, suggesting that additional studies are necessary to specify the physiological effects of this method with respect to the generally used strategies.

11. Exercise Training of Secreted Protein Acidic and Rich in Cysteine (Sparc) KO Mice Suggests That Exercise-Induced Muscle Phenotype Changes Are SPARC-Dependent

The beneficial effects of physical exercise have been well documented, but the molecular basis of these positive outcomes is still unclear. One of the proteins induced by exercise is Secreted Protein Acidic and Rich in Cysteine (SPARC). Ghanemi et al. [10] performed functional studies in *Sparc null* mice, showing that muscle strength and performance are SPARC-dependent. Future studies on the roles of exercise-related proteins in muscle physiology and diseases will be important to clarify the benefits of physical activity for human health. In fact, all these mediator proteins represent potential molecular targets for pharmacological therapy.

12. Effects of High-Impact Weight-Bearing Exercise on Bone Mineral Density and Bone Metabolism in Middle-Aged Premenopausal Women: A Randomized Controlled Trial

Osteoporosis is a serious problem in western countries. High-impact exercise seems to be important for bone mass increase, but the majority of studies were performed in post-menopausal women. Prevention of the onset of osteoporosis would also be important to characterize the effects of high-impact exercise on middle-aged, pre-menopausal women. Kim et al. [11] performed this type of study and showed that a physical activity program (intensity set at 60–80% of maximal heart rate) reduces age-associated changes in bone markers, although it does not increase the bone mineral density.

13. Physical Activity and Redox Balance in the Elderly: Signal Transduction Mechanisms

Reactive Oxygen Species and cellular antioxidant machinery are very important in studies of age-associated diseases. Physical exercise stimulates both these components, creating contrasting effects. The intensity and volume of the exercise, together with the physiological characteristics of the people, seem to be the most important parameters. To better characterize the molecular pathways correlated with the oxidant/antioxidant effects of exercise, Galli et al. [12] reviewed the existent literature on this subject. Although more studies will be necessary to reach a comprehensive view of all the involved pathways, the authors evidenced that, in the future, precision medicine will be able to administer physical activity in a personalized way, transforming wellness in targeted prevention.

14. Pulmonary Effects Due to Physical Exercise in Polluted Air: Evidence from Studies Conducted on Healthy Humans

Air pollution is associated with many chronic diseases (cancer, pulmonary disorders, etc.). However, outdoor physical activity is widely diffused in countries with high levels of pollution. Araneda et al. [13] reviewed the studies conducted on healthy people who performed physical activity in environments with low air quality. The authors concluded that exercise should be performed in safe environmental conditions by reducing pollution, increasing installation of correct filters in gyms and increasing mobile stations for urban races to monitor the load of pollutants.

15. Augmentation Index Is Inversely Associated with Skeletal Muscle Mass, Muscle Strength, and Anaerobic Power in Young Male Adults: A Preliminary Study

Arterial stiffness is correlated with performance parameters such as cardiorespiratory endurance and muscle strength. In fact, the increase in cardiorespiratory endurance reduces body mass index, low-density lipoprotein cholesterol and systolic blood pressure, which represent significant risk factors for cardiovascular disease. In young adults, this correlation is still unclear; thus, Lee et al. [14] investigated the relationship between muscle strength parameters and arterial stiffness in young males. They showed an inverse significant correlation with one of the parameters used to measure arterial stiffness, such as the Augmentation index, suggesting that strength training in young adults contributes to changes in arterial stiffness.

16. The Role of Cholinesterases in Post-Exercise HRV Recovery in University Volleyball Players

Exercise recovery is a complex process that depends on the equilibrium between the sympathetic and the parasympathetic branches of the autonomous nervous system on the heart rate. Notably, the parasympathetic branch slows the heart rate through the increase in acelylcholine release and, therefore, the activation of the Acetylcholinesterase enzyme that is abundant in the sino-atrial node. The levels of Acetylcholinesterase are generally indirectly measured by Cholinesterase in the blood. Hoyos-Flores et al. [15] found a positive correlation between heart rate variability and Cholinesterase levels after long-term and intermittent high-intensity training in volleyball players, suggesting that Cholinesterase and heart rate could be considered as the internal load of the recovery phases after training.

17. Changes in Plasma Bioactive Lipids and Inflammatory Markers during a Half-Marathon in Trained Athletes

After a competitive marathon cytokines, inflammation and oxidative stress increase in athletes. However, the relationship between bioactive lipids and inflammatory mediators is still uncharacterized. Gaggini et al. [16] studied the levels of Ceramides, Diacylglycerols and Sphingomyelin, together with inflammatory markers in athletes, after a half-marathon. Although they did not find a significant correlation between bioactive lipids and inflammatory markers, they observed a significant decrease in lipids after a race, suggesting that these molecules could represent new biomarkers to characterize exercise adaptation and evaluate specific training for different subject categories.

Funding: This research received no external funding.

Acknowledgments: I wish to thank all the authors and the reviewers who have contributed to this Special Issue. Additionally, I wish to thank the Editor in Chief and the editorial office of the journal. Finally, special thanks go to Sara Zhan, my Assistant Editor, who helped me in all the different phases of preparation of this Special Issue.

Conflicts of Interest: The author declares no conflict of interest.

References

1. Kungwengwe, T.; Evans, R. Sana: A Gamified Rehabilitation Management System for Anterior Cruciate Ligament Reconstruction Recovery. *Appl. Sci.* **2020**, *10*, 4868. [CrossRef]
2. Di Credico, A.; Izzicupo, P.; Gaggi, G.; Di Baldassarre, A.; Ghinassi, B. Effect of Physical Exercise on the Release of Microparticles with Angiogenic Potential. *Appl. Sci.* **2020**, *10*, 4871. [CrossRef]
3. Jung, H.; Lee, N.; Kim, Y.; Lee, S. The Effects of Wild Ginseng Extract on Psychomotor and Neuromuscular Performance Recovery Following Acute Eccentric Exercise: A Preliminary Study. *Appl. Sci.* **2020**, *10*, 5839. [CrossRef]
4. Carnevale Pellino, V.; Giuriato, M.; Ceccarelli, G.; Codella, R.; Vandoni, M.; Lovecchio, N.; Nevill, A. Explosive Strength Modeling in Children: Trends According to Growth and Prediction Equation. *Appl. Sci.* **2020**, *10*, 6430. [CrossRef]
5. Sebastia-Amat, S.; Penichet-Tomas, A.; Jimenez-Olmedo, J.; Pueo, B. Contributions of Anthropometric and Strength Determinants to Estimate 2000 m Ergometer Performance in Traditional Rowing. *Appl. Sci.* **2020**, *10*, 6562. [CrossRef]
6. Miyamoto, T.; Shinohara, Y.; Matsui, T.; Kurokawa, H.; Taniguchi, A.; Kumai, T.; Tanaka, Y. Effects of Achilles Tendon Moment Arm Length on Insertional Achilles Tendinopathy. *Appl. Sci.* **2020**, *10*, 6631. [CrossRef]
7. Kim, M.; Park, J. Immediate Effects of an Inverted Body Position on Energy Expenditure and Blood Lactate Removal after Intense Running. *Appl. Sci.* **2020**, *10*, 6645. [CrossRef]
8. Valera-Garrido, F.; Jiménez-Rubio, S.; Minaya-Muñoz, F.; Estévez-Rodríguez, J.; Navandar, A. Ultrasound-Guided Percutaneous Needle Electrolysis and Rehab and Reconditioning Program for Rectus Femoris Muscle Injuries: A Cohort Study with Professional Soccer Players and a 20-Week Follow-Up. *Appl. Sci.* **2020**, *10*, 7912. [CrossRef]
9. Medellín Ruiz, J.; Rubio-Arias, J.; Clemente-Suarez, V.; Ramos-Campo, D. Effectiveness of Training Prescription Guided by Heart Rate Variability Versus Predefined Training for Physiological and Aerobic Performance Improvements: A Systematic Review and Meta-Analysis. *Appl. Sci.* **2020**, *10*, 8532. [CrossRef]
10. Ghanemi, A.; Melouane, A.; Yoshioka, M.; St-Amand, J. Exercise Training of Secreted Protein Acidic and Rich in Cysteine (Sparc) KO Mice Suggests That Exercise-Induced Muscle Phenotype Changes Are SPARC-Dependent. *Appl. Sci.* **2020**, *10*, 9108. [CrossRef]
11. Kim, S.; Seo, M.; Jung, H.; Song, J. Effects of High-Impact Weight-Bearing Exercise on Bone Mineral Density and Bone Metabolism in Middle-Aged Premenopausal Women: A Randomized Controlled Trial. *Appl. Sci.* **2021**, *11*, 846. [CrossRef]
12. Galli, D.; Carubbi, C.; Masselli, E.; Vaccarezza, M.; Presta, V.; Pozzi, G.; Ambrosini, L.; Gobbi, G.; Vitale, M.; Mirandola, P. Physical Activity and Redox Balance in the Elderly: Signal Transduction Mechanisms. *Appl. Sci.* **2021**, *11*, 2228. [CrossRef]
13. Araneda, O.; Kosche-Cárcamo, F.; Verdugo-Marchese, H.; Tuesta, M. Pulmonary Effects Due to Physical Exercise in Polluted Air: Evidence from Studies Conducted on Healthy Humans. *Appl. Sci.* **2021**, *11*, 2890. [CrossRef]
14. Lee, D.; Byun, K.; Hwang, M.; Lee, S. Augmentation Index Is Inversely Associated with Skeletal Muscle Mass, Muscle Strength, and Anaerobic Power in Young Male Adults: A Preliminary Study. *Appl. Sci.* **2021**, *11*, 3146. [CrossRef]
15. Hoyos-Flores, J.; Rangel-Colmenero, B.; Alonso-Ramos, Z.; García-Dávila, M.; Cruz-Castruita, R.; Naranjo-Orellana, J.; Hernández-Cruz, G. The Role of Cholinesterases in Post-Exercise HRV Recovery in University Volleyball Players. *Appl. Sci.* **2021**, *11*, 4188. [CrossRef]
16. Gaggini, M.; Vassalle, C.; Carli, F.; Maltinti, M.; Sabatino, L.; Buzzigoli, E.; Mastorci, F.; Sbrana, F.; Gastaldelli, A.; Pingitore, A. Changes in Plasma Bioactive Lipids and Inflammatory Markers during a Half-Marathon in Trained Athletes. *Appl. Sci.* **2021**, *11*, 4622. [CrossRef]

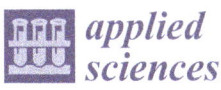

Article

Sana: A Gamified Rehabilitation Management System for Anterior Cruciate Ligament Reconstruction Recovery

Tanaka Kungwengwe * and Richard Evans

College of Engineering, Design and Physical Sciences, Brunel University London, Uxbridge UB8 3PH, UK; richard.evans@brunel.ac.uk
* Correspondence: kungwengwe@outlook.com

Received: 29 June 2020; Accepted: 14 July 2020; Published: 16 July 2020

Abstract: The anterior cruciate ligament (ACL) provides stabilization support for the back and forth motion of the knee joint. ACL ruptures account for 50% of all sports-related knee injuries with approximately 76.6% of them requiring reconstructive surgery, necessitating long-term patient rehabilitation. Compliance with rehabilitation management programs, following ACL reconstruction, is fundamental for the successful restoration of the knee's kinematics and reducing the risk of secondary osteoarthritis. Existing recovery programs are often paper-based and require patients to perform exercises at home, unsupervised, resulting in a low level of self-efficacy; by promoting self-efficacy in home-based settings, rehabilitation outcomes can improve. This paper reports the design development of the Sana system, a mobile and wearable application that adopts behavioral design principles and gamification theory to improve long-term post-operative outcomes for ACL reconstruction recovery. A feasibility study was conducted from 15 October 2019–13 May 2020, employing the double diamond framework and a human-centered design approach (BS EN ISO 9241-210: 2019). Eighteen participants were recruited, including eight domain experts (in fields such as user experience design, human factors, and physiotherapy), and ten representative users who had undergone long-term rehabilitation for musculoskeletal injuries.

Keywords: rehabilitation; compliance; anterior cruciate ligament reconstruction (ACLR); range of motion (ROM); self-efficacy; behavioral design; gamification

1. Introduction

Anterior cruciate ligament (ACL) ruptures account for 50% of all sports-related knee injuries. Approximately 76.6% of them result in reconstructive surgery, requiring long-term patient rehabilitation [1]. ACL tears often occur in activities that involve sudden stops or changes in movement and have profound effects on knee kinematics with recurrent knee instability as the main cause [2]. Anterior cruciate ligament reconstruction (ACLR) surgery is an integral aspect of treatment, but the economic repercussions are significant, with an estimated 15,000 primary ACL reconstructive surgeries performed in the UK annually, at a cost of £63 million [3]. To improve the success rate of recovery treatments, patients must remain compliant and perform exercises correctly. Failure to do so increases the chances of secondary knee osteoarthritis within 10–15 years post-surgery [4].

The digital health device market for ACLR rehabilitation has grown exponentially in recent years. With the emergence of Healthcare 4.0, patient-oriented systems, using the automated capture of patient data and transparent sharing with healthcare providers, can lead to improved healthcare delivery [5]. In the context of home-based physiotherapy (HBPT), following ACL reconstruction, a technological shift from traditional paper-based methods of treatment to automated interventions has occurred, significantly improving physiotherapy services for both patients and caregivers [6]; however, there is an identified need for assistive interventions for post-ACLR recovery patients to ensure optimal recovery.

Non-compliance to HBPT is a significant problem prevalent among patients recovering from musculoskeletal (MSK) injuries, with yearly rates as high as 50–65% [7]. High rates of non-compliance are attributed to the fact that caregivers in public and private healthcare settings continue to administer paper-based treatment procedures. Paper-based procedures fail to provide personalized care and user engagement and, as a result, present barriers to rehabilitation compliance and self-efficacy. Numerous digital rehabilitation interventions exist on the market (e.g., Tracpatch and Re.Flex) that assist in knee surgery rehabilitation, but these are predominantly targeted towards the recovery of total knee replacement surgeries and not ACL injuries. Existing rehabilitation systems typically use augmented reality (AR) and interactive smartphone dashboards to provide patients with real-time feedback on their performance during rehabilitation exercises. Further, they enable caregivers to monitor patients' progress and advise on exercises remotely. Data can also be captured by patients' self-reporting recovery outcomes.

Currently available products and services combine smart mobile applications with wearable hardware devices to allow exercises to be performed and remotely monitored in at-home environments. Through Internet of Things, wireless sensors and biometrics, physiotherapists and doctors can monitor the kinetic and kinematic movements of patients post-surgery. For example, ROMBOT (https://rombot.com/) connects patients with licensed physiotherapists in the United States to create personalized movement programs to assist in pain management, recovery, and the prevention of injuries. Similarly, CyMedica Orthopedics developed e-vive which delivers tele-rehabilitation services connecting clinicians with patients that are undergoing partial and total knee replacement. Gait Up (https://www.gaitup.com/), developed as a spin-off of the University Hospital of Lausanne and the Swiss Institute of Technology of Lausanne, employs sensors, algorithms, and biometrics to convert inertial sensor signals into meaningful motion insights. Finally, physiotherapists at Macquarie University in Australia developed the REPS Recovery Exercises system, a recovery exercise application that allows stroke patients to complete exercises at home as part of a self-maintenance rehabilitation program.

As digital technologies and connectivity improves, rehabilitation management service providers are embedding gamified elements into their core functionality, providing more appealing and personalized experiences to wider audiences. During rehabilitation, gamification provides intrinsic motivation to keep patients on track and allows for provision of immediate feedback, making the process more fun, enjoyable, and interactive. Although numerous products are available for post-surgery rehabilitation management, limitations do exist, including: interfaces tend to be overtly technical and system orientated; they often fail to consider self-efficacy principles mentioned by Magee et al. [8] and Henderson and Cole [9], based on motivation and positive re-enforcement in their interface design. Future ACL recovery systems must (1) measure the quality of patients' adherence to exercise instructions, (2) measure performance through monitoring the quality of pre-determined exercises, and (3) share patient performance data periodically with caregivers to assist in the creation of well-informed, timely treatment decisions. This paper reports on the design development of a HBPT system that aims to improve the long-term post-operative outcomes of ACLR surgery. The platform focuses on addressing phase 1 (initial rehabilitation), where patients are primarily expected to regain their baseline range of motion.

1.1. Post-Operative ACLR Surgery

The time taken to reach full recovery from ACLR surgery varies between patients but can take up to 12 months. During this time, patients are normally provided with a HBPT program, with exercises that are specific to their needs, considering the severity of knee damage and the level of activity a patient is hoping to reobtain [10]. Table 1 provides a breakdown of each phase of rehabilitation, as established by the Royal National Orthopaedic Hospital (National Health Service (NHS) Trust) [11].

Table 1. Rehabilitation guidelines for patients undergoing ACL reconstruction rehabilitation.

Phase 1	Phase 2	Phase 3
Initial Rehabilitation Phase (Duration: 2–6 weeks)	**Recovery Rehabilitation Phase** (Duration: 6–12 weeks)	**Intermediate–Final Rehabilitation Phase** (Duration: 12 weeks–1 year)
<ul><li>Achieve full range of knee extension to 120° flexion.</li><li>Minimal activity related joint effusion.</li><li>Reduce requirement for mobility aids as comfort, swelling, and knee control allows to achieve no gait abnormalities.</li><li>Symmetry on ascending and descending stairs.</li></ul>	<ul><li>Bilaterally equal proprioception tests on single leg stance.</li><li>Bilaterally equal strength of hamstrings, hip adductors, hip abductors, and gastrocnemius.</li></ul>	<ul><li>One Rep Max (RM) single leg press Relative Strength Index (RSI) greater than or equal to 125%.</li><li>Leg Symmetry Index (LSI) 85–100% of knee extensors.</li><li>Symmetry on hop tests.</li><li>Graded return to sport if set as patient goal, when patient has satisfied functional performance testing requirements and when consultant has agreed for patient to return to sport.</li><li>No contact sports for 6 months post-operation.</li><li>Establish long-term maintenance program.</li></ul>

1.2. Related Work

Gamification is defined as the use of game design features and elements in non-game contexts [12]. Extant research has supported the use of gamification in the rehabilitation process for musculoskeletal injuries [13,14] and other health-related conditions [12,15], especially to encourage engagement and increase patients' adherence to exercise programs. Qiu et al. [16] proposed Fun-Knee, a two-dimensional (2D) cartoon-based fishing game designed using UNITY engine. The authors identified that gamification can achieve significant levels of pain distraction, thereby increasing rehabilitation compliance. In their study, patients performed a series of cognitively demanding tasks that diverted their attention away from their injury. Patients could also set the exercise difficulty based on their needs. Egan et al. [17] established that pain and physical discomfort are significant barriers to exercise compliance and determined that pain distraction through gamification is one method that can be adopted to address this. Findings from Qiu et al. [16] showed that gamification methods are useful for enhancing rehabilitation compliance due to their motivating, progress-tracking, and goal-oriented nature. Further, Brown et al. [12] applied motivational principles and game elements to their study, including visualization of progress and automated goal setting activities to enhance engagement and participation. By incorporating these features, adherence and completion rates rose to 97%. Several studies have also shown that the inclusion of concept-based goal setting increases patients' motivation [18,19]. Gunaydin et al. [18] considered three simple game scenarios where the patient accumulated stars according to the correctness of their movement. This feedback was observed to improve the motivation of patients; however, the clinical benefits of the system require further validation using biostatistical analysis before conclusive results can be drawn.

Clausen et al. [19] proposed the GenuSport application, a muscle training program that consists of a strength monitoring unit with three integrated sensors and two primary game modes: maximal strength and flight control. Direct performance feedback was provided after each game. Their findings show that 80% of patients had high levels of compliance, meaning that they trained at least once per day. During the study, none of the patients required face-to-face contact and were able to use the device autonomously after adequate instruction. However, the researchers described seeing an overall decrease in frequency of use during the study and attributed this to the two game modes not developing over time in difficulty. From this, it can be assumed that a limitation of gamification is its need to be continuously evaluated and further developed to maintain long-term engagement.

Qui et al. also expressed similar challenges with regards to sustaining patients' long-term engagement and the fear of exercises becoming routine after initial interest. Deacon et al. [20] proposed a system that utilized the existing architecture of Nintendo Wii Balance with the aim of improving balance controls to reduce the risk of falls in older patients. Feedback provided to the user was focused on positive reinforcement which occurred once the patient had completed an exercise. The benefits of this approach were that it allowed patients to understand when they had completed a task to the best of their ability. The key extrinsic motivational factor was the hope of improved quality of life from using the system. Their results showed a need to implement audible feedback; users stated that they would find this more stimulating and engaging. However, since basic ACLR rehabilitation exercises require the patient to remain in a specific position to ensure accurate knee angle detection, Wii platforms are not ideal for ACLR rehabilitation.

Overall, gamification, like other persuasive architectures has merit, if implemented in the correct manner [12,21]. However, current research has criticized gamification in the healthcare sector. For example, Deloitte [22] described gamification as 'just another over-glorified tech trend', while Bogost [23] considered it a quick fix adopted by innovators to increase and promote engagement. Brown et al. [12] stated that these criticisms likely derive from the belief that "features such as points and leader boards miss the essence and power of games as motivational techniques which have the potential to encourage behavior change or adherence to treatment programs positively". Their study outlined the importance of encouraging engagement to treatment rather than technology, and that designers should consider this when applying gamification methods to contexts where the intention is to alleviate suffering and improve well-being [24]. To date, few studies have implemented gamification strategies to address rehabilitation requirements, specific to ACL reconstruction recovery. Therefore, the aim of this paper is to report the development of mobile system intervention capable of improving long-term post-operative outcomes for patients following ACLR surgery.

2. Methods

To design the proposed system, a feasibility study was conducted over an eight-month period from 15 October 2019–13 May 2020. The double diamond framework was employed to model the investigation, as shown in Figure 1. This consisted of four phases: discover, define, develop, and deliver. Referring to the guidelines outlined in 'BS EN ISO 9241-210: 2019–Part 210 Human-centred design for interactive systems' allowed the authors to ensure that the project adhered to the strict design protocols outlined by the NHS for developing digital health systems [25].

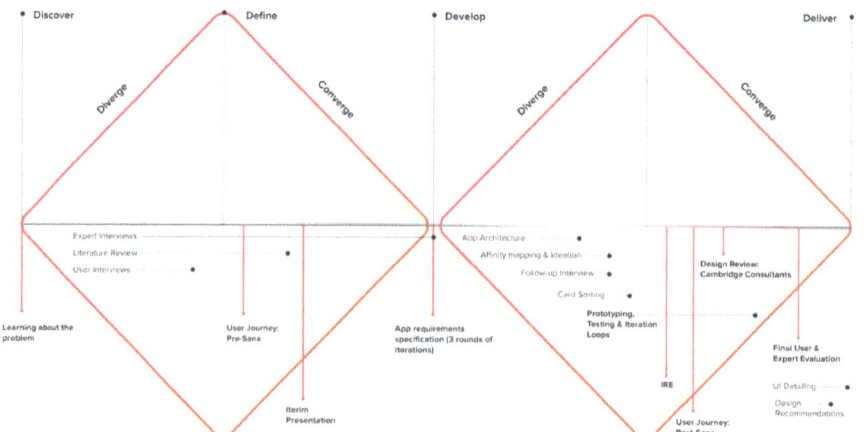

Figure 1. Study design based on the double diamond framework.

2.1. Discover and Define Phases

First, two semi-structured interviews were conducted with one physiotherapist specializing in MSK rehabilitation at multiple stages of the design process. The first interview was conducted during the discovery phase and provided an initial understanding of ACL injuries and a basis for mapping out an initial patient-user journey called pre-Sana. The second follow-up interview was conducted during the define phase and helped validate design assumptions while addressing gaps in the authors' knowledge. The inclusion criteria for the expert interviews were a minimum of 7 years of professional or academic experience in MSK rehabilitation. Second, four representative patients were recruited for semi-structured interviews. This helped identify a range of pain points that patients experienced during HBPT, following total knee reconstruction procedures. The main inclusion criteria were users aged between 21 and 40 who had experienced MSK injury of the knee in the last year and had undergone long-term rehabilitation lasting between 2 and 6 weeks. The primary method used for data collection was voice recording, while insights were transcribed manually. NVivo 12 was used for data analysis. A best-fit approach was employed which ensured that insights were grouped based on their relation to the following themes: education, engagement with caregiver, self-efficacy, and support/education. This criterion was based on prior research conducted in the behavioral design and strong predictors of rehabilitation compliance [8].

2.2. Develop Phase

First, five open-moderated card sorting activities were conducted with representative patients. This user-centered design technique helped uncover the target users' expectations, thereby, allowing the authors to design a system infrastructure that was fit for purpose and delivered an optimal user experience. In the card sorting sessions, participants were tasked with organizing a set of 30 cards that corresponded with predetermined application features and functionalities into groups. The software used for data capture was OptimalSort, which provided qualitative insights that were presented using a dendrogram. Since only five participants were recruited for the study, the best merge method was used for data analysis; this method draws assumptions about more prominent clusters based on individual pair relationships. To obtain qualitative insights, participants were encouraged to think aloud and provide verbal justifications for their pairings. These insights were transcribed and analyzed manually.

Second, a design review with Cambridge Consultants, a technology consultancy with specialisms in medical device development, was conducted to validate the technical and design feasibility of the proposed system. Five participants were recruited who aligned with the specialisms required for the project delivery, including user experience (UX) research, UX design, human factors engineering, and software development. The design review was structured using the approach outlined by Harris [26] with insights categorized as challenges, ideas, likes, and questions.

Finally, online pilot usability tests were conducted over Zoom with two principle UX designers to fine-tune the study design and prototype before user testing. The inclusion criteria for these participants were a minimum of 7 years of professional experience in UX design for medical applications. To ensure that the results were appropriate to use in the final study, participants were recruited who also matched the criteria for the target user demographic of the system. However, since participants were not undergoing rehabilitation at the time of the study, context-setting and role-play instructions were provided during pre-study briefing. Participants were recruited from Cambridge Consultants who had participated in the design review study. The System Usability Scale method, proposed by Lewis and Sauro [27], was used for data analysis. Using the Fibonacci sequence (1–5), 'task criticality' and 'impact' scores were assigned to each task performed in the test. Issue frequency (%) was calculated by dividing the number of occurrences by total participants. The last stage involved calculating the 'severity' of each issue by multiplying the three variables—criticality score, impact score, and issue frequency [28]. The results obtained helped inform decisions regarding usability issues during design and development.

2.3. Deliver Phase

To conclude, one summative evaluation was conducted to assess the overall user experience of the proposed system against design specification and usability heuristics: visibility of system status, provide information feedback, recognition rather than control, aesthetics and minimalist design, and consistency and standards. The inclusion criteria were a minimum of 7 years of professional or academic experience in musculoskeletal rehabilitation. The interview was recorded, with insights being transcribed and analyzed manually.

3. Results

3.1. Discover Phase

The goal of the discovery phase was to establish potential bottlenecks in the patient-user journey. This required interviewing physiotherapists who specialized in MSK rehabilitation and users who had undergone total knee reconstruction surgery followed by long-term rehabilitation. In order to design a solution that effectively addressed users' primary needs, it was first essential to understand the challenges users faced from their point of view and empathize with their experiences. Four user interviews were conducted to gain insights into these challenges and pain points. Through analysis of interview findings, we categorized responses into three core challenges: (1) self-efficacy, (2) education, and (3) engagement with the primary caregiver. Further details are given below.

1. Self-efficacy: Issues related to self-efficacy resulted from patients having an unclear or no indication of progress and improvement during rehabilitation. Patients commonly stated that they often questioned the effectiveness of their therapy and had limited engagement with the exercises they were performing. There was an overall interest in being able to visualize the effects their therapy was having on their recovery and be able to track progress at each stage of rehabilitation. One interviewee stated, "It is easy to notice the pain, but I cannot see the improvement or progress".
2. Education: All interviewees stated that they were issued a paper-based treatment program detailing a summary of their injury and rehabilitation procedure. Users reported limited engagement with this information, reporting that the initial exercise demonstrations provided by their caregivers were more effective in reinforcing the correct exercise technique than static images. One interviewee noted that YouTube videos on exercises were beneficial. Overall, the key takeaway from this was that patients responded better to information that was presented in an engaging manner. Subsequent design concepts must explore ways that this can be achieved. One interviewee stated, "I had no level of engagement with my exercises ... I did not even know if what I was doing was correct."
3. Engagement with the primary caregiver: There was a shared view amongst users that they felt they had just been left to their own devices once discharged from the ward. Feedback would often be provided during patient follow-up; however, this was commonly described as either being 'monotonous', 'disengaging' or 'useless.' One interviewee remarked that something as simple as being told she was making small improvements by her caregiver would have been enough to motivate her to be persistent with therapy. In addition, one interviewee stated, "It would have been nice to have a follow-up with a healthcare specialist who understood the challenges I was having and gave useful advice. The feedback I was provided was often always the same".

3.2. Define Phase

The goal of the define phase was to consolidate the data collected during the discovery phase. A patient-user journey, called pre-Sana, depicting the fundamental pain points and design opportunities of the existing paper-based rehabilitation process was developed, as shown in Figure 2.

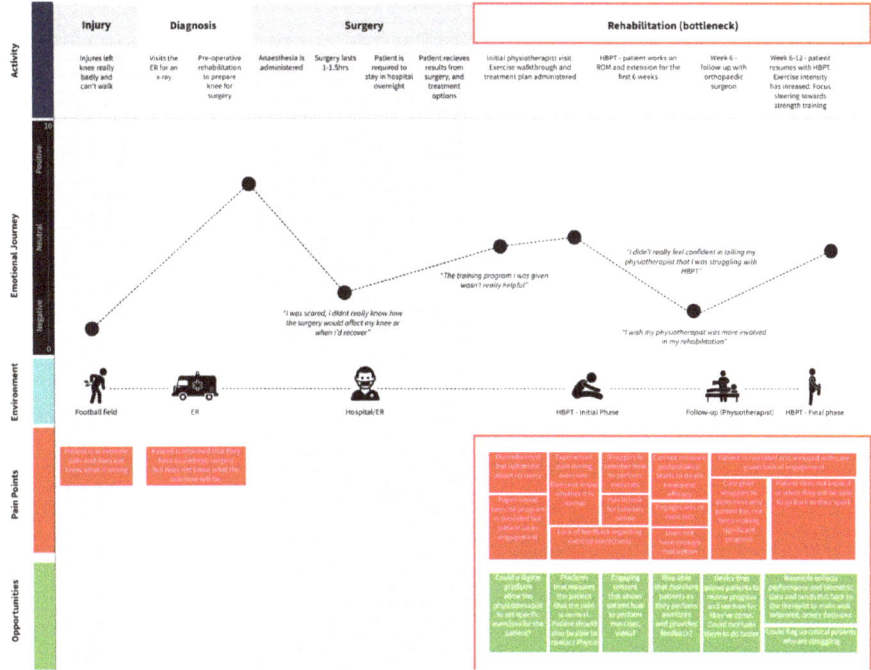

Figure 2. Current paper based anterior cruciate ligament reconstruction (ACLR) rehabilitation procedure: pre-Sana.

3.3. Develop Phase

The development phase focused on creating and refining the iteration flows and digital interface for the proposed system. Engagement with potential users and technical experts was maintained throughout the phase through rapid prototyping, iteration, and testing loops. This helped to ensure that assumptions were being continuously validated against the developed requirements specifications. The first stage in development involved the creation of a Unified Modeling Language (UML) diagram (Figure 3), to visually represent the system's information architecture along with its main actors, roles, and actions. The UML diagram was crucial in defining the initial high-level categories required for conducting the affinity mapping activity. Categories included view profile, therapy and exercises, dashboard, contact physiotherapist, and smart sleeve. These represented the features that patients would primarily interact with when navigating through the system. Considering that caregivers would have an external data collection dashboard, their engagement with the Sana app would primarily be when communicating remotely with the patient via the 'Contact' navigation item.

Once the system architecture was determined, an affinity mapping activity was conducted. The key research findings from the discovery phase were converted into a range of design ideas and potential system functions and features. These were then organized into the following established high-level categories: profile, therapy and exercises, dashboard, and contact. This activity was conducted to identify gaps in the authors' domain knowledge. A list of assumptions and questions was documented (Table 2) which was used to structure a follow-up interview with a physiotherapist (see Table 2).

- Profile: What information, if any, is a patient required to know regarding their injury? How often is a patient called up for follow-up treatment? What kind of advice or medication will a patient be given regarding pain and swelling management?

- Therapy and exercises: Will a patient be provided additional exercise equipment? If so, what are some examples of this equipment? How often do patients engage in exercise? How much input, if any, should a patient have in terms of deciding what exercises? Should patients be given a range of alternative exercises to perform if they are struggling? Is diet something patients need to regularly monitor during rehabilitation?
- Dashboard: What are the different milestones that patients have during phase 1 of rehabilitation? What kind of data do caregivers need to collect about patients? How do patients currently determine whether treatment is working? What are the commonly used metrics to determine a patient's rate of recovery?
- Contact: How much flexibility do patients have in scheduling appointments themselves?

The follow-up interview helped answer the key questions and assumptions identified during the affinity mapping activity. Adjustments to the affinity map were made using insights gathered from the interview. This included disregarding features such as patient appointment scheduling, diet monitoring, and the ability for patients to choose their exercises from a list of approved exercises. From our findings, it was clear that exercise quality, exercise compliance, and pain levels were the most critical metrics caregivers use when completing assessment of whether a patient is successfully recovering.

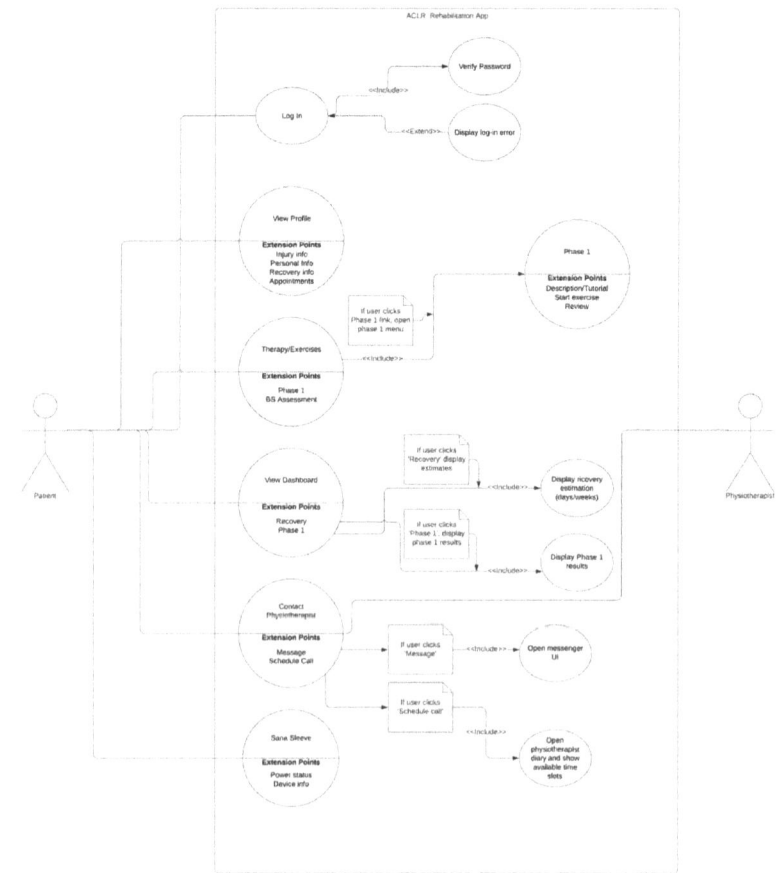

Figure 3. Unified Modeling Language (UML) diagram for the Sana system.

Table 2. Results of the follow-up interview with the physiotherapist.

Question	Comments	Additional Information
What specific information is a patient given regarding the nature of their injury during initial consultation?	Patients will often be given information relating to their goals for that rehabilitation phase and restrictions.	None.
How often are patients called up for follow-up treatment?	Physiotherapists see their patients more frequently during the acute rehabilitation phase (1), and less frequently after that.	Phase 1 is where caregivers need to ensure that the patient is doing everything correctly.
How often do ACL reconstruction patients have to engage in physical therapy?	Patients need to perform exercises consistently during the acute rehabilitation phase.	The type of exercises a patient engages in will depend on the type of injury, severity, and where the tissue is damaged. When physiotherapists are deciding on patient exercises, they need to think about the tissue, healing time frames, and clinical indicators (i.e., adequate quad strength, full range of motion and weight bearing).
What are the various types of equipment that patients will receive to support them with exercises?	This varies depending on the type of injury and the exercises that the physiotherapist wants patients to perform.	None.
Does diet have an impact on a patient's rehabilitation success rate?	Yes.	Diet is subjective. Your system should focus on rehabilitation exercises, improving efficacy, and monitoring the quality of exercises performed.
What type of metrics need to be collected to show that a patient is recovering successfully?	Rotation, extension, bend, velocity, and power are important metrics.	The quantitative metrics we use are strength, range of motion, and swelling. Quality of movement is also important during exercises. Are they weight shifting evenly? It is also useful to keep track of whether a patient's pain levels are going down.
Do patients schedule their own appointments or is this done by the healthcare provider?	No. In private healthcare settings, physiotherapists tend to have a treatment plan; this involves mapping out when the patient will need to visit for follow-up care. Treatment plans are always set in collaboration with the patient during the initial consultation.	None.
What kinds of advice/medication will a patient be given regarding pain and swelling management?	Patients will be given advice regarding swelling management (i.e., how long they need to apply an ice pack on their injury).	In the acute phase, it is important that the patient does not receive too much anti-inflammatory medication.
Are the different phases of recovery fixed for every single post-ACL reconstruction patient?	Depends on the patient's level of injury.	Patients should not push too hard during exercise. It is important to perform exercises correctly rather than too fast and not use correct form.
How do patients monitor their own performance with rehabilitation?	They cannot. They only find out about their performance during follow-up consultation	None.

To determine the most appropriate content to be displayed on the system, we first acknowledged that content is often structured based on what makes sense to the designer, not to the end user. Sherwin [29] highlighted this as the number one usability problem in system design. For the proposed system, usability issues were mitigated by conducting a series of open-moderated card sorting activities. These assisted with the identification of target user demographics mental models and the establishing of the system infrastructure that was representative of these mental models. The data presented in Table 3 shows the key insights extracted from the dendrogram analysis in Figure 4. It highlights the features/cards that participants commonly grouped together and the labels they assigned each grouping during the card sorting activity.

Table 3. Card sort groupings.

Cards/Potential System Features	Groupings and Labels				
	Settings/Wearable Device/FAQs	Exercise/ Rehabilitation/ Therapy	Profile/About Me	Home Page	Dashboard
	Instructions on systems set-up	Providing feedback on my pain levels	Personal details	Setting exercise reminders	My exercise performance
	Syncing my Fitbit/fitness tracker	Guidance on how to complete an exercise	Prescribed medication and dosage information	View my rewards and achievements	Adherence levels to my rehabilitation program
	Detailed product information (e.g., battery life)	Congratulatory message that I have completed an exercise		Summary of my injury and expectations of recovery	
		Real-time performance feedback		Adherence levels to my rehabilitation program	

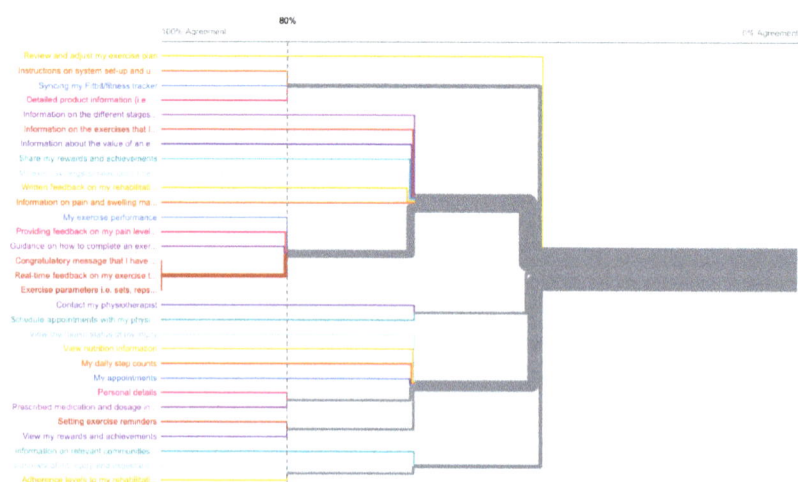

Figure 4. Dendrogram analysis.

Patient User Journey: Post-Sana

To design a new user journey that illustrates how users interact with the proposed system, a design review was conducted with Cambridge Consultants. This critique was crucial for validating the technical and design feasibility of the proposed system. It helped establish which areas required prioritization and refinement with subsequent development. Participants that specialized in UX design, UX research, human factors engineering, and software development participated in the critique. Insights from the affinity mapping and card sorting activities were instrumental for drafting the user interfaces for each stage of the user journey. The final user journey for the proposed system is shown in Figure 5.

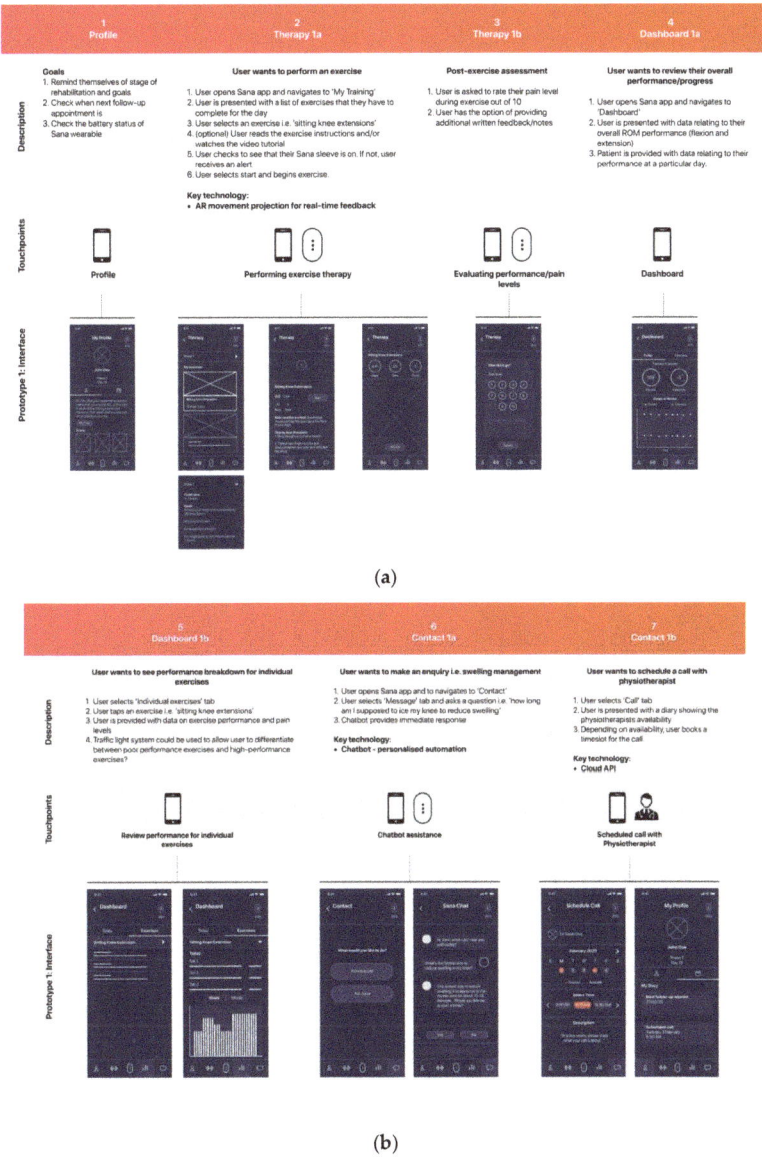

Figure 5. (**a**) User journey for interaction with the proposed system (steps 1–4). (**b**) User journey for interaction with the proposed system (steps 5–7).

From the feedback collected during the design critique, shown in Table 4, it was clear that the focus areas for further development focused on the dashboard and exercise user workflows. As a result, the following actions were established, as shown in Table 4.

- Action 1: Dashboard workflow: Prioritize one dashboard feature for the final system (i.e., exercise reports, range of motion reports or adherence reports) and produce sketch concepts.
- Action 2: Exercise workflow: Refine exercise workflow with an emphasis on AR visualization, gamification, and positive feedback. Feedback on the system's interface was also provided, which was implemented in the next prototype iteration. The comments mainly centered around content hierarchy, navigation, and clarity of information presented within the interface.

Table 4. Feedback collected from the design critique.

Challenges	Ideas and Improvements
<ul><li>Getting patients to wear the device the same way each time without avoiding sensor displacement might be tricky.</li><li>How do you communicate exercise quality to a patient in a way that is actionable? Is this even technically possible? An alternative solution may be to send the exercise quality metrics directly to the caregiver who could use them to teach the patient on how to improve their technique.</li></ul>	<ul><li>Reminder notifications for when to complete exercises.</li><li>Exercise workflow is confusing and needs refinement.</li><li>Gamification features were mentioned in the presentation but could be more clearly represented in the system.</li><li>Research design trends used by sports-related apps (e.g., 'Strava' and 'Adidas Running').</li><li>Could the wearable incorporate haptic feedback?</li><li>Research data visualization techniques.</li><li>The purpose of the dashboard should be to motivate patients.</li></ul>
Likes	**Questions**
<ul><li>The premise of the concept makes sense and addresses the problem well.</li><li>Gamification to encourage engagement with exercises.</li><li>Chat bot functionality is interesting, but feature should be tested with other potential users.</li><li>Using AR to augment movement during an exercise.</li></ul>	<ul><li>How will the device accommodate different body types? (i.e., everyone's definition of quality is different).</li><li>How do you communicate exercise quality to a patient in a way that is actionable?</li><li>System still looks very technical, where is the positive reinforcement feedback?</li></ul>

Following the design critique meeting, the decision was made to prioritize exercise reports when developing the system's dashboard. The justification for this was that the feature directly aligns with the exercise workflow, which is the primary workflow used by patients. A series of sketch concepts were produced to illustrate the process of developing the workflow, as shown in Figure 6.

Similarly, a series of sketch concepts were produced to refine the exercise workflow and address some of the issues raised during the design review, relating to AR visualization, gamification, and positive feedback; these are illustrated in Figure 7.

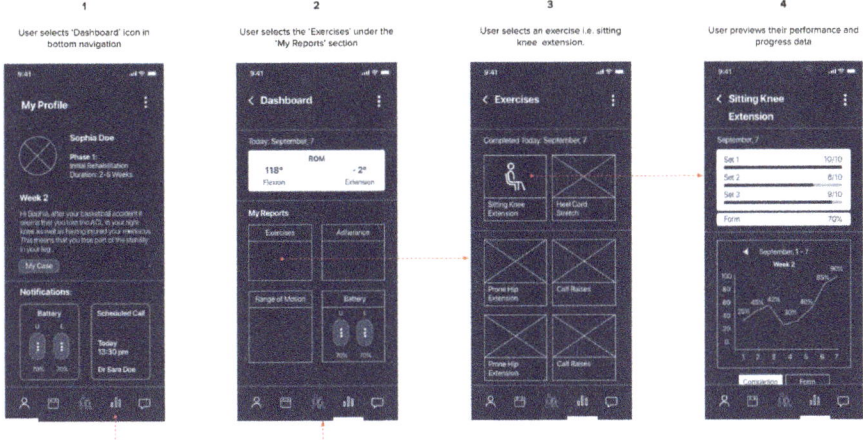

Figure 6. Dashboard workflow.

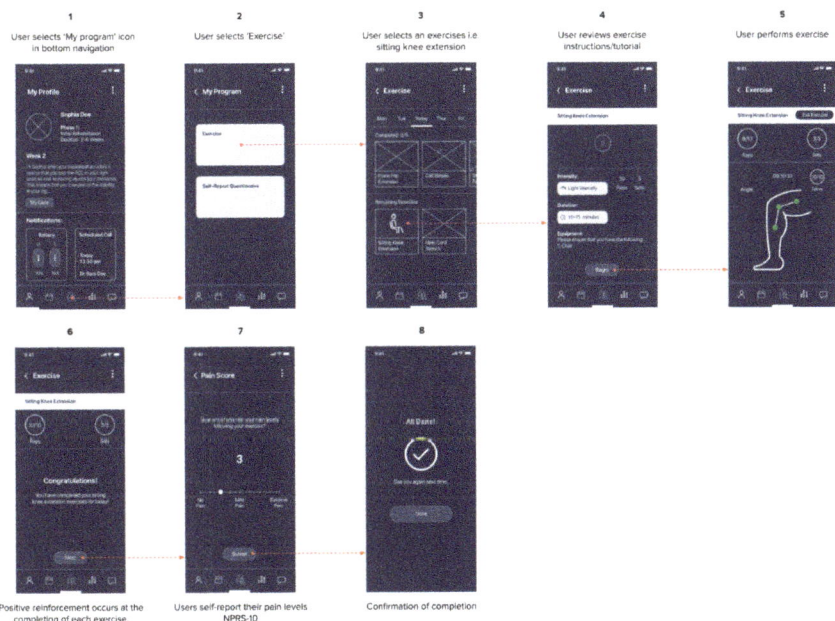

Figure 7. Exercise workflow.

4. The Proposed System: Sana

This chapter presents the developed system that incorporates the three key components of the Sana system, as presented in Figure 8. The system allows users to: (1) assess quality (i.e., measure the quality of adherence to exercise instructions at a specific time), (2) monitor performance (i.e., measure performance by monitoring the quality of a pre-determined set of exercises over time), and (3) share data (i.e., share performance data periodically with caregivers, helping them make well informed and timely treatment decisions). Figure 9 maps the user journey post-Sana development and illustrates the emotions experienced by users during system use.

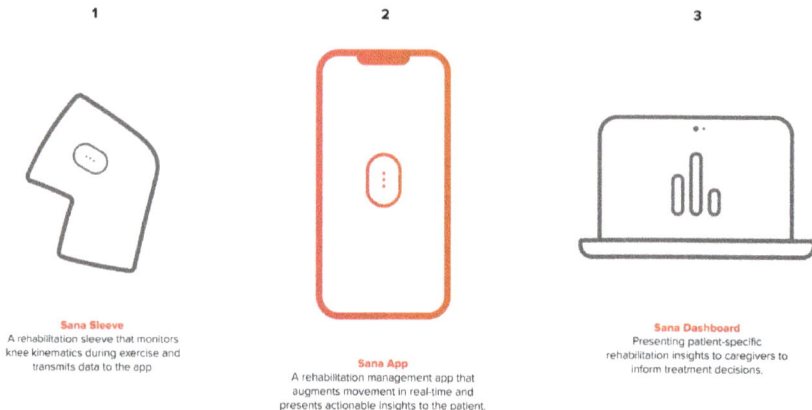

Figure 8. The proposed Sana system.

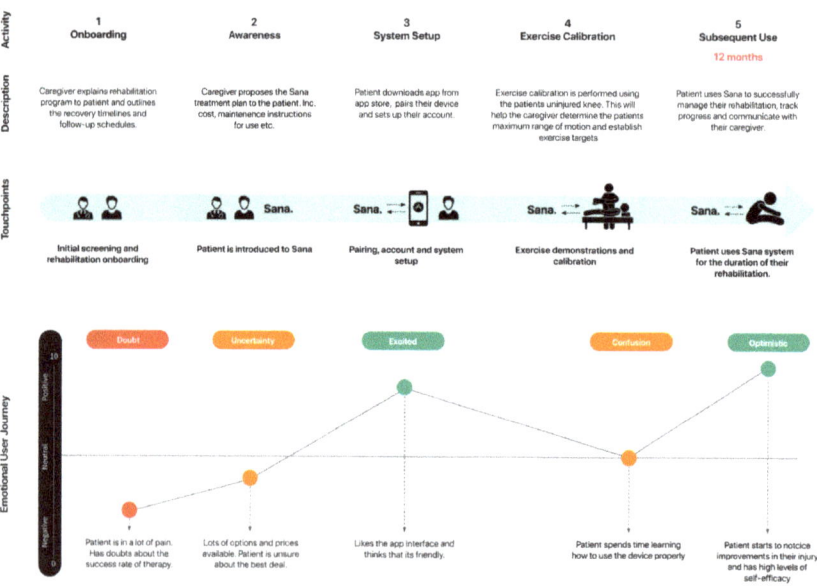

Figure 9. User journey map post-Sana development.

In Figure 10, screen prints of the developed system are shown.

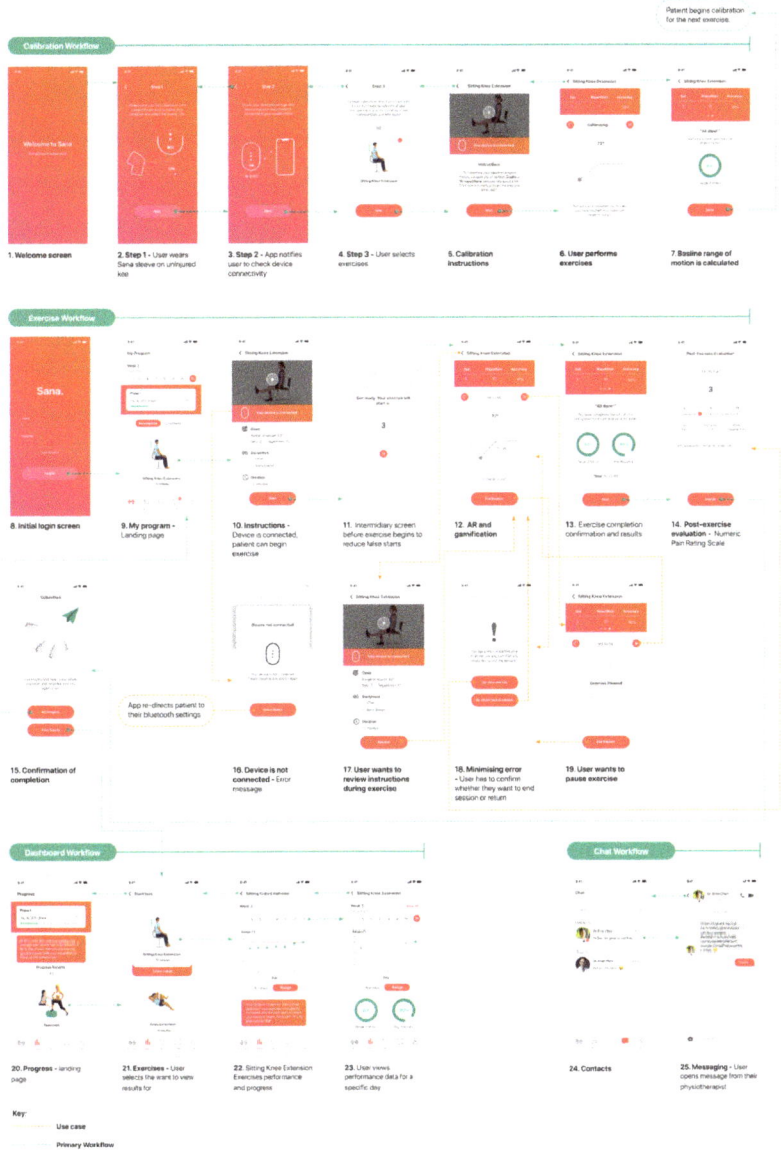

Figure 10. Screen prints of the developed Sana system.

4.1. Exercise Calibration

Setting realistic targets was deemed essential for promoting rehabilitation compliance. To ensure that each rehabilitation plan is optimally personalized to patients' specific needs and that realistic goals are set, patients calibrate their exercises using their uninjured knee during the service onboarding phase. The calibration activity is a crucial aspect of the overall user workflow as it helps physiotherapists to establish a patient's baseline. The baseline is then used as a metric measurement for treatment progression while providing patients with realistic rehabilitation goals. Figure 11 shows the calibration process.

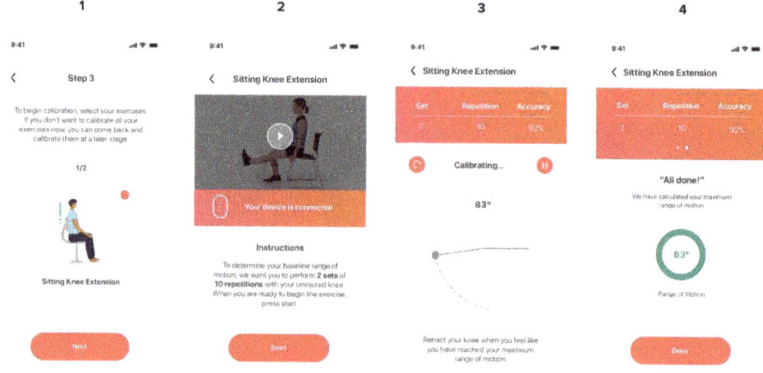

Figure 11. Calibration process.

4.2. Integration of AR and Exercise Gamification

The Sana system builds on the fundamental principles of gamification through goal setting, allowing patients to be more engaged with their exercises. Testament to the validity of implementing this approach, Qiu et al. [16] highlighted how gamification can be an effective method for enhancing rehabilitation compliance due to its motivating, progressive, and goal-oriented nature. The Sana system adopts a simplified gamification approach to minimize the risk of patients pushing themselves too hard and worsening their injury. The patient has one goal: to reach the green circle, as shown in Figure 12, which is set based on their baseline maximum range of motion. Nielsen [30] stated that "sustaining a match between system and the real-world" is a critical usability heuristic; therefore, the Sana system is designed to mimic key aspects of real-life physiotherapy sessions through the use of audio feedback, as the patient progresses through their exercises. The benefits of this could be either positive reinforcement or reminding the patient to stop if they are experiencing pain.

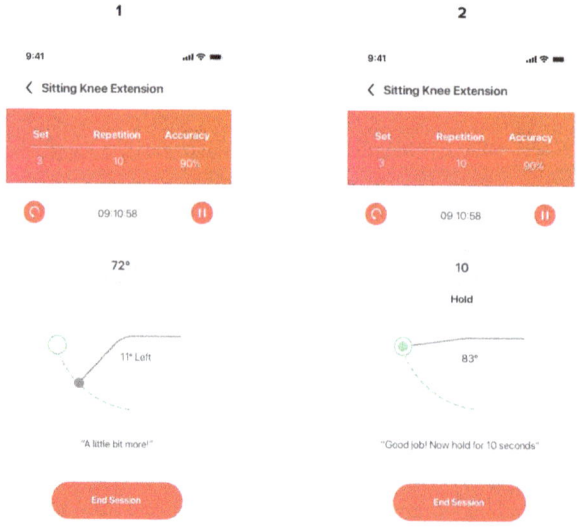

Figure 12. Screen print of the gamification element of the Sana system.

4.3. Progress and Performance Feedback

During the development of the Sana system, the progress dashboard, as shown in Figure 13, had to be thoughtfully designed. While it may be easy to present progress and performance data to a patient through a digital interface only, this had to be achieved in such a way that would continuously keep patients motivated rather than overwhelmed. This is especially important considering that ACLR rehabilitation can take up to 12 months. Progress data are presented simply and unobtrusively via progress bars and colloquial syntax (e.g., "You're 30% there!"). Through this approach, patients perceive the system as friendly and human-oriented, thereby increasing user engagement and long-term adherence to the rehabilitation program. Behavioral design and nudge theory are two fundamental pillars of the dashboard design. Positive reinforcement is used throughout to elicit feelings of personal accomplishment and to boost self-efficacy. Magee et al. [8] highlighted that positive reinforcement methods lead to higher levels of rehabilitation compliance; however, feedback provided by the primary caregiver is irreplaceable. The Sana system facilitates direct patient–caregiver communication by incorporating a chat facility. Magee et al. [8] also stated that patients who are aware of their clinicians' feelings towards their performance and progress are more likely to strive for positive rehabilitation outcomes.

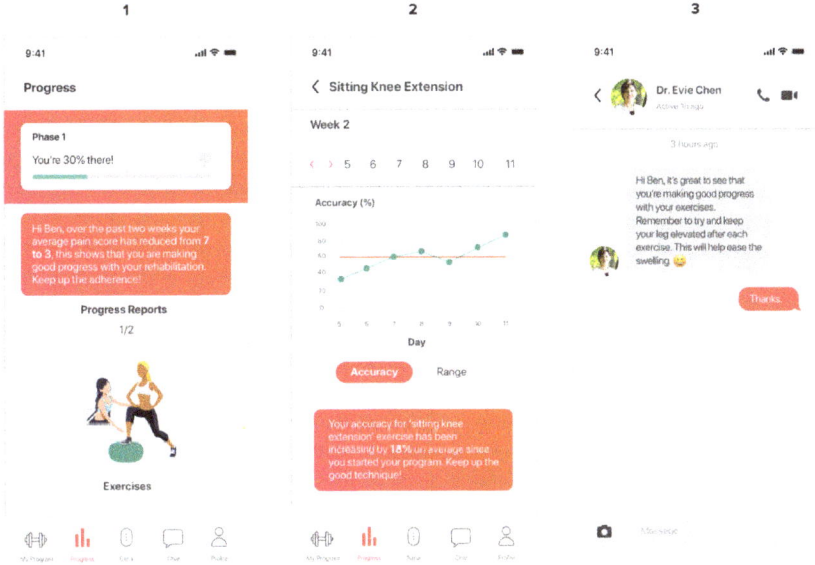

Figure 13. Screen print of the progress and feedback element of the Sana system.

Finally, a summative evaluation was conducted with an occupational therapist to assess the proposed system against the design specification and relevant usability heuristics. Overall, the concept was well-received. The participant stated that being able to review performance remotely was extremely beneficial for rehabilitation purposes. Regarding visual design, the therapist highlighted the simplicity, unobtrusive and friendly nature of the system as favorable characteristics which would lead to high adoption rates. Similarly, the participant did not experience any issues with navigation or performing set tasks, reflecting a good overall user experience. The participant agreed with the idea of using the uninjured knee to calibrate exercises to determine patients' baseline, describing it as "genius", and went on to suggest that they could see applications of this technology in other aspects of rehabilitation, such as shoulder and hand therapy.

5. Conclusions

This paper reports the development of a mobile-based system that improves post-operative outcomes for patients that have undergone long-term rehabilitation for ACLR surgery. The authors developed Sana, a gamified rehabilitation management system with performance monitoring, data sharing, and quality assessment capabilities. Its content is based on rehabilitation guidelines established by the Royal National Orthopaedic Hospital, which incorporates rehabilitation concepts and treatment modalities that are an integral aspect of ACLR rehabilitation. The proposed system builds on the fundamentals of behavioral design and gamification theory to improve patient self-efficacy and engagement during rehabilitation. Findings show that target users found the proposed system to be convenient and unobtrusive, engaging, informative, easy to use, and user-friendly. Additionally, physiotherapists and primary caregivers stated that the proposed system can improve treatment administration and decision-making processes, provide a personalized rehabilitation experience for patients, and facilitate communication between patients and caregivers. These findings suggest that the proposed system is feasible and would make a positive contribution to ACLR rehabilitation and clinical practice.

5.1. Study Limitations

Of course, this study has several limitations. First, time represented a significant limitation. Due to the eight-month constraint of our project, it meant that only one deliverable was feasible, and a longitudinal clinical study could not be conducted to test the efficacy of the system in its intended context and quantify the error of using the system on the opposite leg; this will be conducted as future work. Second, due to limited human resource availability, the authors could not concentrate on all system elements during the time period of the project. Third, although most of the technology required to deliver the proposed system successfully was readily available, there were aspects of the process that would have benefited from additional technical resources, notably, eye-tracking software for user testing; this type of software is widely used in most software development projects and would have provided additional quantitative metrics on visual hierarchy, object weight, and problematic areas within the system's user interface. Using the opposite leg for calibration is a feature that was favored by therapists who participated in the study. Justification being, it aligns with current factors they consider when establishing patient specific rehabilitation goals. However, this feature could present challenges for patients with two injured limbs or those whose opposite leg is significantly weaker than the injured leg, pre-injury. To confirm its efficacy, the platform would need to undergo extensive user testing incorporating different user cases and scenarios. Likewise, it would need to be validated with a wider range of healthcare professionals.

5.2. Future Developments

Overall, the platform was positively received by target users, healthcare specialists, and technologists specializing in medical device development and design alike, which justifies the need to develop research and development further. Throughout our study, questions were raised regarding whether the simplicity of the implemented gamification concept would be enough to provide users with actionable visual feedback, informing them of whether they are performing their exercises correctly and accurately; determining this would require back-end software development. The next phase of the project will involve working with software engineers to develop the platform using Unity engine and testing a fully functional prototype; this will be reported in future research. Development efforts were primarily placed on the exercise, calibration, and progress review workflows, as these were seen as critical components of the proposed system. In the future, other key functionalities of the system, such as chat and my profile will need to be refined to complete the application's service. An integral part of assessing the overall efficacy of the proposed system will involve developing the Sana sleeve and clinician's dashboard and conducting a clinically controlled longitudinal study using the entire system (Sana app, sleeve, and dashboard). Developing the Sana sleeve will require establishing a team consisting of mechanical and material engineers who are specialists in this area. However, academic groups [16,31,32] and commercial organizations, such as Loomia, have developed similar smart textile technologies that could be integrated, reporting high success rates. There is strong evidence to suggest that a smart textile approach is a potential future direction.

Author Contributions: Conceptualization, T.K.; methodology, T.K. and R.E.; validation, T.K.; investigation, T.K.; data curation, T.K.; writing—original draft preparation, T.K.; writing—review and editing, T.K. and R.E.; supervision, R.E.; project administration, T.K. All authors have read and agreed to the published version of the manuscript.

Funding: This research received no external funding.

Acknowledgments: The authors would like to thank Cambridge Consultants, the workshop technicians at Brunel University London for technical support provided during the research, and all those involved in the data collection exercises.

Conflicts of Interest: The authors declare no conflicts of interest. All subjects gave their informed consent for inclusion before they participated in the study. The study was conducted in accordance with the Declaration of Helsinki, and the protocol was approved by the Ethics Committee of Brunel University London (Refs: 19079-LR-Nov/2019- 21331-1 and 19079-LR-Nov/2019- 21331-2).

References

1. Joseph, A.; Collins, C.; Henke, N.; Yard, E.; Fields, S.; Comstock, R. A Multisport Epidemiologic Comparison of Anterior Cruciate Ligament Injuries in High School Athletics. *J. Athl. Train.* **2013**, *48*, 810–817. [CrossRef] [PubMed]
2. Essery, R.; Geraghty, A.; Kirby, S.; Yardley, L. Predictors of adherence to home-based physical therapies: A systematic review. *Disabil. Rehabil.* **2016**, *39*, 519–534. [CrossRef] [PubMed]
3. Comparison of the Clinical and Cost Effectiveness of Two Management Strategies for Non-Acute Anterior Cruciate Ligament (ACL) Injury: Rehabilitation Versus Surgical Reconstruction. Available online: https://ichgcp.net/clinical-trials-registry/NCT02980367 (accessed on 25 April 2020).
4. Pietrosimone, B.; Seeley, M.K.; Johnston, C.; Pfeiffer, S.J.; Spang, J.T.; Blackburn, J.T. Walking Ground Reaction Force Post-ACL Reconstruction: Analysis of Time and Symptoms. *Med. Sci. Sports Exerc.* **2019**, *51*, 246–254. [CrossRef] [PubMed]
5. Tanwar, S.; Parekh, K.; Evans, R. Blockchain-based electronic healthcare record system for healthcare 4.0 applications. *J. Inf. Secur. Appl.* **2020**, *50*, 102407. [CrossRef]
6. Kungwengwe, T. *Business Model. BA Industrial Design and Technology*; Brunel University London: London, UK, 12 May 2020.
7. Adherence to Home Exercise Programs. Available online: https://www.physio-pedia.com/Adherence_to_Home_Exercise_Programs#cite_note-Wright-7 (accessed on 25 April 2020).
8. Magee, D.J.; Zachazewski, J.; Quillen, W.; Manske, R.A. *Pathology and Intervention in Musculoskeletal Rehabilitation*, 2nd ed.; Elsevier Inc.: London, UK, 2016; pp. 16–19.
9. Henderson, K.; Cole, J. The effects of exercise rehabilitation on perceived self-efficacy. *Aust. J. Physiother.* **1992**, *38*, 195–201. [CrossRef]
10. Anterior Cruciate Ligament (ACL) Reconstruction. Available online: https://www.bupa.co.uk/health-information/knee-clinic/treatment-and-care/anterior-cruciate-ligament-acl-reconstruction (accessed on 25 April 2020).
11. Rehabilitation Guidelines for Patients Undergoing Anterior Cruciate Ligament Repair (ACL). Available online: https://www.rnoh.nhs.uk/services/rehabilitation-guidelines (accessed on 17 November 2019).
12. Brown, M.; O'Neill, N.; van Woerden, H.; Eslambolchilar, P.; Jones, M.; John, A. Gamification and Adherence to Web-Based Mental Health Interventions: A Systematic Review. *JMIR Ment. Health* **2016**, *3*, e39. [CrossRef] [PubMed]
13. Tannous, H.; Istrate, D.; Benlarbi-Delai, A.; Sarrazin, J.; Idriss, M.; Tho, M.; Dao, T. Exploring various orientation measurement approaches applied to a serious game system for functional rehabilitation. In Proceedings of the 38th Annual International Conference of the IEEE Engineering in Medicine and Biology Society, Orlando, FL, USA, 16–20 August 2016; IEEE: New York, NY, USA, 2016; p. 16395741.

14. Idriss, M.; Tannous, H.; Istrate, D.; Perrochon, A.; Salle, J.; Ho Ba Tho, M.; Dao, T. Rehabilitation- Oriented Serious Game Development and Evaluation Guidelines for Musculoskeletal Disorders. *JMIR Serious Games* **2017**, *5*, e14. [CrossRef] [PubMed]
15. Mubin, O.; Alnajjar, F.; Jishtu, N.; Alsinglawi, B.; Al Mahmud, A. Exoskeletons with Virtual Reality, Augmented Reality, and Gamification for Stroke Patients' Rehabilitation: Systematic Review. *JMIR Rehabil. Assist. Technol.* **2019**, *6*, e12010. [CrossRef] [PubMed]
16. Qiu, Y.; Man Li, K.; Neoh, E.; Zhang, H.; Khaw, X.; Fan, X.; Miao, C. Fun-Knee™: A Novel Smart Knee Sleeve for Total-Knee-Replacement Rehabilitation with Gamification. In Proceedings of the IEEE 5th International Conference on Serious Games and Applications for Health, Perth, Australia, 2–4 April 2017; IEEE: New York, NY, USA, 2017; p. 16946151.
17. Egan, A.; Mahmood, W.; Fenton, R.; Redziniak, N.; Kyaw Tun, T.; Sreenan, S.; McDermott, J. Barriers to exercise in obese patients with type 2 diabetes. *QJM* **2013**, *106*, 635–638. [CrossRef] [PubMed]
18. Gunaydin, T.; Arslan, R.; Birik, B.; Cirak, Y.; Durustkan Elbasi, N. A Surface Electromyography Based Serious Game for Increasing Patient Participation to Physiotherapy and Rehabilitation Treatment Following Anterior Cruciate and Medial Collateral Ligaments Operations. In Proceedings of the IEEE 31st International Symposium on Computer-Based Medical Systems, Karlstad, Sweden, 18–21 June 2018; IEEE: New York, NY, USA, 2018; p. 17936736.
19. Clausen, J.; Nahen, N.; Horstmann, H.; Lasch, F.; Krutsch, W.; Krettek, C.; Weber-Spickschen, T. Improving Maximal Strength in the Initial Postoperative Phase After Anterior Cruciate Ligament Reconstruction Surgery: Randomized Controlled Trial of an App-Based Serious Gaming Approach. *JMIR Serious Games* **2020**, *8*, e14282. [CrossRef] [PubMed]
20. Deacon, M.; Parsons, J.; Mathieson, S.; Davies, T. Can Wii Balance? Evaluating a Stepping Game for Older Adults. *IEEE Trans. Neural. Syst. Rehabil. Eng.* **2018**, *26*, 1783–1793. [CrossRef] [PubMed]
21. Cugelman, B. Gamification: What It Is and Why It Matters to Digital Health Behavior Change Developers. *JMIR Serious Games* **2013**, *1*, e3. [CrossRef] [PubMed]
22. Tech Trends 2012: Elevate IT for Digital Business. Available online: https://www2.deloitte.com/content/dam/Deloitte/au/Documents/technology/deloitte-au-technology-tech-trends-2012.pdf (accessed on 9 May 2020).
23. Exploitationware: On the Rhetoric of Gamification. From My "Persuasive Games" Column at Gamasutra. Available online: http://bogost.com/writing/exploitationware/ (accessed on 9 May 2020).
24. Gliddon, E.; Lauder, S.; Berk, L.; Cosgrove, V.; Grimm, D.; Dodd, S.; Suppes, T.; Berk, M. Evaluating discussion board engagement in the MoodSwings online self-help program for bipolar disorder: Protocol for an observational prospective cohort study. *BMC Psychiatry* **2015**, *15*. [CrossRef] [PubMed]
25. Digital NHS. Available online: https://digital.nhs.uk/ (accessed on 12 May 2020).
26. How to Conduct Design Review Meetings That don't Get Derailed. Available online: https://uxdesign.cc/how-to-conduct-design-review-meetings-that-dont-get-derailed (accessed on 10 April 2020).
27. Lewis, J.; Sauro, J. Revisiting the Factor Structure of the System Usability Scale. *J. Usability Stud.* **2017**, *12*, 184–192.
28. Turning Usability Testing Data into Action without Going Insane. Available online: https://www.toptal.com/designers/usability/turning-usability-testing-data-into-action (accessed on 25 April 2020).
29. Card Sorting: Uncover Users' Mental Models for Better Information Architecture. Available online: https://www.nngroup.com/articles/card-sorting-definition/ (accessed on 17 January 2020).
30. 10 Usability Heuristics for User Interface Design. Available online: https://www.nngroup.com/articles/ten-usability-heuristics/ (accessed on 10 May 2020).
31. Haladjian, J.; Bredies, K.; Brügge, B. KneeHapp Textile: A Smart Textile System for Rehabilitation of Knee Injuries. In Proceedings of the IEEE 15th International Conference on Wearable and Implantable Body Sensor Networks, Las Vegas, NV, USA, 4–7 March 2018; IEEE: New York, NY, USA, 2018; p. 17681609.
32. Pereira, A.; Folgado, D.; Nunes, F.; Almeida, J.; Sousa, I. Using Inertial Sensors to Evaluate Exercise Correctness in Electromyography-based Home Rehabilitation Systems. In Proceedings of the IEEE International Symposium on Medical Measurements and Applications, Istanbul, Turkey, 26–28 June 2019; IEEE: New York, NY, USA, 2019; p. 18970423.

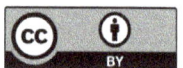

© 2020 by the authors. Licensee MDPI, Basel, Switzerland. This article is an open access article distributed under the terms and conditions of the Creative Commons Attribution (CC BY) license (http://creativecommons.org/licenses/by/4.0/).

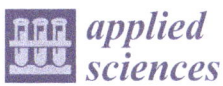

Review

Effect of Physical Exercise on the Release of Microparticles with Angiogenic Potential

Andrea Di Credico, Pascal Izzicupo, Giulia Gaggi, Angela Di Baldassarre * and Barbara Ghinassi

Department of Medicine and Aging Sciences, University "G. D'Annunzio" of Chieti-Pescara, 66100 Chieti, Italy; andrea.dicredico@unich.it (A.D.C.); izzicupo@unich.it (P.I.); giulia.gaggi@unich.it (G.G.); b.ghinassi@unich.it (B.G.)
* Correspondence: angela.dibaldassarre@unich.it

Received: 18 June 2020; Accepted: 14 July 2020; Published: 16 July 2020

Abstract: Cellular communication has a fundamental role in both human physiological and pathological states and various mechanisms are involved in the crosstalk between organs. Among these, microparticles (MPs) have an important involvement. MPs are a subtype of extracellular vesicles produced by a variety of cells following activation or apoptosis. They are normally present in physiological conditions, but their concentration varies in pathological states such as cardiovascular disease, diabetes mellitus, or cancer. Acute and chronic physical exercise are able to modify MPs amounts as well. Among various actions, exercise-responsive MPs affect angiogenesis, the process through which new blood vessels grow from pre-existing vessels. Usually, the neo vascular growth has functional role; but an aberrant neovascularization accompanies several oncogenic, ischemic, or inflammatory diseases. In addition, angiogenesis is one of the key adaptations to physical exercise and training. In the present review, we report evidence regarding the effect of various typologies of exercise on circulating MPs that are able to affect angiogenesis.

Keywords: microparticles; microvesicles; extracellular vesicles; molecular markers; cell–cell communication; physical exercise; physical activity; angiogenesis; secretome; paracrine signaling; cellular crosstalk

---

1. Introduction

The capacity to communicate between cells, tissues, and organs is a fundamental requisite to ensure appropriate physiological functions [1]. One of the most important mechanisms governed by cell communication and signaling is represented by the formation of vasculature. It is well known that vascular formation and growth are processes strictly regulated by growth factors and bioactive molecules. Hypoxia represents an important stimulus for angiogenesis: it activates hypoxia-inducible factors (HIFs) that upregulate various angiogenic genes, including vascular endothelial growth factor (VEGF) [2]. On the other hand, other different factors (e.g., thrombospondin-1, statins) are involved in the inhibition of angiogenesis [3].

Neovascular growth can be a physiological (e.g., in injured tissues [4]) or a pathological process, as it occurs in diabetic retinopathy, maculopathy, in tumors, and in many other disorders. Physiological angiogenesis represents the results of an accurate balance between pro-angiogenic and anti-angiogenic signals [5]. In pathological conditions, this balance is compromised and the new vessels do not provide a functional vascular perfusion [6].

Small extracellular vesicles, named microparticles (MPs), can be involved in angiogenic processes [7]. MPs are defined as heterogeneous small membranous vesicular structures derived from different cell types [8]. They are lacking nucleus and ranging in size from 0.1 to 1 µm. The most abundant population of MPs derives from platelets, but also other different cell types release these vesicles into the circulation such as endothelial cells [9], leucocytes [10] erythrocytes [11], epithelial cells [12], muscle cells, and various tumor cell lines [12]. Therefore, MPs express surface protein and antigens deriving by their parental cell as well as cytoplasmic and nuclear content (e.g., proteins, mRNAs, microRNAs, small-interfering RNAs, long non-coding RNAs), that are signature of their cellular origin [13]. MPs are released in response to cellular activation or apoptosis, elicited by a variety of stimuli, such as inflammation, oxidative stress, or mechanical/hemodynamic fluctuations depending on the involved parental cell [14].

Physical exercise can induce modifications in MP concentration [15]. In fact, MP concentration is modified by stimuli such hypoxia and shear stress [16], conditions elicited to a different extent by physical exercise. It has been demonstrated that MPs produced in response to physical exercise have a stimulating effect on new vessels growth [17].

The purpose of this review is to summarize the effects of different patterns of physical exercise on the concentration of circulating MPs with a known angiogenic potential.

2. Vasculogenesis, Arteriogenesis, and Angiogenesis

Vessels can be formed mainly by three processes: vasculogenesis, arteriogenesis, and angiogenesis. Vasculogenesis is the formation of new vessels that occurs in the embryo as well in the fetal annexes involved in the transportation of maternal nutrients: the placental villi and the yolk sac [18]; it derives from the differentiation of mesodermal cells into angioblasts, that proliferate, migrate, and couple to produce a primitive tube-like vessel. Consequently, vessels continue to develop as angioblasts differentiate in endothelial cells, form a vascular lumen, and deposit the basal lamina [19]. Various growth factors are involved in the molecular signaling of vasculogenesis: the fibroblast growth factor (FGF)-2, involved in mesodermal induction as well as in the induction of the angioblasts from the mesoderm [20], VEGFs family, that plays a pivotal role for its stimulating effects, [21], and finally the transforming growth factor-β family (TGF-βs) that contributes to vasculogenesis, with a dose dependent effect (low doses stimulate, while high doses inhibit endothelial cell growth [22]).

Arteriogenesis is the process whereby small pre-existing arterioles are transformed in functional arteries. One of the major stimuli inducing arteriogenesis is represented by shear stress, a mechanical signal able to activate transcription factors such as early growth response protein-1 (erg-1), that in turn lead to gene expression of chemokines like monocyte chemoattractant protein-1 (MCP-1), and adhesion molecules like intercellular adhesion molecule-1 (ICAM-1). These molecules are important for the docking of monocytes on endothelial cells, a fundamental step in arteriogenesis. Moreover, also growth factors such as VEGF, FGF, and TGF-β are involved in this process [23,24].

Lastly, angiogenesis is the process in which new blood vessels rising from pre-existing vessels, and it can occur mainly through mechanisms such as sprouting and intussusception (also known as vessel splitting or non-sprouting angiogenesis) [25]. Angiogenesis is a fundamental process during embryonic, fetal, and adult life and plays a pivotal role in many physiological process (e.g., as in skeletal growth, in wound healing, in pregnancy); however, angiogenesis represents also an important hallmark of pathological processes such as cancer and several noncommunicable diseases. Angiogenesis is governed by a precise balance between angiogenic growth factors and inhibitors. VEGF-A and its tyrosine kinase receptors represent the main and best characterized signaling pathway involved in developmental angiogenesis [26]. However, other molecules play a key role in endothelial cell proliferation and migration. They are represented by FGFs, platelet-derived growth factor (PDGF), and epidermal growth factor (EGF) [27]. Therefore, angiogenesis is a complex process controlled by several molecules and can have useful as well as detrimental effects on human health, and for this reason the various underlying mechanisms are object of great interest.

3. Extracellular Vesicles Classification

Human cells are able to release various types of membrane vesicles in response to different stimuli, generally called extracellular vesicles (EVs). EVs include exosomes, MPs (also called microvesicles), and apoptotic bodies [28] (Table 1).

Table 1. General characteristics of extracellular vesicles (EVs).

EVs Types	Size	Surface Markers	Mechanism of Production	Content
Exosomes	50–100 nm	Phosphatidylserine (PS, Annexin V$^+$), Lysosomal-Associated Membrane Protein 1 (LAMP1), Tumor Susceptibility 101 (TSG101), Granulophysin (CD63), Target of antiproliferative antibody 1 (CD81), Tetraspanin-29 (CD9)	Fusion of late endosomes/multivesicular bodies (MVBs) with the plasma membrane	Proteins, RNAs, miRNAs
Microparticles	100 nm–1 μm	PS * (Annexin V$^+$) markers of parental cell	Budding/blebbing of the plasma membrane	Proteins, RNAs, miRNAs
Apoptotic bodies	500 nm–3 μm	PS (Annexin V$^+$)	Blebbing of cells undergoing apoptosis	Proteins, RNAs, miRNAs, DNA, organelles

* PS = phosphatidylserine.

Exosomes are vesicles surrounded by a double layer of phospholipids and their size ranges between 50 and 100 nm in diameter. They are released in both physiological condition and upon activation by exocytosis of multivesicular bodies (MVBs) [29]. Exosomes can communicate with other cells either through a direct contact between surface proteins or by vesicles–cell membrane fusion or by endocytosis. They expose phosphatidylserine (PS) on the external membrane and various markers such as LAMP1, TSG101, CD63, CD81, and CD9 [30]. The main functions of exosomes include antigen presentation and immunostimulatory activity. In addition, exosomes are able to horizontally transfer mRNA and miRNA as well as oncogenic receptors [31].

MPs, formerly described as "platelet dust", are now well known cell–cell communicators and they act as signaling molecules in physiological homeostatic processes or as a consequence of pathological condition including diabetes, chronic kidney disease, rheumatoid arthritis, multiple sclerosis, and cardiovascular diseases [32]. MPs are found in most body fluids such as plasma, saliva, urine, and cerebrospinal fluid. They represent a heterogeneous population of vesicular-like structures composed by a phospholipid bilayer and their sizes range from 100 nm to 1 μm in diameter; however precise cut-off values remain to be established. MPs found in bloodstream may originate from various vascular cells (e.g., platelets, monocytes, erythrocytes, granulocytes) [33]. However, among all circulating MPs, platelet-derived MPs (Plt-MPs) are the most abundant population, representing 70–90% of the total [34]. They are produced by budding of the plasma membrane, in a process called ectocytosis. After their release, MPs carry proteins that are signature of their cell of origin, and transport various enzymes, RNA, and miRNA [35]. MPs generally expose PS on their outer leaflet (Annexin V$^+$), however some evidence shows that MPs can also be PS negative [36]. In addition, a subpopulation of various phenotypes of MPs expose tissue factor [37]. The release of MPs is induced upon cell activation or apoptosis.

Apoptotic bodies are EVs larger than MPs and exosomes. Their sizes range from 500 nm to 3 μm and they expose PS; however, their outer membrane differs from MPs due to its permeability [38]. Apoptotic bodies are released by membrane blebbing of cells undergoing apoptosis and they may horizontally transfer their content, such as cell organelles, fragmented DNA, and oncogenes.

4. Methods of Detection of Microparticles

Flow cytometry (FC) is one of the most common methods of detection, quantification, and size evaluation of MPs [39]. In addition, FC allows the phenotypic characterization of MPs using fluorescent antibodies against the diverse antigens expressed by the cell of origin [40]. However, FC has some limitations. For example, MPs with a size ranging from 0.1 to 0.4 μm are too undetected by most cytometers [41]. In addition, the type of instrument, settings, and sample preparation procedures can cause a high level of variability of the results [42].

The nanoparticle tracking analysis (NTA), on the other hand, is able to detect vesicles smaller than those recognized by FC. Such type of analysis correlates the speed of movements, tracked using a microscope, with the size of MPs [43]. Nevertheless, NTA is unable to discriminate vesicles derived from cells from other particles of small dimensions such as high-density lipoprotein (HDL) [44]. Fluorescent nanoparticle tracking analysis (F-NTA), diversely from NTA, is based on the fluorescence of the particles [45].

Other techniques to analyze the EVs are based on image analyses obtained by optical and electron microscopy. Optical microscopy permits to assess the size and morphological features of MPs and of apoptotic bodies, while cannot provide information on their phenotype. This kind of information can, anyway, be obtained by fluorescent microscopy labeling MPs with fluorescent probes that recognize specific surface markers [41]. However, this approach does not permit to specify the size of the EVs [41]. An accurate morphological analysis of MPs is obtained by transmission electron microscopy (TEM), that represents the most used method to assess the composition, morphology, size, and membrane structure of MPs [34]. However, TEM requires a considerable amount of time for both preparation and analysis of the sample.

Western blotting (WB) is a commonly used technique that allows to identify the cellular origin of MPs [46]; anyway, this methodological approach presents some important limitations: indeed, it requires a large amount of MPs to be performed and the analysis needs to be completed with complementary methods such as NTA or TEM [47,48].

Finally, another method for MPs detection is the enzyme-linked immunosorbent assay (ELISA). This is also a quantitative analysis, that measures MPs indirectly: indeed, such method relies on the binding of MPs to specific conjugate-antibodies adsorbed to a well plate [49]. ELISA permits the specification of MPs subtypes, but fresh plasma is indispensable, because the freezing-thawing process leads to an increase of annexin-binding MPs [50].

However, is important to note that most of the studies analyzing MPs in exercise settings utilize the flow cytometric approach [17,51–56].

5. Production Mechanisms of MPs

It is well known that MPs can be released upon activation or apoptotic stimuli; however, most cells constitutively shed MPs by ectocytosis and significant concentrations of these vesicles can be detected in the plasma [57]. The common mechanism for the production of MPs is represented by a change in the asymmetry of the phospholipids composing the plasma membrane. The lipid bilayer of normal cells presents an asymmetrical composition of phospholipids [58]. PS and phosphatidylethanolamine (PE) are located in the internal layer of the plasma membrane whereas the external layer is composed of phosphatidylinositol (PI), phosphatidylcoline (PC), sphingomyelin (SM), and other glycolipids. In order to allow MPs formation, this precise distribution is disrupted. Such changes in membrane architecture are controlled by three enzymes: flippase, floppase, and scramblase [59]. Flippase is involved in the maintenance of the phospholipid asymmetry between the membrane layers. Floppase controls the ATP-dependent translocation of PS to the external layer in response to cellular activation. Finally, scramblase is responsible for the membrane randomization allowing phospholipids to flow down their concentration gradients. In resting cells, only flippase is active, contributing to the internalization of negatively charged phospholipids (e.g., PS and PE) and to the maintenance of the physiological membrane asymmetry. Nevertheless, various events providing cellular activation are able to increase intracellular calcium concentration, causing the flippase inhibition and the activation of floppase, scramblase, and other calcium-sensitive enzymes such as calpain and gelsolin, resulting in MPs release [60].

An important mediator of apoptotic MPs production is Rho-associated kinase (ROCK I), a protein kinase activated via caspase-mediated cleavage. ROCK I may allow the phosphorylation of myosin light-chains, triggering cytoskeletal rearrangement and formation of apoptotic MPs through the coupling of actin-myosin filaments to the plasma membrane [61].

6. MPs and Angiogenesis

Vesicle-like structures have recently emerged as important mediators for cellular communication in both physiological and pathological processes [30]; in particular, MPs released by various cell types may play an important role in angiogenesiss [62,63], by modulating the production of proangiogenic factors through changes in the secretome of endothelial cells [64,65]. Like exosomes, MPs can communicate with other cells through ligands on their membrane that interact with specific receptors of the target cells; alternatively, MPs can fuse with the plasma membrane of the target cells, delivering its cytoplasmic content (e.g., proteins, miRNAs, RNAs). In this way, MPs may elicit the synthesis of proangiogenic or antiangiogenic factors and affect the main processes involved in formation of new vessels, such as endothelial cells adhesion, migration, and proliferation [66].

Endothelial cells-derived MPs (E-MPs) are clearly involved in the formation of blood vessels. A pioneer in vitro study highlighted that vesicles released by endothelial cells can transport integrin-$\beta 1$ and active matrix metalloproteinases-2 and 9 (MMP-2 and MMP-9), thus inducing endothelial cells invasion and tube-like structure [67]. In addition, it has been demonstrated that upon stimulation with the proinflammatory interleukin-3, endothelial cells release vesicles containing pro-angiogenic factors such as miR-126-3p and Stat5 [68]. Moreover, another study shows that endothelial MPs are able to transfer miR-126 from endothelial cells to vascular smooth muscle cells, corroborating the angiogenic properties of endothelial MPs [69].

Additionally, Plt-MPs are involved in angiogenesis. These vesicles can promote angiogenic effects by transferring various cytokines, such as PDGF, VEGF, FGF-2, and activating key proteins such as PI3k, ERK, and src kinase [70]. Various studies found that the angiogenic potential of the platelet-derived MPs can have both functional positive and negative effects: when Plt-MPs were infused in a rat model of myocardial ischemia, indeed, they increased the quantity of functional capillaries [70]; on the other hand, MPs shed by platelets can favor angiogenesis involved in tumor progression, upregulating important angiogenic factors, such as VEGF, HGF, and interleukin-8 [71].

7. Angiogenesis Induced by Physical Exercise

Physical activity has beneficial effects on human health [72–75], and regular physical exercise improves health in both physiological and pathological conditions [76–79]. Numerous evidence demonstrates the inverse relationship between regular exercise and cardiovascular diseases, hypertension, stroke, type 2 diabetes mellitus, metabolic syndrome, obesity, osteoporosis, and various types of cancer [76,80–83]. Depending on the type of physical exercise, we can observe different effects on the organism: endurance (or aerobic) exercise is characterized by a high number of muscular contractions, relative low load, and an important involvement of the cardiorespiratory system, whereas resistance exercise is represented by low number of muscular contraction but with relative higher loads and thus it relies mainly on the neuromuscular system [84]. These two types of exercise can be considered two extremes in a line, and between these two, numerous types of exercise exist, based on the modulation of the exercise variables (e.g., intensity, volume, density, rest). Each type of exercise can increase different responses and adaptions, triggering diverse cellular pathways.

Cardiovascular endurance training is the strongest stimulus for exercise-induced angiogenesis; this results in an improved capillary to fiber ratio in the skeletal muscle to provide an enhanced blood flow and oxygen delivery to the exercising muscles [85–89]. Endurance exercise stimulates the angiogenesis activating several pathways (Figure 1). It induces an important reduction of the partial pressure of oxygen that leads to a local tissue hypoxia. This modification in oxygen levels decreases the hydroxylation of HIF-1alpha trough the inhibition of prolyl hydroxylase domain enzymes (PHD); in this way, HIF-1alpha become more stable and translocate into the nucleus, where forms an active complex with HIF-1beta [90] and activates genes involved in angiogenesis such as VEGF [84].

Another key regulator of VEGF synthesis is the peroxisome proliferator-activated receptor gamma co-activator 1-alpha (PGC-1alpha), which is modulated by aerobic exercise in several ways: intense endurance exercise produces an energy deficit and an increase of the AMP/ATP ratio that activate the AMP-activated protein kinase (AMPK) responsible for the PGC-1alpha phosphorylation. Moreover, an acute bout of exercise increases the NAD^+/NADH ratio that promotes the sirtuin (specifically SIRT1) activity and PGC-1alpha deacetylation [91]. Finally, aerobic exercise affects also the estrogen-related receptor gamma (ERR gamma) that controls the skeletal muscle vascularization by modifying the VEGF expression [92].

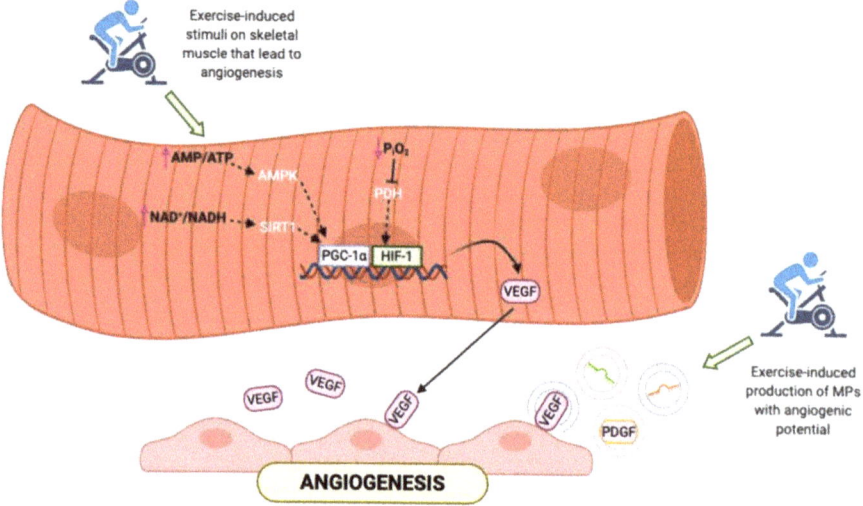

Figure 1. Representation of the main pathways activated in skeletal muscle in response to exercise. In addition to the canonical molecular pathways, aerobic exercise may affect the release of microparticles (MPs) that carry soluble factors involved in angiogenesis. AMP = adenosine monophosphate; ATP = adenosine triphosphate; NAD = nicotinamide adenine dinucleotide; NADH = reduced nicotinamide adenine dinucleotide; PGC-1α = peroxisome proliferator-activated receptor gamma coactivator 1-alpha; HIF = hypoxia-inducible factor; VEGF = vascular endothelial growth factor; PDGF = platelet-derived growth factor.

In the last years it was evidenced that physical exercise induces modification of the MPs release into the bloodstream [93]. These EVs carry various molecules important for the tissues' crosstalk during and post exercise [94,95] and can be also a cargo of soluble factors involved in endothelial cell proliferation, migration, and adhesion. This results in the generation of new vessels in response to exercise.

8. MPs and Physical Exercise

Physical exercise, particularly endurance exercise, is known to stimulate shear stress due to its hemodynamic effects [96]. Intraluminal shear stress has a beneficial effect on vasculature because it is able to ameliorate vascular dilation through mechanisms mediated by nitric oxide [97]. In addition, exercise-induced shear stress can modulate the production of both E-MPs and Plt-MPs. For example, it was seen that high shear stress can reduce the concentration of E-MP while low shear stress is prone to increase such concentration [98]. Moreover, both high and low shear stress can elicit the production of MPs from platelets [99] (Figure 2).

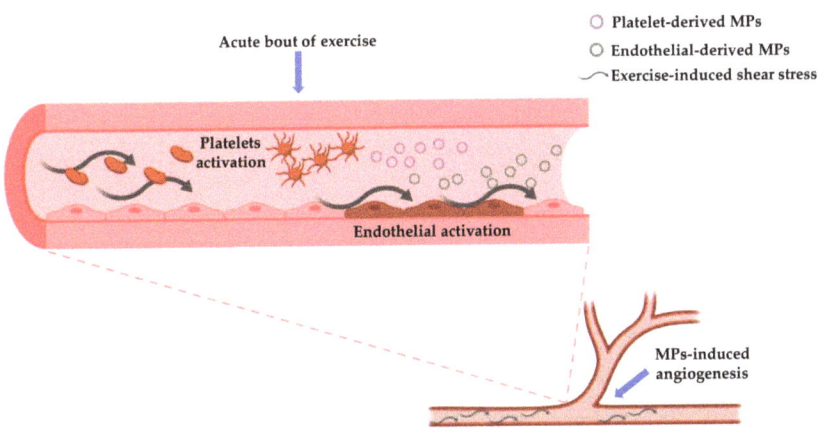

Figure 2. This figure shows the possible mechanisms involved in the production of platelet-derived MPs and endothelial-derived MPs and their role in stimulating angiogenesis. Both platelets and endothelial cells are activated in response to mechanical and chemical stimuli provided by exercise, that in turn elicit the MPs production by ectocytosis. The branching point refers to the site in which MPs stimulate neo-vascularization.

Acute exercise leads to an augmentation of the sympathetic activity, increasing both epinephrine and norepinephrine concentrations [100]. In this regard, studies report that norepinephrine is able to stimulate Plt-MPs release [101]. Along with hormonal response, acute exercise stimulates the secretion of many cytokines from skeletal muscle, named myokines [102]. Among these myokines, IL-6 is released in the bloodstream and elicits multiorgan effects [103]. It has been reported that IL-6 is also able to stimulate Plt-MPs formation [104], thus exercise can be a potent stimulus to enhance such mechanism.

The following sections provide an overview of various studies (summarized in Table 2) investigating the effects of physical exercise and training on MPs concentration, with an emphasis on endothelial and platelet-derived MPs, due to their specific involvement in angiogenesis [17,105–107].

Table 2. Summary of studies that evaluate MPs concentration in relation with physical exercise/exercise training in various populations.

Reference	Participants	Exercise Protocol	MPs Antigen Expression	MPs Collection Time Point	Effects of Exercise on MPs
Bittencourt CRO et al. (2017) [52]	Twenty-five professional half-marathon runners	No experimental protocols, blood was analyzed at rest and compared with that of healthy controls	$CD42^+/CD31^+$ (Plt-MPs)$CD51^+$ (E-MPs)	At rest, after 12 h of fasting	MPs concentration did not differ between runners and controls
Boyle JL et al. (2013) [53]	Eleven healthy men (25 ± 2 year)	5 days of reduced physical activity	$CD31^+/CD42b^-$ (apoptotic E-MPs)$CD62E^+$ (activated E-MPs)	At baseline, days 1, 3, 5 of reduced physical activity	↑ $CD31^+/CD42b^-$ after 5 days ↔ $CD62E^+$ after 5 days
Brahmer A et al. (2019) [108]	Twenty-one healthy male athletes (28.7 ± 4.2)	Incremental cycling test until exhaustion	EVs array including different subtypes	Before, during, and after the exercise test	Among others, ↑ E-MPs and ↑ Plt-MPs
Durrer C et al. (2015) [15]	Overweight/obese males and females	20 min cycling just above VT (HICE) vs. 10×1 min at ≈90% peak aerobic power (HIIE) vs. control	$CD62E^+$ (activated E-MPs)$CD31^+/CD42b^-$ (apoptotic E-MPs)	≈18 h after the three conditions	↓ $CD62E^+$, $CD31^+/CD42b$ in men after both HICE and HIIE↑ $CD62E^+$ in women after HICE↔ $CD31^+/CD42b^-$ in women after both conditions
Guiraud T et al. (2013) [109]	Nineteen males with coronary heart disease (62 ± 11 year)	2×10 min of cycling (15 s at 100% PPO/15 s passive rest) (HIIE) vs. isocaloric MICE session (at 70% PPO)	$CD31^+/CD42b^-$ (apoptotic E-MPs)$CD62E^+$ (activated E-MPs)$CD42b^+$ (Plt-MPs)	10 min before protocols and 20 min, 24 h, and 72 h after protocols	↔ all types of MPs after both exercise protocols
Highton PJ et al. (2019) [110]	Fifteen men (22.9 ± 3.3 year)	1 h of running (70% VO_{2max})	TF^+ Plt-MPS and TF^+ neutrophil MPs	Before exercise, immediately after exercise, 1:30 h post exercise	↓ TF^+ Platelet and TF^+ neutrophil MPs after exercise
Kim JS et al. (2015) [111]	Twenty-one male and female subjects (52.1 ± 1.4)	40 min of aerobic exercise at 65% HR_{max} (3 days/week for 6 months)	$CD31^+/CD42a^-$ (apoptotic E-MPs)$CD62E^+$ (activated E-MPs)	Pre and post exercise intervention	↓ $CD31^+/CD42a^-$ ↓ $CD62E^+$
Kirk RJ et al. (2013) [112]	Seven healthy males (22 ± 3.2 year)	10×15 s at 120% PPO of cycling	$CD105^+$ (E-MPs)$CD106^+$ (E-MPs)	Immediately before and after exercise, 90 min and 180 min post-exercise	↑ $CD105^+$, $CD106^+$ 90 min post-exercise
Kirk RJ et al. (2019) [55]	Eleven women with PCOS (28.00 ± 6.72) and 10 control women (24.26 ± 6.18)	1 h of running on a treadmill at 60% VO_{2max} (3 days/week for 8 weeks)	$CD105^+$ (E-MPs)$CD106^+$ (E-MPs)	Pre, at 4 weeks of the exercise program (mid), and post exercise program	↓ $CD105^+$ in women with PCOS post exercise↔ $CD106^+$ in either groups post exercise
Lansford KA et al. (2015) [51]	Sixteen healthy men (24.5 ± 0.8 year) and 10 healthy women (22.4 ± 0.52 year)	Stationary cycling at 60–70% VO_{2peak} until reaching a total energy expenditure of 598 kcal	$CD62E^+$ (activated E-MPs)$CD34^+$ (hematopoietic cell derived MPs)$CD31^+/CD42b^-$ (apoptotic E-MPs)	At baseline and within 5 min of completing the exercise protocol	↑ $CD62E^+$ in men only↔ $CD31^+/CD42b$ ↑ $CD34^+$ in women only
Rafiei H et al. (2019) [54]	Fifteen overweight/obese women (48.9 ± 10.7)	2 weeks (10 sessions) of progressive HIIT or MICT on a cycle ergometer	$CD62E^+$ (activated E-MPs)$CD31^+/CD42b^-$ (apoptotic E-MPs)	Pre and post exercise protocols	↓ $CD62^+$ for both HIIT and MICT↔ $CD31^+/CD42b$ for both HIIT and MICT

Table 2. Cont.

Reference	Participants	Exercise Protocol	MPs Antigen Expression	MPs Collection Time Point	Effects of Exercise on MPs
Rakobowchuk M et al. (2017) [56]	Twelve healthy men (29.2 ± 6.1 year)	45 min of eccentric or concentric cycling	$CD62E^+$ (activated E-MPs)/$CD41^+$ (Plt-MPs)	Pre and post exercise protocols	↑ $CD41^+$ after both exercise modalities↔ $CD62E^+$
Rigamonti AE et al. (2020) [113]	Fifteen obese (21.2 ± 8.8) and eight normal weight subjects (26.2 ± 7.2) male and female	Moderate intensity (60% VO_{2max}) treadmill to exhaustion	$CD14^+$ (monocyte/macrophage derived -MPs), $CD61^+$ (Plt-MPs), $CD62E^+$ (activated E-MPs), $CD105^+$ (E-MPs), $SCGA^+$ (skeletal muscle derived MPs), $FABP^+$ (adipocyte derived MPs)	1 h before, at the end, 3 h, and 24 h after exercise	Changes were tissue, sex, and BMI specific, ↓ $CD61^+$ immediately and 24 h post exercise
Schwarz V et al. (2017) [114]	Ninety marathon runners (49 ± 6 year)	Marathon run (i.e., 42 km run)	$CD144^+$ (E-MPs), $CD62E^+$ (activated E-MPs), $CD31^+$ $CD62P^+$ (Plt-MPs), $CD42b^+$ (Plt-MPs) $CD14^+$ (monocyte derived MPs), $CD45^+$ (leukocyte derived MPs)	Three days before, immediately after, within 2 days after the marathon run	↑$CD144^+$, $CD62E^+$, $CD31^+$↑ $CD62P^+$, $CD42b^+$ ↓ $CD14^+$, $CD45^+$
Serviente C et al. (2019) [115]	Thirty-six healthy active women (40-65 year)	30 min of treadmill exercise at 60–64% VO_{2peak}	$CD62E^+$ (activated E-MPs) $CD31^+/CD42b^-$ (apoptotic E-MPs)	At baseline, and 30 min after the exercise protocol	↓ $CD62E^+$ ↓ $CD31^+/CD42b^-$
Shill DD et al. (2018) [116]	Ten healthy men (23.6 ± 3.27) and 10 healthy women (23.6 ± 5.58)	HIIE (10 × 1 min ≈95% VO_{2max}/75 s active recovery) vs. MICE (energy-matched continuous bout at 65% VO_{2max})	$CD34^+$ (hematopoietic cell derived MPs) $CD62E^+$ (activated E-MPs)	At baseline, half exercise, immediately after exercise, 30, 60, 90, 120 min after exercise	Changes in $CD62E^+$ and $CD34^+$ were intensity dependent, and sex specific
Whal P et al. (2014) [117]	Twelve men triathletes/cyclists (24.7 ± 3.4)	130 min at 55% PPO vs. 4 × 4 min at 95% PPO vs. 4 × 30 s all-out	$CD31^+/CD42b^-$ (apoptotic E-MPs)	Before exercise, and 0, 30, 60, 180 min post-exercise	↓ $CD31^+/CD42b^-$ after all three exercise protocols
Wilhelm EN et al. (2016) [17]	Nine healthy young men (25 ± 1 year)	1 h of moderate (46 ± 2% VO_{2max}) vs. heavy (67 ± 2% VO_{2max}) intensity semirecumbent cycling	$CD62E^+$ (apoptotic E-MPs) $CD41^+$ (Plt-MPs)	At baseline, 30, 60, 80, 100, 120, 150, 180, and 240 min of the protocol	↔ $CD62E^+$ for both MI and HI↑ $CD41^+$ at 30 and 60 min of HI exercise

↑ = increased concentration, ↓ = decreased concentration, ↔ unaltered concentration; E-MPs = endothelial cell-derived MPs; Plt-MPs = platelets derived MPs; TF$^+$ = tissue factor positive; VT = ventilatory threshold; HICE = high-intensity continuous exercise; HIIE = high-intensity interval exercise; HIIT = high-intensity interval training; MICT = moderate-intensity continuous training; PPO = peak power output.

8.1. The Effect of Physical Exercise on MPs with Angiogenic Potential in Athletes

Endurance athletes have the characteristics to present greater adaptation of the cardiorespiratory and neuromuscular systems resulting in the increase of the delivery and the consumption of oxygen [118]. Two of the sports that highly rely on these adaptations are marathon and half-marathon. Bittencourt et al. compared the amounts of E-MPs and Plt-MPs in a group of half-marathon runners with a control group of gender-matched healthy controls showing that $CD51^+$ E-MPs and $CD42^+/CD31^+$ Plt-MPs did not significantly differ between the two groups [52]. This data suggests that athletes exposed to chronic endurance training can benefit from exercise effects but that such type of training does not lead to further decrease in MPs compared with a healthy non-athlete population. On the other hand, E-MPs and Plt-MPs significantly increase following a marathon run and return to baseline values within 2 days; conversely, leukocyte and monocyte-derived MPs decrease after such run [114].

Like long distance running, road cycling and triathlon are two sports heavily relying on cardiorespiratory endurance [119]. In triathletes/cyclists, high-volume (2 h at 55% of peak power output) and high intensity (four sets of minutes at 90–95% of peak power output interspersed by 3 min of active recovery or four sets of 30 s at maximal effort separated by 7:30 of active recovery) trials on cycle ergometer, significantly decrease $CD31^+/CD42b^-$ apoptotic E-MPs 60 and 180 min after the termination of the trials [117]. It seems that such decrease was due to an increased uptake of MPs by cells. Indeed, triathletes/cyclists' serum collected 180 min after high intensities exercises promote the uptake of $CD31^+/CD42b^-$ apoptotic E-MPs in endothelial cells in vitro [117]. Another recent study involving male athletes showed that an incremental cycling protocol until exhaustion determined a significant increase of $CD105^+$, $CD146^+$ E-MPs, and $CD62P^+$ Plt-MPs at the peak of the exercise session [108].

8.2. The Effect of Physical Exercise on MPs with Angiogenic Potential in Healthy Subjects

The physical exercise performed in a regular manner elicits beneficial effects that include improved cardiorespiratory fitness, body composition, decreased risk of noncommunicable diseases and of all-cause mortality [76,120–124].

Data on the effects of aerobic exercise on E-MPs and Plt-MPs are controversial. After 1 h of treadmill run at 70% of VO_{2max}, a decrease in TF^+ Plt-MPs and neutrophil-derived MPs in healthy men [110] has been observed; moreover, a single session of 30 min of moderate intensity aerobic exercise (60–64% of their VO_{2peak}) reduces the number of $CD62E^+$ activated E-MPs and $CD31^+/CD42b^-$ apoptotic E-MPs [115]. On the other hand, in prehypertensive male and female, aerobic exercise performed at 65% of predicted maximal heart rate for a duration of 6 months, with a frequency of three times per week, decreases the blood concentration of $CD62E^+$ E-MPs and $CD31^+/CD42a^-$ E-MPs [111]. Some authors also evidenced a possible sex/gender effect on the MPs release: indeed, an acute bout of aerobic exercise at 60–70% of the VO_{2peak} produced a significant increase in $CD62E^+$ E-MPs in men, and an increase in $CD34^+$ MPs in women [51]. However, results of study involving both male and female are inconclusive. Indeed, another study showed $CD62E^+$ E-MPs decrease both during and after moderate intensity continuous exercise (65% of VO_{2max}) in women but not in men [116].

One of the factors that must be taken into account analyzing the effects of physical exercise on the MPs is the timing of the analysis. In response to low to moderate intensity (33% of VO_{2max}) concentric or eccentric cycling, men show higher concentration of $CD41^+$ Plt-MPs 5 min following exercise, but these levels returned to baseline levels after 40 min of recovery, while $CD62E^+$ E-MPs do not show modifications [56]. Another experimental study performed in young males showed that $CD41^+$ Plt-MPs and $CD62E^+$ E-MPs were unaffected by 1 h of cycling at $\approx 46\%$ of VO_{2max}, while when the intensity were set $\approx 67\%$ of VO_{2max} an increase of $CD41^+$ Plt-MPs was observed [17]. Interestingly, the MPs released in response to such type of exercise enhanced endothelial proliferation, migration, and tubule-like formation in vitro, compared with MPs present in resting conditions [17].

Another modality of training that is of increasing interest in research is high intensity interval training (HIIT). HIIT is a useful exercise modality to enhance cardiorespiratory endurance, and such type of training can be performed also at strenuous intensities [125,126]. Supramaximal sprint cycling protocol consisting of 10 bouts of 15 s at 120% of peak power output separated by 45 s of active recovery lead to a significant increase of circulating CD105$^+$ and CD106$^+$ E-MPs 90 min after the exercise session, whereas at 180 min post-exercise MPs returned towards resting values [112]. On the other hand, no changes in endothelial MPs concentration was observed after a high intensity interval exercise (95% of VO$_{2max}$) [116].

Physical inactivity and sedentary behaviors have detrimental effects on vasculature state, contributing to the development of cardiovascular and metabolic diseases [127–129]. After 5 days of reduced physical activity (<5000 steps/day), significant increase of CD31$^+$/CD42b$^-$ apoptotic E-MPs was registered, whereas CD62E$^+$ activated E-MPs remained unchanged, suggesting that inactivity fosters vascular dysfunction increasing endothelial apoptosis in recreationally active men [53].

8.3. The Effect of Physical Exercise on MPs with Angiogenic Potential in Pathologic Subjects

Physical exercise is a fundamental stimulus for improving metabolic and cardiovascular health. Among the various typology, HIIT has the same, or superior capacity to improve health status in pathological subjects (e.g., presenting diabetes, cardiovascular diseases, or cancer) [130,131]. In overweight/obese men, high-intensity continuous exercise (20 min of cycling at just above the subjective ventilatory threshold) and high-intensity interval exercise (10 bouts of 1 min at ≈90% peak aerobic power) reduce E-MPs concentration 18 h following exercise; different results were observed in overweight/obese women in which high-intensity continuous exercise increased activated CD62E$^+$ E-MPs, leaving unaffected CD31$^+$/CD42b$^-$ apoptotic E-MPs, regardless the intensity [15]. However, the chronic exposure of overweight/obese subjects to exercise (2 weeks of HIIT or moderate intensity continuous training) lowered the concentration of activated CD62E$^+$ E-MPs [54]. The effect of exercise on MPs release may also depend on the intensity of the physical activity. Indeed, in a recent study involving both over and normal weight subjects, a bout of moderate intensity (60% of their VO$_{2max}$) aerobic exercise, reduced the total EVs in the MPs range (130–700 nm); however, the release of MPs in normal weight subjects was higher than in obese and in females than in males. [113].

Polycystic ovary syndrome (PCOS) is an endocrine disorder in which endothelial dysfunction and altered angiogenesis are common. Eight weeks of aerobic training consisting of three sessions per week of 1 h of running on a treadmill at 60% VO$_{2max}$ led to a significant decrease in CD105$^+$ MPs in women with PCOS compared with a control group of healthy women, while did not have an effect on the amount of CD106$^+$ E-MPs [55].

Coronary artery diseases determine a diminished myocardial perfusion that may result in angina, myocardial infarction, and heart failure [132]. In stable coronary heart disease patients, neither moderate-intensity continuous exercise (28.7 min at 70% of peak power output) nor a single bout of high-intensity interval exercise (10 min session with work interval of 15 s at 100% of peak power output interspersed with 15 s of passive recovery) have an effect on the concentration of circulating E-MPs and Plt-MPs [109].

Overall, the numerous studies show contrasting results regarding the qualitative and quantitative changes of MPs in response to acute physical exercise and to exercise training as well. Such divergent conclusions could be due to the heterogeneity of the studies, as they involved different samples in terms of age, sex, training status, possible pharmacological therapies [133], and pathologies [93] (Figure 3). More standardized and harmonized procedures are needed to compare the studies and obtain definitive data on the release of MPs with angiogenic potential in response to physical exercise.

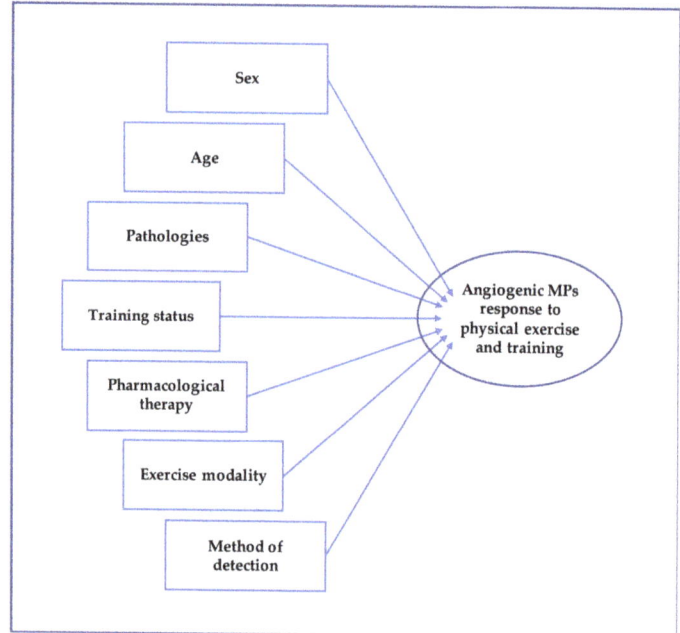

Figure 3. This figure shows the potential influencing factors affecting MPs following physical exercise and training.

9. Conclusions

Various modalities of cardiovascular endurance-based exercise can modify blood concentration of E-MPs and Plt-MPs, known to affect angiogenic processes. It is well known that physical exercise, among different adaptations, can lead to a functional angiogenesis resulting in a wider vascular bed that increases the blood flow to exercising muscles. Results regarding the effect of exercise on MPs are divergent, but it seems that acute exercise results in an increase of MPs while chronic exposure to exercise results in a decrease in most cases. In addition, MPs sensitivity to exercise can be affected by the training status, sex, age, as well as mode of exercise (e.g., run on a treadmill, road run, cycle ergometer), pharmacological therapies, diseases, and method of detection. While only one study directly showed the pro-angiogenic effects of MPs produced following exercise [17], numerous studies highlight the potential of E-MPs and Plt-MPs in communicating with other cells and stimulating angiogenesis [69,105–107]. Thus, future evidence regarding the effect of both acute exercise and training on MPs affecting angiogenesis will be useful to add important insights on the mechanisms by which exercise elicits vascular adaptations and to design specific training programs for various populations.

Author Contributions: A.D.C., P.I., G.G., A.D.B. and B.G. conceived of and designed the outline of the manuscript and examined and ensured the consistency and validity of the contents. A.D.B. and B.G. revised the final version of the manuscript. All authors have read and agreed to the published version of the manuscript.

Funding: This research was supported by the Italian Ministry of Education, University and Research (Ministero dell'Istruzione, dell'Università e della Ricerca-MIUR), grant number PRIN 2017ATZ2YK_003.

Conflicts of Interest: The authors declare no conflict of interest.

References

1. Nair, A.; Chauhan, P.; Saha, B.; Kubatzky, K.F. Conceptual Evolution of Cell Signaling. *Int. J. Mol. Sci.* **2019**, *20*, 3292. [CrossRef]
2. Carmeliet, P. Angiogenesis in health and disease. *Nat. Med.* **2003**, *9*, 653–660. [CrossRef] [PubMed]
3. Volpert, O.V.; Stellmach, V.; Bouck, N. The modulation of thrombospondin and other naturally occurring inhibitors of angiogenesis during tumor progression. *Breast Cancer Res. Treat.* **1995**, *36*, 119–126. [CrossRef] [PubMed]
4. Hanahan, D.; Folkman, J. Patterns and Emerging Mechanisms of the Angiogenic Switch during Tumorigenesis. *Cell* **1996**, *86*, 353–364. [CrossRef]
5. Bergers, G.; Benjamin, L.E. Tumorigenesis and the angiogenic switch: Angiogenesis. *Nat. Rev. Cancer* **2003**, *3*, 401–410. [CrossRef] [PubMed]
6. Gowdak, L.H.W.; Krieger, J.E. Vascular Growth Factors, Progenitor Cells, and Angiogenesis. In *Endothelium and Cardiovascular Diseases*; Elsevier: Amsterdam, The Netherlands, 2018; pp. 49–62.
7. Mezentsev, A.; Merks, R.M.H.; O'Riordan, E.; Chen, J.; Mendelev, N.; Goligorsky, M.S.; Brodsky, S.V. Endothelial microparticles affect angiogenesis in vitro: Role of oxidative stress. *Am. J. Physiol. Heart Circ. Physiol.* **2005**, *289*, H1106–H1114. [CrossRef] [PubMed]
8. Van Niel, G.; D'Angelo, G.; Raposo, G. Shedding light on the cell biology of extracellular vesicles. *Nat. Rev. Mol. Cell Biol.* **2018**, *19*, 213–228. [CrossRef]
9. Deng, F.; Wang, S.; Zhang, L. Endothelial microparticles act as novel diagnostic and therapeutic biomarkers of circulatory hypoxia-related diseases: A literature review. *J. Cell. Mol. Med.* **2017**, *21*, 1698–1710. [CrossRef]
10. He, Z.; Tang, Y.; Qin, C. Increased circulating leukocyte-derived microparticles in ischemic cerebrovascular disease. *Thromb. Res.* **2017**, *154*, 19–25. [CrossRef] [PubMed]
11. Rautou, P.; Bresson, J.; Sainte-Marie, Y.; Vion, A.; Paradis, V.; Renard, J.; Devue, C.; Heymes, C.; Letteron, P.; Elkrief, L.; et al. Abnormal Plasma Microparticles Impair Vasoconstrictor Responses in Patients with Cirrhosis. *Gastroenterology* **2012**, *143*, 166–176. [CrossRef]
12. Batool, S. Microparticles and their Roles in Inflammation: A Review. *Open Immunol. J.* **2013**, *6*, 1–14. [CrossRef]
13. Chen, Y.; Li, G.; Liu, M.-L. Microvesicles as Emerging Biomarkers and Therapeutic Targets in Cardiometabolic Diseases. *Genom. Proteom. Bioinform.* **2018**, *16*, 50–62. [CrossRef] [PubMed]
14. Yuana, Y.; Sturk, A.; Nieuwland, R. Extracellular vesicles in physiological and pathological conditions. *Blood Rev.* **2013**, *27*, 31–39. [CrossRef] [PubMed]
15. Durrer, C.; Robinson, E.; Wan, Z.; Martinez, N.; Hummel, M.L.; Jenkins, N.T.; Kilpatrick, M.W.; Little, J.P. Differential Impact of Acute High-Intensity Exercise on Circulating Endothelial Microparticles and Insulin Resistance between Overweight/Obese Males and Females. *PLoS ONE* **2015**, *10*, e0115860. [CrossRef]
16. Ayers, L.; Nieuwland, R.; Kohler, M.; Kraenkel, N.; Ferry, B.; Leeson, P. Dynamic microvesicle release and clearance within the cardiovascular system: Triggers and mechanisms. *Clin. Sci.* **2015**, *129*, 915–931. [CrossRef]
17. Wilhelm, E.N.; González-Alonso, J.; Parris, C.; Rakobowchuk, M. Exercise intensity modulates the appearance of circulating microvesicles with proangiogenic potential upon endothelial cells. *Am. J. Physiol. Heart Circ. Physiol.* **2016**, *311*, H1297–H1310. [CrossRef]
18. Gaggi, G.; Izzicupo, P.; Di Credico, A.; Sancilio, S.; Di Baldassarre, A.; Ghinassi, B. Spare Parts from Discarded Materials: Fetal Annexes in Regenerative Medicine. *Int. J. Mol. Sci.* **2019**, *20*, 1573. [CrossRef]
19. Patan, S. Vasculogenesis and angiogenesis as mechanisms of vascular network formation, growth and remodeling. *J. Neurooncol.* **2000**, *50*, 1–15. [CrossRef]
20. Cox, C.M.; Poole, T.J. Angioblast differentiation is influenced by the local environment: FGF-2 induces angioblasts and patterns vessel formation in the quail embryo. *Dev. Dyn.* **2000**, *218*, 371–382. [CrossRef]
21. Lampropoulou, A.; Ruhrberg, C. Neuropilin regulation of angiogenesis. *Biochem. Soc. Trans.* **2014**, *42*, 1623–1628. [CrossRef]
22. Hofer, E.; Schweighofer, B. Signal transduction induced in endothelial cells by growth factor receptors involved in angiogenesis. *Thromb. Haemost.* **2007**, *97*, 355–363. [PubMed]
23. Schaper, W.; Scholz, D. Factors Regulating Arteriogenesis. *Arterioscler. Thromb. Vasc. Biol.* **2003**, *23*, 1143–1151. [CrossRef] [PubMed]

24. D'amico, M.A.; Ghinassi, B.; Izzicupo, P.; Di Ruscio, A.; Di Baldassarre, A. IL-6 Activates PI3K and PKCζ Signaling and Determines Cardiac Differentiation in Rat Embryonic H9c2 Cells: IL-6 and cardiac differentiation of H9c2 cells. *J. Cell. Physiol.* **2016**, *231*, 576–586. [CrossRef] [PubMed]
25. Mentzer, S.J.; Konerding, M.A. Intussusceptive angiogenesis: Expansion and remodeling of microvascular networks. *Angiogenesis* **2014**, *17*, 499–509. [CrossRef]
26. Ferrara, N.; Kerbel, R.S. Angiogenesis as a therapeutic target. *Nature* **2005**, *438*, 967–974. [CrossRef]
27. Carmeliet, P. Mechanisms of angiogenesis and arteriogenesis. *Nat. Med.* **2000**, *6*, 389–395. [CrossRef] [PubMed]
28. Théry, C.; Ostrowski, M.; Segura, E. Membrane vesicles as conveyors of immune responses. *Nat. Rev. Immunol.* **2009**, *9*, 581–593. [CrossRef] [PubMed]
29. Stoorvogel, W.; Kleijmeer, M.J.; Geuze, H.J.; Raposo, G. The biogenesis and functions of exosomes. *Traffic* **2002**, *3*, 321–330. [CrossRef] [PubMed]
30. György, B.; Szabó, T.G.; Pásztói, M.; Pál, Z.; Misják, P.; Aradi, B.; László, V.; Pállinger, É.; Pap, E.; Kittel, Á.; et al. Membrane vesicles, current state-of-the-art: Emerging role of extracellular vesicles. *Cell. Mol. Life Sci.* **2011**, *68*, 2667–2688. [CrossRef] [PubMed]
31. Valadi, H.; Ekström, K.; Bossios, A.; Sjöstrand, M.; Lee, J.J.; Lötvall, J.O. Exosome-mediated transfer of mRNAs and microRNAs is a novel mechanism of genetic exchange between cells. *Nat. Cell Biol.* **2007**, *9*, 654–659. [CrossRef] [PubMed]
32. Hargett, L.A.; Bauer, N.N. On the Origin of Microparticles: From "Platelet Dust" to Mediators of Intercellular Communication. *Pulm. Circ.* **2013**, *3*, 329–340. [CrossRef] [PubMed]
33. Flaumenhaft, R.; Dilks, J.R.; Richardson, J.; Alden, E.; Patel-Hett, S.R.; Battinelli, E.; Klement, G.L.; Sola-Visner, M.; Italiano, J.E. Megakaryocyte-derived microparticles: Direct visualization and distinction from platelet-derived microparticles. *Blood* **2008**, *113*, 1112–1121. [CrossRef] [PubMed]
34. Burnouf, T.; Goubran, H.A.; Chou, M.-L.; Devos, D.; Radosevic, M. Platelet microparticles: Detection and assessment of their paradoxical functional roles in disease and regenerative medicine. *Blood Rev.* **2014**, *28*, 155–166. [CrossRef]
35. Diehl, P.; Fricke, A.; Sander, L.; Stamm, J.; Bassler, N.; Htun, N.; Ziemann, M.; Helbing, T.; El-Osta, A.; Jowett, J.B.M.; et al. Microparticles: Major transport vehicles for distinct microRNAs in circulation. *Cardiovasc. Res.* **2012**, *93*, 633–644. [CrossRef] [PubMed]
36. Connor, D.E.; Exner, T.; Ma, D.D.F.; Joseph, J.E. The majority of circulating platelet-derived microparticles fail to bind annexin V, lack phospholipid-dependent procoagulant activity and demonstrate greater expression of glycoprotein Ib. *Thromb. Haemost.* **2010**, *103*, 1044–1052. [PubMed]
37. Zwicker, J.I.; Trenor, C.C.; Furie, B.C.; Furie, B. Tissue Factor–Bearing Microparticles and Thrombus Formation. *Arterioscler. Thromb. Vasc. Biol.* **2011**, *31*, 728–733. [CrossRef] [PubMed]
38. Dignat-George, F.; Boulanger, C.M. The Many Faces of Endothelial Microparticles. *Arterioscler. Thromb. Vasc. Biol.* **2011**, *31*, 27–33. [CrossRef]
39. Orozco, A.F.; Lewis, D.E. Flow cytometric analysis of circulating microparticles in plasma. *Cytom. Part A* **2010**, *77A*, 502–514. [CrossRef]
40. Inglis, H.C.; Danesh, A.; Shah, A.; Lacroix, J.; Spinella, P.C.; Norris, P.J. Techniques to improve detection and analysis of extracellular vesicles using flow cytometry: Accuracy and Efficiency of EV Detection Using FCM. *Cytom. Part A* **2015**, *87*, 1052–1063. [CrossRef]
41. Van Der Pol, E.; Hoekstra, A.G.; Sturk, A.; Otto, C.; Van Leeuwen, T.G.; Nieuwland, R. Optical and non-optical methods for detection and characterization of microparticles and exosomes: Detection and characterization of microparticles and exosomes. *J. Thromb. Haemost.* **2010**, *8*, 2596–2607. [CrossRef]
42. Burger, D.; Schock, S.; Thompson, C.S.; Montezano, A.C.; Hakim, A.M.; Touyz, R.M. Microparticles: Biomarkers and beyond. *Clin. Sci.* **2013**, *124*, 423–441. [CrossRef] [PubMed]
43. Gradziuk, M.; Radziwon, P. Methods for detection of microparticles derived from blood and endothelial cells. *Acta Haematol. Pol.* **2017**, *48*, 316–329. [CrossRef]
44. van der Pol, E.; Böing, A.N.; Gool, E.L.; Nieuwland, R. Recent developments in the nomenclature, presence, isolation, detection and clinical impact of extracellular vesicles. *J. Thromb. Haemost.* **2016**, *14*, 48–56. [CrossRef] [PubMed]

45. Dragovic, R.A.; Gardiner, C.; Brooks, A.S.; Tannetta, D.S.; Ferguson, D.J.P.; Hole, P.; Carr, B.; Redman, C.W.G.; Harris, A.L.; Dobson, P.J.; et al. Sizing and phenotyping of cellular vesicles using Nanoparticle Tracking Analysis. *Nanomed. Nanotechnol. Biol. Med.* **2011**, *7*, 780–788. [CrossRef] [PubMed]
46. Fritzsching, B.; Schwer, B.; Kartenbeck, J.; Pedal, A.; Horejsi, V.; Ott, M. Release and Intercellular Transfer of Cell Surface CD81 via Microparticles. *J. Immunol.* **2002**, *169*, 5531–5537. [CrossRef] [PubMed]
47. Berezin, A.E.; Mokhnach, R.E. The approaches to none-invasive detection of cell-derived extracellular vesicles. *Biol. Markers Guid. Ther.* **2016**, *3*, 155–175. [CrossRef]
48. Barteneva, N.S.; Fasler-Kan, E.; Bernimoulin, M.; Stern, J.N.; Ponomarev, E.D.; Duckett, L.; Vorobjev, I.A. Circulating microparticles: Square the circle. *BMC Cell Biol.* **2013**, *14*, 23. [CrossRef]
49. Hnasko, R. *ELISA: Methods and Protocols*; Humana Press: New York, NY, USA, 2015.
50. Nomura, S.; Shouzu, A.; Taomoto, K.; Togane, Y.; Goto, S.; Ozaki, Y.; Uchiyama, S.; Ikeda, Y. Assessment of an ELISA Kit for Platelet-Derived Microparticles by Joint Research at Many Institutes in Japan. *J. Atheroscler. Thromb.* **2010**, *16*, 878–887. [CrossRef]
51. Lansford, K.A.; Shill, D.D.; Dicks, A.B.; Marshburn, M.P.; Southern, W.M.; Jenkins, N.T. Effect of acute exercise on circulating angiogenic cell and microparticle populations: Exercise, circulating angiogenic cell and microparticle populations. *Exp. Physiol.* **2016**, *101*, 155–167. [CrossRef]
52. Bittencourt, C.R.d.O.; Izar, M.C.d.O.; França, C.N.; Schwerz, V.L.; Póvoa, R.M.d.S.; Fonseca, F.A.H. Effects of Chronic Exercise on Endothelial Progenitor Cells and Microparticles in Professional Runners. *Arq. Bras. Cardiol.* **2017**, *108*, 212–216. [CrossRef]
53. Boyle, L.J.; Credeur, D.P.; Jenkins, N.T.; Padilla, J.; Leidy, H.J.; Thyfault, J.P.; Fadel, P.J. Impact of reduced daily physical activity on conduit artery flow-mediated dilation and circulating endothelial microparticles. *J. Appl. Physiol.* **2013**, *115*, 1519–1525. [CrossRef] [PubMed]
54. Rafiei, H.; Robinson, E.; Barry, J.; Jung, M.E.; Little, J.P. Short-term exercise training reduces glycaemic variability and lowers circulating endothelial microparticles in overweight and obese women at elevated risk of type 2 diabetes. *Eur. J. Sport Sci.* **2019**, *19*, 1140–1149. [CrossRef] [PubMed]
55. Kirk, R.J.; Madden, L.A.; Peart, D.J.; Aye, M.M.; Atkin, S.L.; Vince, R.V. Circulating Endothelial Microparticles Reduce in Concentration Following an Exercise Programme in Women with Polycystic Ovary Syndrome. *Front. Endocrinol.* **2019**, *10*, 200. [CrossRef] [PubMed]
56. Rakobowchuk, M.; Ritter, O.; Wilhelm, E.N.; Isacco, L.; Bouhaddi, M.; Degano, B.; Tordi, N.; Mourot, L. Divergent endothelial function but similar platelet microvesicle responses following eccentric and concentric cycling at a similar aerobic power output. *J. Appl. Physiol.* **2017**, *122*, 1031–1039. [CrossRef]
57. Angelillo-Scherrer, A. Leukocyte-Derived Microparticles in Vascular Homeostasis. *Circ. Res.* **2012**, *110*, 356–369. [CrossRef]
58. Manno, S.; Takakuwa, Y.; Mohandas, N. Identification of a functional role for lipid asymmetry in biological membranes: Phosphatidylserine-skeletal protein interactions modulate membrane stability. *Proc. Natl. Acad Sci. USA* **2002**, *99*, 1943–1948. [CrossRef]
59. Daleke, D.L. Regulation of transbilayer plasma membrane phospholipid asymmetry. *J. Lipid Res.* **2003**, *44*, 233–242. [CrossRef]
60. Morel, O.; Jesel, L.; Freyssinet, J.-M.; Toti, F. Cellular Mechanisms Underlying the Formation of Circulating Microparticles. *Arterioscler. Thromb. Vasc. Biol.* **2011**, *31*, 15–26. [CrossRef]
61. Coleman, M.L.; Sahai, E.A.; Yeo, M.; Bosch, M.; Dewar, A.; Olson, M.F. Membrane blebbing during apoptosis results from caspase-mediated activation of ROCK I. *Nat. Cell Biol.* **2001**, *3*, 339–345. [CrossRef]
62. Deregibus, M.C.; Cantaluppi, V.; Calogero, R.; Lo Iacono, M.; Tetta, C.; Biancone, L.; Bruno, S.; Bussolati, B.; Camussi, G. Endothelial progenitor cell derived microvesicles activate an angiogenic program in endothelial cells by a horizontal transfer of mRNA. *Blood* **2007**, *110*, 2440–2448. [CrossRef]
63. Todorova, D.; Simoncini, S.; Lacroix, R.; Sabatier, F.; Dignat-George, F. Extracellular Vesicles in Angiogenesis. *Circ. Res.* **2017**, *120*, 1658–1673. [CrossRef]
64. Soleti, R.; Benameur, T.; Porro, C.; Panaro, M.A.; Andriantsitohaina, R.; Martinez, M.C. Microparticles harboring Sonic Hedgehog promote angiogenesis through the upregulation of adhesion proteins and proangiogenic factors. *Carcinogenesis* **2009**, *30*, 580–588. [CrossRef]
65. Ramakrishnan, D.P.; Hajj-Ali, R.A.; Chen, Y.; Silverstein, R.L. Extracellular Vesicles Activate a CD36-Dependent Signaling Pathway to Inhibit Microvascular Endothelial Cell Migration and Tube Formation. *Arterioscler. Thromb. Vasc. Biol.* **2016**, *36*, 534–544. [CrossRef] [PubMed]

66. Zernecke, A.; Bidzhekov, K.; Noels, H.; Shagdarsuren, E.; Gan, L.; Denecke, B.; Hristov, M.; Köppel, T.; Jahantigh, M.N.; Lutgens, E.; et al. Delivery of microRNA-126 by apoptotic bodies induces CXCL12-dependent vascular protection. *Sci. Signal.* **2009**, *2*, ra81. [CrossRef] [PubMed]
67. Taraboletti, G.; D'Ascenzo, S.; Borsotti, P.; Giavazzi, R.; Pavan, A.; Dolo, V. Shedding of the Matrix Metalloproteinases MMP-2, MMP-9, and MT1-MMP as Membrane Vesicle-Associated Components by Endothelial Cells. *Am. J. Pathol.* **2002**, *160*, 673–680. [CrossRef]
68. Lombardo, G.; Dentelli, P.; Togliatto, G.; Rosso, A.; Gili, M.; Gallo, S.; Deregibus, M.C.; Camussi, G.; Brizzi, M.F. Activated Stat5 trafficking via Endothelial Cell-derived Extracellular Vesicles Controls IL-3 Pro-angiogenic Paracrine Action. *Sci. Rep.* **2016**, *6*, 1–14. [CrossRef] [PubMed]
69. Wahl, P.; Wehmeier, U.F.; Jansen, F.J.; Kilian, Y.; Bloch, W.; Werner, N.; Mester, J.; Hilberg, T. Acute Effects of Different Exercise Protocols on the Circulating Vascular microRNAs -16, -21, and -126 in Trained Subjects. *Front. Physiol.* **2016**, *7*, 643. [CrossRef]
70. Brill, A.; Dashevsky, O.; Rivo, J.; Gozal, Y.; Varon, D. Platelet-derived microparticles induce angiogenesis and stimulate post-ischemic revascularization. *Cardiovasc. Res.* **2005**, *67*, 30–38. [CrossRef]
71. Janowska-Wieczorek, A.; Wysoczynski, M.; Kijowski, J.; Marquez-Curtis, L.; Machalinski, B.; Ratajczak, J.; Ratajczak, M.Z. Microvesicles derived from activated platelets induce metastasis and angiogenesis in lung cancer. *Int. J. Cancer* **2005**, *113*, 752–760. [CrossRef]
72. Warburton, D.E.R.; Bredin, S.S.D. Health benefits of physical activity: A systematic review of current systematic reviews. *Curr. Opin. Cardiol.* **2017**, *32*, 541–556. [CrossRef]
73. Di Blasio, A.; Izzicupo, P.; Di Baldassarre, A.; Gallina, S.; Bucci, I.; Giuliani, C.; Di Santo, S.; Di Iorio, A.; Ripari, P.; Napolitano, G. Walking training and cortisol to DHEA-S ratio in postmenopause: An intervention study. *Women Health* **2018**, *58*, 387–402. [CrossRef]
74. Condello, G.; Capranica, L.; Migliaccio, S.; Forte, R.; Di Baldassarre, A.; Pesce, C. Energy Balance and Active Lifestyle: Potential Mediators of Health and Quality of Life Perception in Aging. *Nutrients* **2019**, *11*, 2122. [CrossRef] [PubMed]
75. Forte, R.; Pesce, C.; Di Baldassarre, A.; Shea, J.; Voelcker-Rehage, C.; Capranica, L.; Condello, G. How Older Adults Cope with Cognitive Complexity and Environmental Constraints during Dual-Task Walking: The Role of Executive Function Involvement. *Int. J. Environ. Res. Public Health* **2019**, *16*, 1835. [CrossRef] [PubMed]
76. Garber, C.E.; Blissmer, B.; Deschenes, M.R.; Franklin, B.A.; Lamonte, M.J.; Lee, I.-M.; Nieman, D.C.; Swain, D.P. Quantity and Quality of Exercise for Developing and Maintaining Cardiorespiratory, Musculoskeletal, and Neuromotor Fitness in Apparently Healthy Adults: Guidance for Prescribing Exercise. *Med. Sci. Sports Exerc.* **2011**, *43*, 1334–1359. [CrossRef]
77. Condello, G.; Forte, R.; Monteagudo, P.; Ghinassi, B.; Di Baldassarre, A.; Capranica, L.; Pesce, C. Autonomic Stress Response and Perceived Effort Jointly Inform on Dual Tasking in Aging. *Brain Sci.* **2019**, *9*, 290. [CrossRef] [PubMed]
78. Pedrinolla, A.; Venturelli, M.; Tamburin, S.; Fonte, C.; Stabile, A.M.; Galazzo, I.B.; Ghinassi, B.; Venneri, M.A.; Pizzini, F.B.; Muti, E.; et al. Non-Aβ-Dependent Factors Associated with Global Cognitive and Physical Function in Alzheimer's Disease: A Pilot Multivariate Analysis. *J. Clin. Med.* **2019**, *8*, 224. [CrossRef] [PubMed]
79. Condello, G.; Forte, R.; Falbo, S.; Shea, J.B.; Di Baldassarre, A.; Capranica, L.; Pesce, C. Steps to Health in Cognitive Aging: Effects of Physical Activity on Spatial Attention and Executive Control in the Elderly. *Front. Hum. Neurosci.* **2017**, *11*, 107. [CrossRef]
80. Di Mauro, M.; Gallina, S.; D'Amico, M.A.; Izzicupo, P.; Lanuti, P.; Bascelli, A.; Di Fonso, A.; Bartoloni, G.; Calafiore, A.M.; Di Baldassarre, A. Functional mitral regurgitation. *Int. J. Cardiol.* **2013**, *163*, 242–248. [CrossRef]
81. Di Francescomarino, S.; Sciartilli, A.; Di Valerio, V.; Di Baldassarre, A.; Gallina, S. The Effect of Physical Exercise on Endothelial Function. *Sports Med.* **2009**, *39*, 797–812. [CrossRef]
82. Morena, F.; Argentati, C.; Trotta, R.; Crispoltoni, L.; Stabile, A.; Pistilli, A.; di Baldassarre, A.; Calafiore, R.; Montanucci, P.; Basta, G.; et al. A Comparison of Lysosomal Enzymes Expression Levels in Peripheral Blood of Mild- and Severe-Alzheimer's Disease and MCI Patients: Implications for Regenerative Medicine Approaches. *Int. J. Mol. Sci.* **2017**, *18*, 1806. [CrossRef]

83. Filardi, T.; Ghinassi, B.; Di Baldassarre, A.; Tanzilli, G.; Morano, S.; Lenzi, A.; Basili, S.; Crescioli, C. Cardiomyopathy Associated with Diabetes: The Central Role of the Cardiomyocyte. *Int. J. Mol. Sci.* **2019**, *20*, 3299. [CrossRef] [PubMed]
84. Egan, B.; Zierath, J.R. Exercise Metabolism and the Molecular Regulation of Skeletal Muscle Adaptation. *Cell Metab.* **2013**, *17*, 162–184. [CrossRef] [PubMed]
85. Kissane, R.W.; Egginton, S. Exercise-mediated angiogenesis. *Curr. Opin. Physiol.* **2019**, *10*, 193–201. [CrossRef]
86. Izzicupo, P.; D'Amico, M.A.; Di Blasio, A.; Napolitano, G.; Nakamura, F.Y.; Di Baldassarre, A.; Ghinassi, B. Aerobic Training Improves Angiogenic Potential Independently of Vascular Endothelial Growth Factor Modifications in Postmenopausal Women. *Front. Endocrinol.* **2017**, *8*, 363. [CrossRef]
87. Izzicupo, P.; D'Amico, M.A.; Di Blasio, A.; Napolitano, G.; Di Baldassarre, A.; Ghinassi, B. Nordic walking increases circulating VEGF more than traditional walking training in postmenopause. *Climacteric* **2017**, *20*, 533–539. [CrossRef]
88. Izzicupo, P.; Ghinassi, B.; D'Amico, M.A.; Di Blasio, A.; Gesi, M.; Napolitano, G.; Gallina, S.; Di Baldassarre, A. Effects of ACE I/D Polymorphism and Aerobic Training on the Immune–Endocrine Network and Cardiovascular Parameters of Postmenopausal Women. *J. Clin. Endocrinol. Metab.* **2013**, *98*, 4187–4194. [CrossRef]
89. Di Mauro, M.; Izzicupo, P.; Santarelli, F.; Falone, S.; Pennelli, A.; Amicarelli, F.; Calafiore, A.M.; Di Baldassarre, A.; Gallina, S. ACE and AGTR1 Polymorphisms and Left Ventricular Hypertrophy in Endurance Athletes. *Med. Sci. Sports Exerc.* **2010**, *42*, 915–921. [CrossRef]
90. Taylor, C.T. Mitochondria and cellular oxygen sensing in the HIF pathway. *Biochem. J.* **2008**, *409*, 19–26. [CrossRef]
91. Oliveira, A.N.; Hood, D.A. Exercise is mitochondrial medicine for muscle. *Sports Med. Health Sci.* **2019**, *1*, 11–18. [CrossRef]
92. Gorski, T.; De Bock, K. Metabolic regulation of exercise-induced angiogenesis. *Vasc. Biol.* **2019**, *1*, H1–H8. [CrossRef]
93. Highton, P.J.; Martin, N.; Smith, A.C.; Burton, J.O.; Bishop, N.C. Microparticles and Exercise in Clinical Populations. *Exerc. Immunol. Rev.* **2018**, *24*, 46–58. [PubMed]
94. Whitham, M.; Parker, B.L.; Friedrichsen, M.; Hingst, J.R.; Hjorth, M.; Hughes, W.E.; Egan, C.L.; Cron, L.; Watt, K.I.; Kuchel, R.P.; et al. Extracellular Vesicles Provide a Means for Tissue Crosstalk during Exercise. *Cell Metab.* **2018**, *27*, 237–251. [CrossRef] [PubMed]
95. Trovato, E.; Di Felice, V.; Barone, R. Extracellular Vesicles: Delivery Vehicles of Myokines. *Front. Physiol.* **2019**, *10*, 522. [CrossRef] [PubMed]
96. Thijssen, D.H.J.; Dawson, E.A.; Black, M.A.; Hopman, M.T.E.; Cable, N.T.; Green, D.J. Brachial Artery Blood Flow Responses to Different Modalities of Lower Limb Exercise. *Med. Sci. Sports Exerc.* **2009**, *41*, 1072–1079. [CrossRef]
97. Woodman, C.R.; Price, E.M.; Laughlin, M.H. Shear stress induces eNOS mRNA expression and improves endothelium-dependent dilation in senescent soleus muscle feed arteries. *J. Appl. Physiol.* **2005**, *98*, 940–946. [CrossRef]
98. Vion, A.-C.; Ramkhelawon, B.; Loyer, X.; Chironi, G.; Devue, C.; Loirand, G.; Tedgui, A.; Lehoux, S.; Boulanger, C.M. Shear Stress Regulates Endothelial Microparticle Release. *Circ. Res.* **2013**, *112*, 1323–1333. [CrossRef]
99. Chen, Y.-W.; Chen, J.-K.; Wang, J.-S. Strenuous exercise promotes shear-induced thrombin generation by increasing the shedding of procoagulant microparticles from platelets. *Thromb. Haemost.* **2010**, *104*, 293–301. [CrossRef]
100. Fisher, J.P.; Young, C.N.; Fadel, P.J. Autonomic Adjustments to Exercise in Humans. In *Comprehensive Physiology*; Terjung, R., Ed.; John Wiley & Sons, Inc.: Hoboken, NJ, USA, 2015; pp. 475–512.
101. Tschuor, C.; Asmis, L.M.; Lenzlinger, P.M.; Tanner, M.; Härter, L.; Keel, M.; Stocker, R.; Stover, J.F. In vitro norepinephrine significantly activates isolated platelets from healthy volunteers and critically ill patients following severe traumatic brain injury. *Crit. Care* **2008**, *12*, R80. [CrossRef]
102. Pedersen, B.K. Muscles and their myokines. *J. Exp. Biol.* **2011**, *214*, 337–346. [CrossRef]
103. Ellingsgaard, H.; Hojman, P.; Pedersen, B.K. Exercise and health—Emerging roles of IL-6. *Curr. Opin. Physiol.* **2019**, *10*, 49–54. [CrossRef]

104. Nomura, S.; Imamura, A.; Okuno, M.; Kamiyama, Y.; Fujimura, Y.; Ikeda, Y.; Fukuhara, S. Platelet-Derived Microparticles in Patients with Arteriosclerosis Obliterans. *Thromb. Res.* **2000**, *98*, 257–268. [CrossRef]
105. Varon, D.; Shai, E. Role of platelet-derived microparticles in angiogenesis and tumor progression. *Discov. Med.* **2009**, *8*, 237–241.
106. Lacroix, R.; Sabatier, F.; Mialhe, A.; Basire, A.; Pannell, R.; Borghi, H.; Robert, S.; Lamy, E.; Plawinski, L.; Camoin-Jau, L.; et al. Activation of plasminogen into plasmin at the surface of endothelial microparticles: A mechanism that modulates angiogenic properties of endothelial progenitor cells in vitro. *Blood* **2007**, *110*, 2432–2439. [CrossRef] [PubMed]
107. Kim, H.K.; Song, K.S.; Chung, J.-H.; Lee, K.R.; Lee, S.-N. Platelet microparticles induce angiogenesis in vitro. *Br. J. Haematol.* **2004**, *124*, 376–384. [CrossRef]
108. Brahmer, A.; Neuberger, E.; Esch-Heisser, L.; Haller, N.; Jorgensen, M.M.; Baek, R.; Möbius, W.; Simon, P.; Krämer-Albers, E.-M. Platelets, endothelial cells and leukocytes contribute to the exercise-triggered release of extracellular vesicles into the circulation. *J. Extracell. Vesicles* **2019**, *8*, 1615820. [CrossRef] [PubMed]
109. Guiraud, T.; Gayda, M.; Juneau, M.; Bosquet, L.; Meyer, P.; Théberge-Julien, G.; Galinier, M.; Nozza, A.; Lambert, J.; Rhéaume, E.; et al. A Single Bout of High-Intensity Interval Exercise Does Not Increase Endothelial or Platelet Microparticles in Stable, Physically Fit Men with Coronary Heart Disease. *Can. J. Cardiol.* **2013**, *29*, 1285–1291. [CrossRef] [PubMed]
110. Highton, P.J.; Goltz, F.R.; Martin, N.; Stensel, D.J.; Thackray, A.E.; Bishop, N.C. Microparticle Responses to Aerobic Exercise and Meal Consumption in Healthy Men. *Med. Sci. Sports Exerc.* **2019**, *51*, 1935–1943. [CrossRef]
111. Kim, J.-S.; Kim, B.; Lee, H.; Thakkar, S.; Babbitt, D.M.; Eguchi, S.; Brown, M.D.; Park, J.-Y. Shear stress-induced mitochondrial biogenesis decreases the release of microparticles from endothelial cells. *Am. J. Physiol. Heart Circ. Physiol.* **2015**, *309*, H425–H433. [CrossRef]
112. Kirk, R.J.; Peart, D.J.; Madden, L.A.; Vince, R.V. Repeated supra-maximal sprint cycling with and without sodium bicarbonate supplementation induces endothelial microparticle release. *Eur. J. Sport Sci.* **2014**, *14*, 345–352. [CrossRef]
113. Rigamonti, A.E.; Bollati, V.; Pergoli, L.; Iodice, S.; De Col, A.; Tamini, S.; Cicolini, S.; Tringali, G.; De Micheli, R.; Cella, S.G.; et al. Effects of an acute bout of exercise on circulating extracellular vesicles: Tissue-, sex-, and BMI-related differences. *Int. J. Obes.* **2020**, *44*, 1108–1118. [CrossRef]
114. Schwarz, V.; Düsing, P.; Liman, T.; Werner, C.; Herm, J.; Bachelier, K.; Krüll, M.; Brechtel, L.; Jungehulsing, G.J.; Haverkamp, W.; et al. Marathon running increases circulating endothelial- and thrombocyte-derived microparticles. *Eur. J. Prev. Cardiol.* **2018**, *25*, 317–324. [CrossRef] [PubMed]
115. Serviente, C.; Burnside, A.; Witkowski, S. Moderate-intensity exercise reduces activated and apoptotic endothelial microparticles in healthy midlife women. *J. Appl. Physiol.* **2019**, *126*, 102–110. [CrossRef] [PubMed]
116. Shill, D.D.; Lansford, K.A.; Hempel, H.K.; Call, J.A.; Murrow, J.R.; Jenkins, N.T. Effect of exercise intensity on circulating microparticles in men and women. *Exp. Physiol.* **2018**, *103*, 693–700. [CrossRef] [PubMed]
117. Wahl, P.; Jansen, F.; Achtzehn, S.; Schmitz, T.; Bloch, W.; Mester, J.; Werner, N. Effects of High Intensity Training and High Volume Training on Endothelial Microparticles and Angiogenic Growth Factors. *PLoS ONE* **2014**, *9*, e96024. [CrossRef] [PubMed]
118. Hackney, A.C. Molecular and Physiological Adaptations to Endurance Training. In *Concurrent Aerobic and Strength Training*; Schumann, M., Rønnestad, B.R., Eds.; Springer International Publishing: Cham, Switzerland, 2019; pp. 19–34.
119. O'Toole, M.L.; Douglas, P.S. Applied Physiology of Triathlon. *Sports Med.* **1995**, *19*, 251–267. [CrossRef] [PubMed]
120. Izzicupo, P.; D'Amico, M.A.; Bascelli, A.; Di Fonso, A.; D'Angelo, E.; Di Blasio, A.; Bucci, I.; Napolitano, G.; Gallina, S.; Di Baldassarre, A. Walking training affects dehydroepiandrosterone sulfate and inflammation independent of changes in spontaneous physical activity. *Menopause J. N. Am. Menopause Soc.* **2012**, 1. [CrossRef]
121. Martelli, F.; Ghinassi, B.; Lorenzini, R.; Vannucchi, A.M.; Rana, R.A.; Nishikawa, M.; Partamian, S.; Migliaccio, G.; Migliaccio, A.R. Thrombopoietin Inhibits Murine Mast Cell Differentiation. *Stem Cells* **2008**, *26*, 912–919. [CrossRef]

122. Ghinassi, B.; Ferro, L.; Masiello, F.; Tirelli, V.; Sanchez, M.; Migliaccio, G.; Whitsett, C.; Kachala, S.; Riviere, I.; Sadelain, M.; et al. Recovery and Biodistribution of Ex Vivo Expanded Human Erythroblasts Injected into NOD/SCID/IL2R γ null mice. *Stem Cells Int.* **2011**, *2011*, 1–13. [CrossRef] [PubMed]
123. Gallina, S.; Di Francescomarino, S.; Di Mauro, M.; Izzicupo, P.; D'Angelo, E.; D'Amico, M.A.; Pennelli, A.; Amicarelli, F.; Di Baldassarre, A. NAD(P)H oxidase p22phox polymorphism and cardiovascular function in amateur runners. *Acta Physiol.* **2012**, *206*, 20–28. [CrossRef]
124. Izzicupo, P.; Di Valerio, V.; D'Amico, M.A.; Di Mauro, M.; Pennelli, A.; Falone, S.; Alberti, G.; Amicarelli, F.; Miscia, S.; Gallina, S.; et al. Nad(P)H Oxidase and Pro-Inflammatory Response during Maximal Exercise: Role of C242T Polymorphism of the P22PHOX Subunit. *Int. J. Immunopathol. Pharmacol.* **2010**, *23*, 203–211. [CrossRef]
125. Buchheit, M.; Laursen, P.B. High-Intensity Interval Training, Solutions to the Programming Puzzle: Part I: Cardiopulmonary Emphasis. *Sports Med.* **2013**, *43*, 313–338. [CrossRef] [PubMed]
126. Di Blasio, A.; Izzicupo, P.; Tacconi, L.; Di Santo, S.; Leogrande, M.; Bucci, I.; Ripari, P.; Di Baldassarre, A.; Napolitano, G. Acute and delayed effects of high intensity interval resistance training organization on cortisol and testosterone production. *J. Sports Med. Phys. Fit.* **2016**, *56*, 192–199.
127. Kohl, H.W.; Craig, C.L.; Lambert, E.V.; Inoue, S.; Alkandari, J.R.; Leetongin, G.; Kahlmeier, S. The pandemic of physical inactivity: Global action for public health. *Lancet* **2012**, *380*, 294–305. [CrossRef]
128. Izzicupo, P.; Di Blasio, A.; Di Credico, A.; Gaggi, G.; Vamvakis, A.; Napolitano, G.; Ricci, F.; Gallina, S.; Ghinassi, B.; Di Baldassarre, A. The Length and Number of Sedentary Bouts Predict Fibrinogen Levels in Postmenopausal Women. *Int. J. Environ. Res. Public Health* **2020**, *17*, 3051. [CrossRef]
129. Biswas, A.; Oh, P.I.; Faulkner, G.E.; Bajaj, R.R.; Silver, M.A.; Mitchell, M.S.; Alter, D.A. Sedentary Time and Its Association with Risk for Disease Incidence, Mortality, and Hospitalization in Adults: A Systematic Review and Meta-analysis. *Ann. Intern. Med.* **2015**, *162*, 123. [CrossRef]
130. Ross, L.M.; Porter, R.R.; Durstine, J.L. High-intensity interval training (HIIT) for patients with chronic diseases. *J. Sport Health Sci.* **2016**, *5*, 139–144. [CrossRef]
131. Lee, K.; Kang, I.; Mack, W.J.; Mortimer, J.; Sattler, F.; Salem, G.; Dieli-Conwright, C.M. Effect of High Intensity Interval Training on Matrix Metalloproteinases in Women with Breast Cancer Receiving Anthracycline-Based Chemotherapy. *Sci. Rep.* **2020**, *10*, 1–7. [CrossRef]
132. Sanchis-Gomar, F.; Perez-Quilis, C.; Leischik, R.; Lucia, A. Epidemiology of coronary heart disease and acute coronary syndrome. *Ann. Transl. Med.* **2016**, *4*, 256. [CrossRef]
133. Suades, R.; Padró, T.; Alonso, R.; Mata, P.; Badimon, L. Lipid-lowering therapy with statins reduces microparticle shedding from endothelium, platelets and inflammatory cells. *Thromb. Haemost.* **2013**, *110*, 366–377. [CrossRef]

© 2020 by the authors. Licensee MDPI, Basel, Switzerland. This article is an open access article distributed under the terms and conditions of the Creative Commons Attribution (CC BY) license (http://creativecommons.org/licenses/by/4.0/).

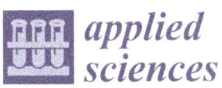

Article

The Effects of Wild Ginseng Extract on Psychomotor and Neuromuscular Performance Recovery Following Acute Eccentric Exercise: A Preliminary Study

Hyun Chul Jung [1], Nan Hee Lee [2], Young Chan Kim [3] and Sukho Lee [2,*]

1. Department of Coaching, College of Physical Education, Kyung Hee University-Global Campus, 1732 Deokyoungdaero, Giheung-gu, Yongin-si, Gyeonggi-do 17014, Korea; jhc@khu.ac.kr
2. Department of Counseling, Health, and Kinesiology, College of Education and Human Development, Texas A&M University-San Antonio One University Way, San Antonio, TX 78224, USA; nanhee.lee@biosci.gatech.edu
3. Korea Food Research Institute, 245, Nongsaengmyeong-ro, Iseo-myeon, Wanju-gun, Jeollabuk-do 55365, Korea; yckim@kfri.re.kr
* Correspondence: slee@tamusa.edu; Tel.: +(1)210-784-2537

Received: 30 July 2020; Accepted: 21 August 2020; Published: 23 August 2020

Abstract: To examine the efficacy of wild ginseng extract (WGE) on psychomotor and neuromuscular performance recovery following acute eccentric exercise. This study was a double-blind, crossover, and placebo-controlled design with a 14-day washout period. Ten male adults, aged 27.1 ± 4.33 years old, voluntarily participated in the study. Subjects were assigned to one of two parallel conditions (WGE or placebo) in a counterbalanced manner. Subjects consumed two packs of WGE (350 mg/package) or placebo drink immediately after acute eccentric exercise and the following four days. The eccentric exercise consisted of 20 min of downhill running at 60% of VO_{2peak} and five sets (of 20) of drop jump exercise. Computer-based cognitive function test and neuromuscular performance tests, including straight leg raise, vertical jump, isometric leg strength, and anaerobic power test were administered four times, at baseline, 2 h, 48 h, and 96 h after acute exercise. The interleukin-6 (IL-6), myoglobin, cortisol, total antioxidant capacity (TAC), and perceived muscle soreness were also assessed at each time point. A significance level was set at 0.05. No significant differences between the WGE and the placebo groups were observed in psychomotor and neuromuscular performance variables. Blood markers, including IL-6 ($p = 0.013$), myoglobin ($p < 0.001$), and cortisol level ($p = 0.047$) were changed significantly across the time. A post-hoc test revealed that a significant increase in IL-6 was observed only in the placebo group ($p = 0.014$), while no significant changes found in the WGE condition. The perceived muscle soreness was not different between the WGE and the placebo conditions. The administration of WGE immediately after acute eccentric exercise and the following four days have no benefits on psychomotor and neuromuscular performance recovery in healthy adults. However, the acute WGE supplementation may attenuate the eccentric exercise-induced inflammatory process, such as IL-6, but future study with a large sample size is required to clarify the anti-inflammation process in response to acute eccentric exercise.

Keywords: ginseng; performance; recovery; eccentric exercise; inflammation

---

1. Introduction

Ginseng is a popular selling product among herbal medicines and it has a long history concerning its efficacy on adaptogenic properties, such as stress management and fatigue recovery among Asian countries [1,2]. Various ginsengs, such as Cultivated Ginseng, Mountain Cultivated Ginseng, and Wild Ginseng have been introduced based on the grown environment and harvest methods [3]. Wild ginseng is grown in nature for an extended period to propagate in the mountain, while other ginsengs cultivate within 5–6 years in a farmland or mountain [3]. Chemical components of ginseng are also varied, depending on cultivation methods and curing processes [4]. One of the active ingredients, known as ginsenosides, plays an essential role in anti-inflammatory agents [5], and supplementation of these ingredients has been used to address the risk factors of cardiovascular diseases (CVDs) [6]. Over 40 different kinds of ginsenosides, such as Rb1, Rb2, Rc, Rd, Re, Rf, Rg1, Rg2, Rg3, Rh1, Rh2 have been identified to date, and the ginsenosides are determined by their positions on thin-layer chromatograms [5]. It has been reported that ginseng extract improves brain function, neuromuscular strength, and endurance [7–10]. Additionally, a decrease in anxiety and depression [11], as well as an increase in cognitive function [12] have been observed following ginseng supplementation. For these reasons, ginseng has been administrated not only for natural herb medicines but also for health supplements [13,14]. Recently, it is believed that ginseng may act as an ergogenic aid or recovery facilitator [15]. However, the ergogenic effects on physical performance is still unclear due to inconsistent results from the previous studies [2,16].

Participating in regular exercise and physical activity improves physical performance and immune function [17,18]. However, acute strenuous exercise or intense eccentric exercise can cause the disturbance of intracellular pro-oxidant-antioxidant homeostasis that leads to an increase in the accumulation of inflammation [19]. For instance, Banerjee et al. reported that an acute bout of exercise and/or prolonged intense exercise may cause a transient reduction and damage of various body tissues due to the augment exercise-induced oxidative stress [20]. In other words, performing one-off intense exercise can cause physiological imbalances, and this imbalanced physiological function is linked to immune dysfunction, lipid peroxidation, and free radical production. One of the common symptoms following intense or eccentric exercise is muscle soreness. Particularly, repetitive eccentric contraction exercise causes severe muscular pain 2–3 days later, which is known as Delayed Onset Muscle Soreness (DOMS) [21]. This acute muscle soreness is initially identified at the muscle/tendon junction, and then is gradually widespread to the entire muscle group [21]. An increase in muscle damage and soreness following intense or eccentric exercise affects performance recovery [22] as well as cognitive function [23].

Nutritional supplementation, such as ginseng, may be one feasible nutritional option to attenuate exercise-induced inflammation, as well as to facilitate performance recovery. Previous studies have reported that ginseng supplementation improves endurance performance [24–26], but fewer studies have been examined in other performance areas, such as neuromuscular performance. Pumpa et al. reported that ginseng supplementation following downhill running exercise was not associated with jump performance recovery in well-trained males [27]. Recently, a meta-analysis study demonstrated that there was a significant effect on fatigue recovery following ginseng supplementation, but the author pointed out that insufficient literature may not guarantee its efficacy on fatigue recovery [2]. We believe that well-designed studies are necessary to clarify the efficacy of ginseng supplementation on performance recovery, especially neuromuscular performance in healthy adults. Therefore, the purpose of this study was to examine the effects of wild ginseng extract on psychomotor and neuromuscular performance recovery following acute eccentric exercise.

2. Materials and Methods

2.1. Subjects

Subjects were randomly recruited by flyer and oral presentation in the university. Inclusion criteria of subjects were a) male adults aged from 18 to 40 years old, b) have no health problems, including skeletomuscular injuries, cardiovascular or pulmonary diseases, and c) have no experience using any ginseng supplementations. Subjects who were a) not able to participate in the physical activity or b) take any herbal-related medications were excluded from the study. Initially, 12 subjects agreed to participate the study, but only 10 subjects completed all procedures. Two participants voluntarily dropped out of the study for personal reasons (i.e., lack of interest, personal reason). All subjects received oral explanations, including the study procedure, possible risk, and benefits. Participants completed a physical activity readiness questionnaire (PAR-Q) and a written risk stratification screening form. When participants reported no issues with exercise, resting heart rate and blood pressure were taken, according to the American College of Sports Medicine (ACSM) guidelines. A written consent form approved by the Institutional Review Board of Texas A&M University, San Antonio, (#2015-126), was obtained from each subject.

2.2. Experimental Design

This study was a double-blind, randomized crossover design. All subjects participated in the pre-tests baseline measurements for their basic characteristics, including body weight, height, resting blood pressure, body composition, and peak oxygen uptake (VO_2peak). Then, subjects visited the laboratory three times (1st, 3rd, 5th day) to complete the first supplementation trial. Subjects performed the acute eccentric exercise, including 20 min of downhill running and five sets of 20 drop-jump exercises. The wild ginseng extract (WGE) or placebo drink was given to subjects immediately after the acute eccentric exercise and the following 4-day period. The WGE and placebo drink were in the identical packs manufactured by the Korea Food Research Institute. The dependent variables, including computer-based cognitive function test, physical performance test, blood analysis, and perceived muscle soreness were measured four times, at baseline, 2 h, 48 h, and 96 h after the acute eccentric exercise. The second trial was conducted after a 14 days washout period. The procedure for the second trial was the same as the first trial, with different supplement. All tests were performed at the Human Performance Laboratory in the university. The time points of each measurement are presented in Table 1.

Table 1. The time points of measurements.

Variables	Base	Eccentric Exercise	2 h	24 h	48 h	72 h	96 h
• Psychomotor Performance • Neuromuscular Performance • Blood Analyses • Perceived Muscle Soreness	✓	Downhill Running and Drop Jump Exercise	✓		✓		✓

2.3. Supplementation

The WGE used in this study was 350 mg of cultivated wild ginseng extract in 140 mL packages. Subjects took two packs of WGE (WGE powder 350 mg/package) a day for five days after acute eccentric exercise. The ingredients of WGE drinks were composed of 13.8% of Korea wild ginseng, 1.5% of soy powder, 1.5% of almond paste, 1.75% of isomaltooligosaccharide, 1.75% of fructooligosaccharide, 0.05% of refined salt, 0.05% of scented almond, 0.025% of xanthan gum, 0.19% of sodium bicarbonate, 0.05% of grapefruit seed extract, and 79.335% of water. The placebo drink was manufactured to be identical in appearance and content, except the ginseng extract. The placebo contained 0.25% of scented ginseng, 1.5% of soy powder, 1.5% of almond paste, 1.75% of isomaltooligosaccharide, 1.75% of fructooligosaccharide, 0.05% of refined salt, 0.05% of scented almond, 0.025% of xanthan gum, 0.19% of sodium bicarbonate, 0.05% of grapefruit seed extract, and 92.885% of water. The WGE and placebo drink were provided by Korea Food Research Institute. Supplements were given to subjects in a counterbalanced manner to minimize the order effect. Subjects were asked not to consume any caffeine-containing (i.e., coffee, energy drink) or herbal-containing beverages during the intervention.

2.4. Pre-tests

The pre-tests included body weight, height, resting blood pressure, body composition, and VO2peak test. Subjects' body height and weight were measured by a wall stadiometer (PAT #290237,

Novel Products, Rockton, USA) and a digital weight scale (HD-366, Tanita, Tokyo, Japan). Then, resting blood pressure was measured using an autonomic device (BP79IT, Omron, Japan). Systolic blood pressure, diastolic blood pressure, and resting heart rate were recorded. Three sites of skinfold thickness, including chest, abdominal, and thigh were measured with a skinfold caliper (PAT #3008239, Beta Technology, Santa Cruz, USA) to estimate body composition. Each site was measured three times by the trained technician and an average value was recorded. The body density and body fat percentage was estimated by Jackson and Pollock and Siri's equation, respectively [28,29]. The VO_2peak test was performed to accurately prescribe the exercise intensity for downhill running. The subject sat on the chair and wore a mask that connected with a metabolic cart (TrueOne 2400, Medics, USA). When the subject's respiratory exchange ratio (RER) dropped below 0.75, the graded exercise test begun on the treadmill. The Bruce protocol was applied at a speed of 2.74 km/h and a 10% grade. The speed and grade gradually increased every 3 min until subjects reached exhaustion. The VO_2peak test was terminated when subjects met at least two of the following conditions: (a) showed signs of intense effort (heavy breathing, facial flushing, unsteady gait, and sweating), (b) respiratory exchange ratio (RER), 1.15, (c) rating of perceived exertion (RPE) $\geq$ 19 (Borg 6–20 scale), or (d) volitional fatigue.

2.5. Acute Eccentric Exercise

The acute eccentric exercise program consisted of downhill running and drop jump exercise. The exercise program was modified based on the previous studies [30,31]. Prior to exercise, subjects performed jogging for 5 min on the 0-graded treadmill. Then, subjects performed downhill running for 20 min on a treadmill with a grade lowered to −10°. The speed of downhill running was set at 60% of the subject's VO_2peak. The average speed of downhill running was 6.4 ± 1.11 km/hour. After the downhill running, subjects performed drop jump exercises—five sets of 20 maximal drop jumps from the height of a 60 cm box. There was a 2-min rest interval between sets.

2.6. Psychomotor and Physical Performance Tests

Psychomotor performance test: to assess the subject's psychomotor performance, the computer-based cognitive function test was performed. Prior to the test, subjects performed one trial for the familiarization during the pre-test. The test included psychomotor vigilance task (PVT) and delayed-match-to-sample task (DMS). The PVT test was composed of 40 trials for 5 min to assess mean reaction time while the DMS test consisted of 20 trials 20 min to assess memory ability [32].

Physical performance test: the physical performance test included straight leg raise, vertical jump performance, isometric leg strength, and anaerobic power. The straight leg raise was measured with a goniometer (Baseline stainless steel goniometers, USA) to evaluate the range of motion. The subjects lay on the medical bed in a supine position. Then, the subject raised the dominant leg as high as possible with the knee fully extended while the opposite leg remained on the bed firmly without movement [33]. Each subject performed two trials and the best score was recorded. Vertical jump performance was measured to evaluate the explosive power. The subject raised the dominant arm, fully extended, on the measuring board, and the point was marked as an initial point. Then, subjects performed a countermovement jump as high as possible and marked the highest point. The vertical jump performance (VJP)was calculated from the maximal jump height minus the initial point. Each subject performed three times with one-minute interval between trials, and the best score was recorded [33]. Isometric leg strength was measured by a hand-held dynamometer (Lafayette Instruments, Lafayette, USA). The device was validated in previous studies [34–36] and has been used to measure isometric muscle strength in healthy subjects [37]. Subjects were seated on the table in a supine position, and the knee and hip were positioned 90 degrees. The handheld dynamometer force pad was placed just proximal to the ankle joint area and the subject's knee extensor and flexor strength was recorded in kilogram force. All subjects performed two maximal isometric leg extension and flexions, holding for 3 to 5 s with a minute rest interval between trials. The highest score was recorded. Lastly, subjects performed anaerobic power tests measured by an Automatic Power Cycle

(Power Cycle, Austin, TX, USA). The device has been validated in previous studies [36]. First, subjects performed 2 min of warm-up cycling at 100 to 120 rpm with power of 100 to 120 Watt. Then, subjects performed cycling maximally for approximately 5 s. Each subject performed four trials with one-minute intervals between trials, and the highest peak and mean power were recorded [37]. Standardized verbal encouragement was applied to all subjects for their maximal performance.

2.7. Blood Analyses

Blood sample was collected four times at baseline, 2 h, 48 h, and 96 h after acute exercise to analyze the markers of inflammation (interleukin 6; IL-6) and muscle damage (cortisol, myoglobin) as well as antioxidant capacity (total antioxidant capacity). Moreover, 3 mL of blood sample was withdrawn from an antecubital vein at each time point by the trained phlebotomist. The collected blood samples were drawn into a tube containing ethylenediaminetetraacetic acid (EDTA) to prevent coagulation. Then, the blood samples were centrifuged at 3000 rpm for 10 min. The upper layer of plasma was transferred into a conical tube and stored at −80 °C. Inflammation and muscle damage markers, including IL-6, myoglobin, and cortisol were analyzed by the enzyme-linked immunosorbent assay (ELISA) method using a commercially available Human ELISA IL-6 kit (EMD Millipore, Germany), myoglobin kit (EIA, Biocheck, USA), and cortisol kit (ELISA, DRG, USA). Total antioxidant capacity (TAC) was analyzed with the ELISA method using an antioxidant assay kit (total antioxidant, USA). All measurements were performed in duplicate. The coefficient variation (CV) of all blood analyses were below 10%.

2.8. Perceived Muscle Soreness

Perceived muscle soreness was measured by a Visual Analogue Scale (VAS). The scale was distributed from 0 to 10 scales where '0' indicated not sore at all, and '10' indicated maximal soreness. Subjects were asked to point the score four times, at baseline, 2 h, 48 h, and 96 h after the acute eccentric exercise.

2.9. Data Analysis

All data analyses were performed by a computer software program (SPSS version 25.0, SPSS Inc., Chicago, IL, USA). Prior to the data analyses, a Kolmogorov–Smirnov test was applied to check the normality of data. All variables exhibited normal distribution. Descriptive statistics, including mean, standard deviation (SD), and 95% confidence interval were computed for all variables. The repeated analysis of variances (ANOVAs) for conditions (WGE vs. placebo) by time (baseline, 2 h, 48 h, 96 h after acute exercise) were applied to assess the effects of WGE on dependent variables. If any significant interaction or main effects were identified, paired test for condition effects and repeated ANOVA with least significant difference (LSD) post-hoc test for time effects were applied. The effect size was presented as a partial eta-squared (η_p^2) value. The effect size can be considered as "large effect", if the value is 0.14 or higher [38]. The level of statistical significance was set at 0.05.

3. Results

3.1. Basic Characteristics

All participants underwent pre-examination, including height, weight, resting blood pressure, heart rate, body fat percentage, and VO$_2$peak tests. The results are presented in Table 2.

3.2. Psychomotor and Neuromuscular Performance

The results of psychomotor performance are shown in Table 3. No significant interaction effects for condition by time were observed in the psychomotor performance, including psychomotor vigilance task (PVT) and delayed-match-to-sample task (DMS). However, the DMS correction (F = 8.844, p = 0.019, η_p^2 = 0.317) and DMS time (F = 4.961, p = 0.025, η_p^2 = 0.355) were significantly reduced across the time in both conditions. Regarding neuromuscular performance, no significant interaction effects for group by time were also identified in all performance variables. However, there was a significant time effect on straight leg raise (F = 4.100, p = 0.030, η_p^2 = 0.313) where the straight leg raise value was significantly greater at 96 h compared to 2 h after exercise. The results of physical performance are presented in Table 4.

Table 2. Participants' basic characteristics.

Variables	Mean (SD)
Age (year)	27.1 (4.33)
Height (cm)	174.8 (9.39)
Weight (kg)	78.0 (13.70)
Resting Systolic Blood Pressure (mmHg)	117.8 (17.84)
Resting Diastolic Blood Pressure (mmHg)	73.4 (9.42)
Resting Heart Rate (beats/min)	65.4 (7.96)
Body fat (%)	12.7 (4.43)
VO_2peak (ml/kg/min)	44.9 (7.48)

Table 3. The results of psychomotor performance following acute eccentric exercise.

Variables	Group	Base	2 h	48 h	96 h	p-Value G	T	G × T
PVT Correctness (score)	Placebo (SD) 95% CI	36.7 −3.91 33.9–39.5	37.7 −2.16 36.2–39.2	37.7 −2.21 36.1–39.3	37.3 −5.17 33.6–41.0	0.568	0.498	0.969
	WGE (SD) 95% CI	37.2 −3.77 34.5–39.9	37.9 −3.21 35.6–40.2	38.1 −2.77 36.1–40.1	37.5 −4.17 34.5–40.5			
PVT reaction time (msec)	Placebo (SD) 95% CI	335.3 −34.07 311.0–359.7	338.8 −28.4 318.5–359.1	340 −26.07 321.4–358.7	346.1 −32 323.2–369.0	0.073	0.355	0.626
	WGE (SD) 95% CI	345.2 −32.12 322.3–368.2	350.3 −34.29 325.7–374.8	345.8 −33.24 322.0–369.6	349.2 −39.13 321.2–377.2			
DMS correctness (score)	Placebo (SD) 95% CI	26.5 −2.68 24.6–28.4	25.2 * −3.68 22.6–27.8	26.7 −3.68 24.1–29.3	26.7 −3.56 24.2–29.2	0.136	0.019	0.768
	WGE (SD) 95% CI	27.3 −3.27 25.0–29.6	26.0 * −4 23.1–28.9	27.2 −3.19 24.9–29.5	26.6 −4.67 23.3–29.9			
DMS time (msec)	Placebo (SD) 95% CI	2942.1 −1948.13 1548.5–4335.7	2533.5 * −1747.26 1283.5–3783.4	2598.9 * −1495.75 1528.9–3668.9	2283.9 * −1524.06 1193.7–3374.2	0.272	0.025	0.416
	WGE (SD) 95% CI	3335.8 −1948.13 1846.8–4824.7	2507.6 * −1390.8 1512.7–3502.5	2806.3 * −1849.86 1483.0–4129.6	2908.4 * −1535.01 1810.3–4006.5			
DMS reaction time (msec)	Placebo (SD) 95% CI	1784.9 −715.58 1273.0–2296.8	1740.9 −790.94 1175.1–2306.7	1711.7 −516.6 1342.1–2081.2	1533.2 −518.58 1162.3–1904.2	0.139	0.061	0.412
	WGE (SD) 95% CI	1905.1 −351.92 1653.3–2156.8	1693.3 −366.75 1431.6–1954.9	1881.8 −759.4 1338.5–2425.0	1823.8 −629.23 1373.7–2274.0			

Note. * p < 0.05, indicate a significant different compared to baseline. DMS, delayed-match-to-sample task; G, group; G × T, group × time; msec, millisecond; PVT, psychomotor vigilance task; T, time; WGE, wild ginseng extract.

Table 4. The results of physical performance following acute eccentric exercise.

Variables	Group	Base	2 h	48 h	96 h	p-Value G	p-Value T	p-Value G × T
Straight leg raise (°)	Placebo (SD) 95% CI	71.2 −7.13 65.5–77.1	69.2 −8.82 61.7–75.9	69.1 −11.49 59.2–77.7	75.4 * −7.23 69.6–81.3	0.29	0.03	0.412
	WGE (SD) 95% CI	67.5 7.32 62.3–72.7	66.7 −5.44 62.8–70.6	69.8 −7.13 64.7–74.9	72.6 * −4.5 69.4–75.8			
Vertical Jump (cm)	Placebo (SD) 95% CI	53.5 −6.93 47.4–57.9	50.4 −7.92 43.5–56.1	51.5 −9.12 43.5–57.7	51.1 −6.62 45.4–56.0	0.205	0.324	0.307
	WGE (SD) 95% CI	50.6 −8.62 44.4–56.7	50.1 −7.06 45.1–55.2	49.8 −6.76 44.9–54.6	51.2 −7.79 45.6–56.8			
Isometric Leg extension (kg)	Placebo (SD) 95% CI	44.1 −9.3 37.5–50.8	40.9 −9.49 34.1–47.7	43.2 −11.1 35.2–51.1	43.3 −11.9 34.8–51.8	0.818	0.259	0.832
	WGE (SD) 95% CI	44.9 −11.04 37.0–52.8	42.1 −13.04 32.8–51.4	42.2 −9.02 35.7–48.7	43.3 −9.75 36.3–50.2			
Isometric Leg Flexion (kg)	Placebo (SD) 95% CI	35.5 −8.77 29.2–41.8	34.8 −7.54 29.4–40.2	36.8 −7.48 31.4–42.1	36.2 −6.99 31.2–41.2	0.671	0.173	0.911
	WGE (SD) 95% CI	35.5 −8.21 29.6–41.4	33.5 −6.81 28.6–38.4	36.5 −8.9 30.2–42.9	35.5 −6.39 30.9–40.0			
Mean Power (Watts/kg)	Placebo (SD) 95% CI	13.9 −1.11 13.1–14.7	13.9 −1.71 12.7–15.1	13.6 −1.58 12.4–14.7	13.9 −1.36 12.9–14.9	0.45	0.447	0.389
	WGE (SD) 95% CI	12.7 −4.33 9.6–15.8	13.8 −1.56 12.7–14.9	13.8 −1.34 12.9–14.8	14.2 −1.36 13.2–15.1			
Peak Power (Watts/kg)	Placebo (SD) 95% CI	14.1 −1.15 13.3–14.9	14.1 −1.73 12.9–15.3	13.7 −1.62 12.5–14.9	14 −1.33 13.1–15.0	0.583	0.452	0.786
	WGE (SD) 95% CI	14.1 −1.63 13.0–15.3	14 −1.56 12.9–15.1	14 −1.31 13.0–14.9	14.3 −1.35 13.3–15.3			

Note. * $p < 0.05$, significantly greater compared to 2 h after acute eccentric exercise. WGE, wild ginseng extract; G, group; T, time; G × T, group × time.

3.3. Blood Analyses

In this study, IL-6, cortisol, myoglobin, and total antioxidant capacity were analyzed to evaluate the changes of inflammation and muscle damage markers as well as antioxidant capacity following the acute eccentric exercise. There were no significant differences in all blood variables between the WGE and the placebo conditions. However, IL-6 (F = 5.671, p = 0.013, η_p^2 = 0.387), myoglobin (F = 23.309, p < 0.001, η_p^2 = 0.744) and cortisol levels changed significantly across the time (F = 3.553, p = 0.047, η_p^2 = 0.282). Especially, a significant increase in IL-6 was observed only in the placebo condition (F = 5.995, p = 0.014, η_p^2 = 0.400) while no significant difference found in the WGE condition. The results of blood analyses are presented in Figure 1.

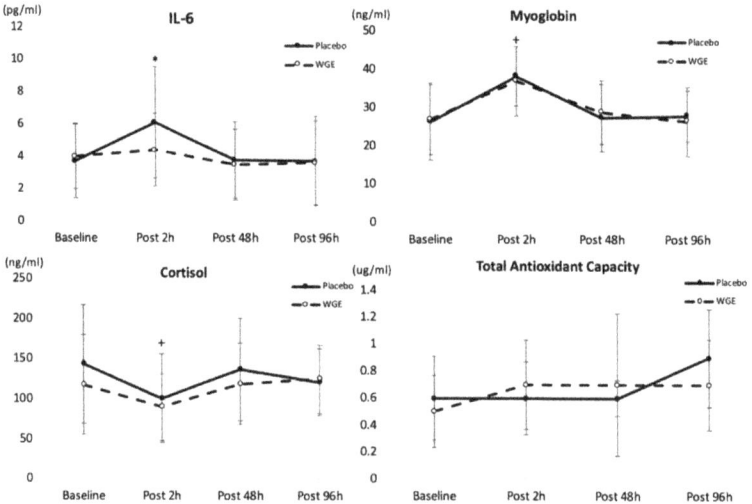

Note. *p < 0.05, significantly increased only in the placebo trial at post 2 h
+ p < 0.05, significantly different compared to baseline, 48h, and 96 h in both trials
WGE, wild ginseng extract

Figure 1. The results of blood markers of muscle damage.

3.4. Perceived Muscle Soreness

There was no significant interaction effect for group by time on perceived muscle soreness measured by VAS. However, the increased in perceived muscle soreness was observed both the WGE and the placebo conditions after 2 h of acute eccentric exercise (F = 9.236, p = 0.001, η_p^2 = 0.506). The results are shown in Table 5.

Table 5. The results of perceived muscle soreness following acute eccentric exercise.

Variables	Group	Base	2 h	48 h	96 h	p-Value		
						G	T	G × T
Perceived Muscle Soreness	Placebo (SD) 95% CI	0.6 (0.70) 0.1–1.1	3.0 * (2.16) 1.5–4.5	2.3 (1.89) 0.9–3.7	0.8 (1.03) 0.1–1.5	0.922	0.001	0.462
	WGE (SD) 95% CI	0.4 (0.47) 0.0–0.7	3.5 * (2.34) 1.8–5.2	1.8 (1.75) 0.5–3.0	1.2 (1.69) 0.0–2.4			

Note. * p < 0.05, significantly different compared to baseline, 48 h, and 96 h in both trials. WGE, wild ginseng extract; G, group; T, time; G × T, group × time.

4. Discussion

The present study examined the efficacy of WGE on psychomotor and neuromuscular performance recovery following acute eccentric exercise in male adults. Our findings showed that the administration of WGE immediately after acute eccentric exercise and the following four days have no benefits on psychomotor and neuromuscular performance recovery. However, a favoring trend has been identified that a significant increase in IL-6 was observed only in the placebo condition, while no significant changes were found in the WGE condition.

4.1. Psychomotor Performance

We examined the computer-based cognitive function test including PVT and DMS task to evaluate psychomotor performance during recovery. The supplementation of WGE following acute eccentric exercise did not provide a benefit on psychomotor performance in male adults. Consistent results have been identified in the previous study that 14 days of Korean ginseng (GINST15) supplementation prior to resistance exercise were not associated with the improvement of cognitive performance (i.e., quick board reaction time test) in healthy male and female adults [39]. A single dose of Panax ginseng (G115) for eight days also did not improve the working memory process in healthy subjects [40]. In contrast to our findings, Reay et al. reported that a single dose of Panax Ginseng (200 mg, G115) improves cognitive performance, such as serial seven task in healthy adults, but high dosages (400 mg, G115) and placebo conditions did not improve the cognitive performance [41]. Other Ginseng studies also demonstrated that cognitive functions, such as speed of the attention task [42], and secondary memory performance of cognitive research battery [43], improved following a single dose of Panax Ginseng (200 mg, 400 mg, respectively). Some possible explanations, such as the modulation of blood glucose and nitric oxide (NO) production have been proposed as potential mechanisms that may contribute to the improvement of cognitive performance [41]. It was believed that one of the active ingredients, ginsenosides, contributes to the enhancement of NO synthesis [44], and it modulates the glucose metabolism and insulin secretion in patients with type II diabetes mellitus [45]. Although some possible mechanisms, as well as benefits on cognitive function, have been demonstrated in the previous studies, our study confirms that five days of ginseng supplementation following acute eccentric exercise does not provide benefits on psychomotor performance recovery in male adults. In the present study, the DMS task correction and total time were significantly reduced across the time both in WGE and placebo conditions. We assume that decreased DMS correction partially related to 'speed accuracy trade-off'. Therefore, it is difficult to confirm that a decrease in cognitive function, such as DMS correction, was due to acute eccentric exercise.

4.2. Neuromuscular Performance

In the present study, straight leg raise, vertical jump performance, isometric leg strength, and anaerobic power were measured as indicators of neuromuscular performance. We found that WGE supplementation has no benefit on neuromuscular performance recovery. Ginseng supplementation has long been believed to improve stamina or fatigue recovery, but it is unclear whether the apoptogenic properties can facilitate the performance recovery or not. In particular, the discrepancy among literature to confirm the roles as an ergogenic aid may be limited. While the favoring results have been found mostly in animal studies [15,16], the literature with human studies are limited. Pumpa et al. reported that five days of Panax Notoginseng supplementation, before and after downhill running exercise, did not show significant improvement in jump performance [27]. A recent study showed the 14 days of Korean Ginseng supplementation (GINST15, high dose: 960 mg/day, low dose: 160 mg/day) following acute resistance exercise (5 sets of 12 repetitions at 70% one-repetition maximum (1RMmax)) had no benefit on peak power in healthy adults [39]. However, authors pointed out an important consideration about the responder and non-responder effect in the supplementation research. Although this approach is not a novel concept, Cadwell et al. reported that the responders among high dose trials showed greater peak power compared to low dose and placebo trials [39]. Relatively long-term treatment (> 8 weeks) also demonstrated no benefits on neuromuscular performance, such as anaerobic peak power and mean power in active women [46]. As opposed to the current study, Liang et al. reported that 30 days of Panax notoginseng (1350 mg/day) supplementation have contributed to improve endurance performance time by >7 min in young adults [24]. Supplementation of ginseng saponin complex mixed with taurine and other substances for 15 days improved free fatty acid utilization during exhaustive cycling tests, which resulted in improving endurance performance by average 2.94 min in male adults [26]. Interestingly, the efficacy of ginseng supplementation has been observed in the particular area of performance, such as endurance performance [24–26]. A recent study reported

12-week administration of high-dose ginsenoside complex (500 mg/day) improved maximal oxygen consumption, but the efficacy was not found in muscle strength [25]. It has been proposed that ginseng supplementation improves energy utilization [15]. Although it is difficult to explain the outcomes of the animal study directly into human studies, Ma et al. reported that the administration of Panax ginseng extract improves glucose uptake, fatty acid utilization, and lower the lactate concentration that possibly contributed to the improvement of endurance swimming performance [15]. We assumed that if ginseng or active ingredients, such as ginsenosides, modulate the energy metabolism, such as glucose and free fatty acid utilization during exercise, the improvement of neuromuscular performance that predominantly utilized the energy through ATP–PCr and glycolytic energy system may be limited. In summary, we confirm that the administration of WGE immediately after an eccentric exercise, and the following four days, have no benefit on neuromuscular performance recovery, such as muscle strength and anaerobic power. Further studies may be needed to clarify whether WGE could act as a potential ergogenic aid for endurance performance.

4.3. Inflammation Markers of Muscle Damage

Acute intense or eccentric exercise changes markers of muscle damage and inflammation resulted in inducing delayed-onset muscle soreness [19]. Various nutritional approaches have been introduced to attenuate the inflammation process or facilitate the recovery from muscle damages [47]. In this study, blood markers, including IL-6, myoglobin, cortisol, and TAC were not significantly different between the WGE and the placebo conditions following acute eccentric exercise. However, a favoring trend has been found that the serum IL-6 level significantly increased only in the placebo condition during 2 h recovery, whereas this value did not significantly change in the WGE condition. Similar results have been reported in previous studies [48–50]. Jung et al. reported that 7 days of Panax ginseng supplementation (20 g/d) prior to the uphill treadmill running (45 min at 10 km/h speed with a 15 degree) attenuated the increment of IL-6 level during 2 h and 3 h recovery period in young adults [48]. Another study also demonstrated that administrations of ginseng-based steroid Rg1 (5 mg) one night and one hour before 60-min cycling exercise suppressed the exercise-induced expression of IL-10 mRNA in quadriceps muscle [49]. Recently, Pumpa et al. reported that the level of serum IL-6 declined after downhill running in the ginseng group whereas the placebo group increased up to 4 h [27]. However, their findings revered 24 h after downhill running where the placebo group demonstrated a rapid return to baseline compared to the ginseng group. Interestingly, the placebo condition in this study also returned the IL-6 level to near baseline 24 h after eccentric exercise. A question arises based on the present and the previous studies whether the benefits of acute ginseng administration only valid during the first 2–4 h after eccentric exercise. However, this question should be approached carefully in the future study because the present and the previous data demonstrated inconsistent patterns from 24 h to 96 h after acute eccentric exercise. Although our study revealed a favoring trend at the first 2 h after the exercise, the benefit is not guaranteed until future research with a large sample size is conducted to clarify the anti-inflammation process in response to acute eccentric exercise.

Myoglobin is a muscle protein that is released from the damaged muscle following high intense eccentric exercise [19]. In the present study, the myoglobin level increased two hours after acute eccentric exercise, but no difference was found between the conditions. Lin et al. reported 12 weeks of Panax ginseng supplementation did not change inflammation adaptation, including muscle damage, oxidative, and inflammatory biomarkers to eccentric exercise training [51]. Pumpa et al. applied 5 bouts of 8 min downhill running at 80% of maximal heart rate (HRmax) with lowered −10° and participants received Panax notoginseng capsule (4000 mg/day) or placebo for 5 times (at 1 h prior to exercise and the following four days) in a crossover design. The author reported that myoglobin significantly increased after downhill running, but no significant differences were observed between conditions that support our result [27]. Cortisol is a glucocorticoid hormone that regulates energy metabolism during exercise [52]. It also interacts with inflammatory markers and nutritional supplementation, such as carbohydrates, and has been shown to lower cortisol levels after intense exercise [53]. In the present study, there were no difference in serum cortisol level between the WGE and placebo conditions. Youl et al. reported that a single bout of ginseng root extract (20 g) administered following a standardized exercise did not make a significant difference in cortisol levels [54]. Thus, it is confirmed that cortisol response following eccentric exercise was not influenced by ginseng supplement.

There are some strengths and limitations in the present study that need to be considered when interpreting the data. This study was well designed with randomized, double-blinded, placebo controlled, and crossover design. It assessed a wide range of markers of muscle damage and neuromuscular performance variables assessing effect of WGE in response to the eccentric exercise. However, small sample size may impact the statistical significance of the findings. Secondly, the outcomes can result differently by exercise protocols. The exercise protocol in this study was modified from the previous literature that was performed with healthy adults [30,31]. Although the current eccentric exercise protocol demonstrated a change of markers of muscle damage, such as myoglobin, IL-6, and cortisol, no significant changes in neuromuscular performance were observed after acute eccentric exercise. These results may tell us that the exercise protocol used in the present study may be insufficient to induce the delayed onset of muscle soreness.

5. Conclusions

Our findings indicate that the administration of WGE (700 mg/day) immediately after eccentric exercise and the following four days have no benefits on psychomotor and neuromuscular performance recovery in male adults. However, the acute WGE supplementation may attenuate the eccentric exercise-induced inflammatory process, such as IL-6, but a future study with a large sample size is required to clarify the anti-inflammation process in response to acute eccentric exercise.

Author Contributions: Conceptualization, H.C.J. and S.L.; Formal analysis, H.C.J. and S.L.; investigation, H.C.J., N.H.L., Y.C.K., and S.L.; methodology, H.C.J., N.H.L., Y.C.K., and S.L.; Project administration, S.L.; Supervision, S.L. writing—original draft preparation, H.C.J.; writing—review and editing, H.C.J., S.L. All authors have read and agreed to the published version of the manuscript.

Funding: This research received no external funding.

Acknowledgments: All authors wish to thank the participants who participated in this study.

Conflicts of Interest: The authors declare no conflict of interest.

References

1. Provino, R. The role of adaptogens in stress management. *Aus. J. Med. Herbal.* **2010**, *22*, 41.
2. Bach, H.V.; Kim, J.; Myung, S.K.; Cho, Y. Efficacy of Ginseng supplements on fatigue and physical performance: A meta-analysis. *J. Kor. Med. Sci.* **2016**, *31*, 1879–1886. [CrossRef] [PubMed]
3. Liu, D.; Li, Y.G.; Xu, H.; Sun, S.Q.; Wang, Z.T. Differentiation of the root of cultivated ginseng, mountain cultivated ginseng and mountain wild ginseng using FT-IR and two-dimensional correlation IR spectroscopy. *J. Mol. Struc.* **2008**, *883*, 228–235. [CrossRef]
4. Murthy, H.N.; Dandin, V.S.; Park, S.Y.; Paek, K.Y. Quality, safety and efficacy profiling of ginseng adventitious roots produced in vitro. *Appl. Microbiol. Biotechnol.* **2018**, *102*, 7309–7317. [CrossRef]
5. Park, J.S.; Park, E.M.; Kim, D.H.; Jung, K.; Jung, J.S.; Lee, E.J.; Hyun, J.W.; Kang, H.S.; Kim, H.S. Anti-inflammatory mechanism of ginseng saponins in activated microglia. *J. Neuroimmunol.* **2009**, *209*, 40–49. [CrossRef]
6. Lee, C.H.; Kim, J.H. A review on the medicinal potentials of ginseng and ginsenosides on cardiovascular diseases. *J. Ginseng. Res.* **2014**, *38*, 161–166. [CrossRef]
7. Sohn, E.H.; Yang, Y.J.; Koo, H.J.; Park, D.W.; Kim, Y.J.; Jang, K.H.; Namkoong, K.H.; Kang, S.C. Effects of Korean ginseng and wild simulated cultivation ginseng for muscle strength and endurance. *Kor. J. Plant. Res.* **2012**, *25*, 657–663. [CrossRef]

8. Chang, W.H.; Tsai, Y.L.; Huang, C.Y.; Hsieh, C.C.; Chaunchaiyakul, R.; Fang, Y.; Lee, S.D.; Kuo, C.H. Null effect of ginsenoside Rb1 on improving glycemic status in men during a resistance training recovery. *J. Int. Soc. Sports Nutr.* **2015**, *12*, 34. [CrossRef]
9. Cheng, Y.; Shen, L.H.; Zhang, J.T. Anti-amnestic and anti-aging effects of ginsenoside Rg1 and Rb1 and its mechanism of action. *Acta. Pharm. Sin.* **2005**, *26*, 143–149. [CrossRef]
10. Nah, S.Y.; Kim, D.H.; Rhim, H. Ginsenosides: Are any of them candidates for drugs acting on the central nervous system? *CNS Drug Rev.* **2007**, *13*, 381–404. [CrossRef] [PubMed]
11. Lee, B.; Kim, H.; Shim, I.; Lee, H.; Hahm, D.H. Wild ginseng attenuates anxiety-and depression-like behaviors during morphine withdrawal. *J. Microbiol. Biotechnol.* **2011**, *21*, 1088–1096. [CrossRef] [PubMed]
12. Lee, S.T.; Chu, K.; Sim, J.Y.; Heo, J.H.; Kim, M. Panax ginseng enhances cognitive performance in Alzheimer disease. *Alzheimer Dis. Assoc. Disord.* **2008**, *22*, 222–226. [CrossRef] [PubMed]
13. Kim, J.; Kang, D.I. A descriptive statistical approach to the Korean pharmacopuncture therapy. *J. Acupunct. Meridian Stud.* **2010**, *3*, 141–149. [CrossRef]
14. Bahrke, M.S.; Morgan, W.P. Evaluation of the ergogenic properties of ginseng. *Sports Med.* **2000**, *29*, 113–133. [CrossRef]
15. Ma, G.D.; Chiu, C.H.; Hsu, Y.J.; Hou, C.W.; Chen, Y.M.; Huang, C.C. Changbai Mountain ginseng (Panax ginseng CA Mey) extract supplementation improves exercise performance and energy utilization and decreases fatigue-associated parameters in mice. *Molecules* **2017**, *22*, 237. [CrossRef]
16. Oliynyk, S.; Oh, S. Actoprotective effect of ginseng: Improving mental and physical performance. *J. Ginseng Res.* **2013**, *37*, 144. [CrossRef]
17. Gleeson, M. Immune function in sport and exercise. *J. Appl. Physiol.* **2007**, *103*, 693–699. [CrossRef]
18. Matthews, C.E.; Ockene, I.S.; Freedson, P.S.; Rosal, M.C.; Merriam, P.A.; Hebert, J.R. Moderate to vigorous physical activity and risk of upper-respiratory tract infection. *Med. Sci. Sports Exerc.* **2002**, *34*, 1242–1248. [CrossRef]
19. Sayers, S.P.; Clarkson, P.M. Short-term immobilization after eccentric exercise. Part II: Creatine kinase and myoglobin. *Med. Sci. Sports Exerc.* **2003**, *35*, 762–768. [CrossRef]
20. Banerjee, A.K.; Mandal, A.; Chanda, D.; Chakraborti, S. Oxidant, antioxidant and physical exercise. *Mol. Cell Biochem.* **2003**, *253*, 307–312. [CrossRef]
21. Cheung, K.; Hume, P.A.; Maxwell, L. Delayed onset muscle soreness. *Sports Med.* **2003**, *33*, 145–164. [CrossRef] [PubMed]
22. Nottle, C.; Nosaka, K. Changes in power assessed by the Wingate Anaerobic Test following downhill running. *J. Strength Cond. Res.* **2007**, *21*, 145–150. [CrossRef] [PubMed]
23. Skurvydas, A.; Brazaitis, M.; Kamandulis, S.; Sipaviciene, S. Muscle damaging exercise affects isometric force fluctuation as well as intraindividual variability of cognitive function. *J. Motor Behav.* **2010**, *42*, 179–186. [CrossRef] [PubMed]
24. Liang, M.T.; Podolka, T.D.; Chuang, W.J. *Panax* notoginseng supplementation enhances physical performance during endurance exercise. *J. Strength Cond. Res.* **2005**, *19*, 108. [CrossRef] [PubMed]
25. Lee, E.S.; Yang, Y.J.; Lee, J.H.; Yoon, Y.S. Effect of high-dose ginsenoside complex (UG0712) supplementation on physical performance of healthy adults during a 12-week supervised exercise program: A randomized placebo-controlled clinical trial. *J. Ginseng Res.* **2018**, *42*, 192–198. [CrossRef] [PubMed]
26. Yeh, T.S.; Chan, K.H.; Hsu, M.C.; Liu, J.F. Supplementation with soybean peptides, taurine, Pueraria isoflavone, and ginseng saponin complex improves endurance exercise capacity in humans. *J. Med. Food* **2011**, *14*, 219–225. [CrossRef]
27. Pumpa, K.L.; Fallon, K.E.; Bensoussan, A.; Papalia, S. The effects of Panax notoginseng on delayed onset muscle soreness and muscle damage in well-trained males: A double blind randomised controlled trial. *Complement. Ther. Med.* **2013**, *21*, 131–140. [CrossRef]
28. Jackson, A.S.; Pollock, M.L. Generalized equations for predicting body density of men. *Br. J. Nutr.* **2004**, *91*, 161–168. [CrossRef]
29. Siri, W.E. Body composition from fluid spaces and density: Analysis of methods. 1961. *Nutrition* **1993**, *9*, 480–491.
30. Peake, J.M.; Suzuki, K.; Wilson, G.; Hordern, M.; Nosaka, K.; Mackinnon, L.; Coombes, J.S. Exercise-induced muscle damage, plasma cytokines, and markers of neutrophil activation. *Med. Sci. Sports Exerc.* **2005**, *37*, 737–745. [CrossRef]

31. Kirby, T.J.; Triplett, N.T.; Haines, T.L.; Skinner, J.W.; Fairbrother, K.R.; McBride, J.M. Effect of leucine supplementation on indices of muscle damage following drop jumps and resistance exercise. *Amino Acids* **2012**, *42*, 1987–1996. [CrossRef] [PubMed]
32. Hwang, J.; Castelli, D.M.; Gonzalez-Lima, F. The positive cognitive impact of aerobic fitness is associated with peripheral inflammatory and brain-derived neurotrophic biomarkers in young adults. *Physiol. Behav.* **2017**, *179*, 75–89. [CrossRef] [PubMed]
33. Jung, H.C.; Lee, N.H.; Lee, S. Jumping exercise restores stretching-induced power loss in healthy adults. *Mont. J. Sports Sc. Med.* **2018**, *7*, 55–62. [CrossRef]
34. Abizanda, P.; Navarro, J.L.; García-Tomás, M.I.; López-Jiménez, E.; Martínez-Sánchez, E.; Paterna, G. Validity and usefulness of hand-held dynamometry for measuring muscle strength in community-dwelling older persons. *Arch. Gerontol. Geriatr.* **2012**, *54*, 21–27. [CrossRef]
35. Arnold, C.M.; Warkentin, K.D.; Chilibeck, P.D.; Magnus, C.R. The reliability and validity of handheld dynamometry for the measurement of lower-extremity muscle strength in older adults. *J. Strength Cond. Res.* **2010**, *24*, 815–824. [CrossRef]
36. Martin, J.C.; Diedrich, D.; Coyle, E.F. Learning effects associated with maximal power testing: Implications for validity. *Int. J. Sports Med.* **2000**, *21*, 485–487. [CrossRef]
37. Lee, N.H.; Jung, H.C.; Ok, G.; Lee, S. Acute effects of Kinesio taping on muscle function and self-perceived fatigue level in healthy adults. *Eur. J. Sport Sci.* **2017**, *17*, 757–764. [CrossRef]
38. Lakens, D. Calculating and reporting effect sizes to facilitate cumulative science: A practical primer for t-tests and ANOVAs. *Front. Psychol.* **2013**, *4*, 863. [CrossRef]
39. Caldwell, L.K.; DuPont, W.H.; Beeler, M.K.; Post, E.M.; Barnhart, E.C.; Hardesty, V.H.; Anders, J.P.; Borden, E.C.; Volek, J.S.; Kraemer, W.J. The effects of a Korean ginseng, GINST15, on perceptual effort, psychomotor performance, and physical performance in men and women. *J. Sports Sci. Med.* **2018**, *17*, 92.
40. Reay, J.L.; Scholey, A.B.; Kennedy, D.O. Panax ginseng (G115) improves aspects of working memory performance and subjective ratings of calmness in healthy young adults. *Hum. Psychopharmacol.* **2010**, *25*, 462–471. [CrossRef]
41. Reay, J.L.; Kennedy, D.O.; Scholey, A.B. Single doses of Panax ginseng (G115) reduce blood glucose levels and improve cognitive performance during sustained mental activity. *J. Psychopharmacol.* **2005**, *19*, 357–365. [CrossRef] [PubMed]
42. Kennedy, D.O.; Haskell, C.F.; Wesnes, K.A.; Scholey, A.B. Improved cognitive performance in human volunteers following administration of guarana (Paullinia cupana) extract: Comparison and interaction with Panax ginseng. *Pharmacol. Biochem. Behav.* **2004**, *79*, 401–411. [CrossRef] [PubMed]
43. Kennedy, D.O.; Scholey, A.B.; Wesnes, K.A. Modulation of cognition and mood following administration of single doses of Ginkgo biloba, ginseng, and a ginkgo/ginseng combination to healthy young adults. *Physio. Behav.* **2002**, *75*, 739–751. [CrossRef]
44. Chen, X.; Lee, T.J.F. Ginsenosides-induced nitric oxide-mediated relaxation of the rabbit corpus cavernosum. *Br. J. Pharmacol.* **1995**, *115*, 15–18. [CrossRef]
45. Vuksan, V.; Sievenpiper, J.L.; Koo, V.Y.; Francis, T.; Beljan-Zdravkovic, U.; Xu, Z.; Vidgen, E. American ginseng (Panax quinquefolius L) reduces postprandial glycemia in nondiabetic subjects and subjects with type 2 diabetes mellitus. *Arch. Intern. Med.* **2000**, *160*, 1009–1013. [CrossRef]
46. Engels, H.J.; Kolokouri, I.; Cieslak, T.J., II; Wirth, J.C. Effects of ginseng supplementation on supramaximal exercise performance and short-term recovery. *J. Strength Cond. Res.* **2001**, *15*, 290–295.
47. Hennigar, S.R.; McClung, J.P.; Pasiakos, S.M. Nutritional interventions and the IL-6 response to exercise. *FASEB J.* **2017**, *31*, 3719–3728. [CrossRef]
48. Jung, H.L.; Kwak, H.E.; Kim, S.S.; Kim, Y.C.; Lee, C.D.; Byurn, H.K.; Kang, H.Y. Effects of Panax ginseng supplementation on muscle damage and inflammation after uphill treadmill running in humans. *Am. J. Chin. Med.* **2011**, *39*, 441–450. [CrossRef]
49. Hou, C.W.; Lee, S.D.; Kao, C.L.; Cheng, I.S.; Lin, Y.N.; Chuang, S.J.; Chen, C.Y.; Ivy, J.L.; Haung, C.Y.; Kuo, C.H. Improved inflammatory balance of human skeletal muscle during exercise after supplementations of the ginseng-based steroid Rg1. *PLoS ONE* **2015**, *10*. [CrossRef]
50. Flanagan, S.D.; DuPont, W.H.; Caldwell, L.K.; Hardesty, V.H.; Barnhart, E.C.; Beeler, M.K.; Post, E.M.; Vlek, J.S.; Kraemer, W.J. The effects of a Korean ginseng, GINST15, on hypo-pituitary-adrenal and oxidative activity induced by intense work stress. *J. Med. Food* **2018**, *21*, 104–112. [CrossRef]

51. Lin, H.F.; Chou, C.C.; Chao, H.H.; Tanaka, H. Panax ginseng and Salvia miltiorrhiza supplementation during eccentric resistance training in middle-aged and older adults: A double-blind randomized control trial. *Complement. Ther. Med.* **2016**, *29*, 158–163. [CrossRef] [PubMed]
52. Papanicolaou, D.A.; Petrides, J.S.; Tsigos, C.; Bina, S.; Kalogeras, K.T.; Wilder, R.; Gold, P.W.; Deuster, G.P.; Chrousos, G.P. Exercise stimulates interleukin-6 secretion: Inhibition by glucocorticoids and correlation with catecholamines. *Am. J. Physiol.* **1996**, *271*, E601–E605. [CrossRef] [PubMed]
53. Nehlsen-Cannarella, S.L.; Fagoaga, O.R.; Nieman, D.C.; Henson, D.A.; Butterworth, D.E.; Schmitt, R.L.; Bailey, E.M.; Warren, B.J.; Utter, A.; Davis, J.M. Carbohydrate and the cytokine response to 2.5 h of running. *J. Appl. Physiol.* **1997**, *82*, 1662–1667. [CrossRef] [PubMed]
54. Youl, H.K.; Hwan, S.K.; Jun, W.L.; Byrne, H.K. Effects of ginseng ingestion on growth hormone, testosterone, cortisol, and insulin-like growth factor 1 responses to acute resistance exercise. *J. Strength Cond. Res.* **2002**, *16*, 179–183. [CrossRef]

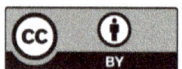

© 2020 by the authors. Licensee MDPI, Basel, Switzerland. This article is an open access article distributed under the terms and conditions of the Creative Commons Attribution (CC BY) license (http://creativecommons.org/licenses/by/4.0/).

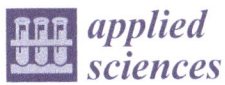

Article

Explosive Strength Modeling in Children: Trends According to Growth and Prediction Equation

Vittoria Carnevale Pellino [1,2,†], Matteo Giuriato [3,†], Gabriele Ceccarelli [4,*], Roberto Codella [5,6], Matteo Vandoni [1], Nicola Lovecchio [1,5] and Alan M. Nevill [7]

1. Laboratory of Adapted Motor Activity (LAMA), Department of Public Health, Experimental Medicine & Forensic Science, University of Pavia, 27100 Pavia, Italy; vittoria.carnevalepellino@unipv.it (V.C.P.); matteo.vandoni@unipv.it (M.V.); nicola.lovecchio@unipv.it (N.L.)
2. Department of Industrial Engineering, University of TorVergata, 00133 Rome, Italy
3. Department of Neurosciences, Biomedicine and Movement Sciences, Università di Verona, 37129 Verona, Italy; matteo.giuriato@univr.it
4. Human Anatomy Institute, Department of Public Health, Experimental Medicine & Forensic Science, University of Pavia, 27100 Pavia, Italy
5. Department of Biomedical Science for Health, Università degli Studi di Milano, 20133 Milano, Italy; roberto.codella@unimi.it
6. Department of Endocrinology, Nutrition and Metabolic Diseases, IRCCS MultiMedica, 20138 Milano, Italy
7. Faculty of Education, Health and Wellbeing, University of Wolverhampton, Walsall WV1 1SB, UK; a.m.nevill@wlv.ac.uk
* Correspondence: gabriele.ceccarelli@unipv.it; Tel.: +39-0382987661
† These authors contribute equally to this work.

Received: 26 August 2020; Accepted: 11 September 2020; Published: 15 September 2020

Abstract: Lower limb explosive strength has been widely used to evaluate physical fitness and general health in children. A plethora of studies have scoped the practicality of the standing broad jump (SBJ), though without accounting for body dimensions, which are tremendously affected by growth. This study aimed at modeling SBJ-specific allometric equations, underlying an objectively predictive approach while controlling for maturity offset (MO). A total of 7317 children (8–11 years) were tested for their SBJs; demographics and anthropometrics data were also collected. The multiplicative model with allometric body size components, MO, and categorial differences were implemented with SBJ performance. The log-multiplicative model suggested that the optimal body shape associated with SBJs is ectomorphic (H = −0.435; M = 1.152). Likewise, age, sex, and age–sex interactions were revealed to be significant ($p < 0.001$). Our results confirmed the efficacy of the allometric approach to identify the most appropriate body size and shape in children. Males, as they mature, did not significantly augment their performances, whereas females did, outperforming their peers. The model successfully fit the equation for SBJ performance, adjusted for age, sex, and MO. Predictive equations modeled on developmental factors are needed to interpret appropriately the performances that are used to evaluate physical fitness.

Keywords: allometry; standing broad jump; children; growth; maturity offset

1. Introduction

The relevance of muscular strength and power is well recognized in human performance [1,2] and contributes to bone health across different age groups [3]. Several reviews highlighted health outcomes associated with muscular strength and showed that poor muscular strength in children and adolescents is associated with cardiovascular disease, metabolic profiles, skeletal health, and adiposity [4,5]. Other studies have shown that high muscular strength in youths is associated with better lipid metabolic profiles, independent of cardiorespiratory fitness [3]. Ideally, muscular power (or explosive strength, as it is known in practical context) should be measured in lab settings [6], yielding valid values of muscular outcomes. Nevertheless, sometimes this may lack feasibility, and therefore field tests like the standing broad jump (SBJ) are preferable, since they are recognized as acceptable alternatives to lab assessments [7]. In addition, musculoskeletal fitness evaluation may enrich individual feedback to students and athletes, providing comparisons to international references on performance and health. For this reason, several youth fitness batteries [7–9] incorporated SBJ testing into their evaluation panel. Normative values for children and adolescents were created from these validation studies, proposing 50th percentiles as a proper medium level of performance that one could refer to. However, this procedure seems to have some limitations. For example, in Tomkinson et al. [10], the SBJ showed a mean improvement of 9 cm between 9–10 and 10–11 years (both males and females), while no information was obtained about changes in body mass and height, which differ according to age group and sex.

This stratification is useful for primarily surveillance purposes [11], but not for accurately monitoring training or developmental aspects. Moreover, childhood is a crucial period for detecting sensitive increases in performance (+10–15% per year) [12,13]. In children 7–8 years of age, SBJ performance is strictly dependent on body mass and height [14]. Although Body Mass Index (BMI) is the parameter summarizing the two variables, it does not represent a proper predictor of authentic performance [15,16]. Indeed, growth does not reflect parallel increases in this developmental pattern; while height increases by 3–4% per year, body mass increases by 8–10% [17]. Furthermore, a commonly used ratio scaling—the power-to-body mass ratio—may be a misleading index [18]. An alternative could be represented by the stratification of performance according to social condition [19] or BMI categories [16]. However, as mentioned earlier, this could result in a partial analysis. To convey these conceptual bottlenecks to a convincing ground of discussion, it is necessary to scale for maturity differences and determine the role of body size on performance [20], which is the allometric model. The objective of scaling is to normalize the performance for anthropometric characteristics [21]. In this framework, it is crucial to consider an adjunct polynomial model to analyze data and appropriately interpret them, discerning the contribution of developmental growth and maturation, among other factors, considering the exponential trend of human growth [22,23]. In the performance evaluation, another critical assessment item during the child growing phase could be the maturity offset (MO) at the peak of maturity. To this end, the peak high velocity (PHV) is capable of capturing a peculiar significance of speed and power results throughout growth, as well as the MO in strength (explosive strength) [16] or endurance outcomes [15]. In particular, the strength outcome depends on the developmental stage of the physiological determinants, whereas the peak of strength corresponds to the PHV [24]. Indeed, absolute values of specific strength actions, such as jumping or changing directions, are differently positioned in peak performance velocity curves as to PHV [25]. As such, controlling maturity is of paramount importance [26].

This study aims to model strength test-specific allometric equations, considering multiple individual factors such as height, body mass, sex, and age. Predictive equations will enforce a robust reliable indication of fitness per the structure and maturation levels of children (8–11 years old).

2. Materials and Methods

2.1. Experimental Approach to the Problem

During childhood, manifold factors could ameliorate performance, especially age and sex, according to the MO. In particular, the strength outcome depends on the developmental stage of the physiological determinants, whereas the peak of strength corresponds to PHV, where absolute values of specific strength actions are differently positioned in the peak performance velocity curves as compared with PHV. In this study, we decided to investigate the muscular power related to actual children's maturity, taking into account multiple individual proxies such as height, body mass, sex, and age. Children performed an SBJ as per the field test guidelines. The biological maturation (MO) was estimated using the somatic maturation method proposed by Werneck et al. [27]. Then, the age of PHV was determined by subtracting the MO from the chronological age. Participants were classified as late, early, or on time through the one-SD method derived from the current sample.

2.2. Subjects

This cross-sectional study involved 7317 children (3627 girls) aged 8–11 years, recruited from 119 Northeast Italian primary schools (third, fourth, and fifth grade). Children with known chronic cardiac, respiratory, neurological, or musculoskeletal disorders were excluded. All the described measures were taken during physical education classes as scheduled in the morning activities (8:00–12:00 a.m.). The study protocol, including each feature of the experimental design, was approved by the ethical boards of the enrolled schools in accordance with the World Medical Association Declaration of Helsinki, as revised in 1983. All participants were free to withdraw their participation at any time. Written informed consent was obtained from the parents or legal guardians, while verbal assent was obtained from the children prior to participation.

2.3. Procedures

Data collection included demographic and anthropometric information (sex, age, mass, and height) measured before the test sessions using standardized techniques (Table 1). Height was measured using a portable stadiometer with a precision of ± 1 mm (Stadiometer Seca 213, Intermed S.r.l. Milan, Italy) with children in an upright position, with bare feet placed slightly apart, arms extended, and head positioned in the Frankfort plane. Body mass was assessed using a beam scale with a precision of ±100 g (Seca 813, Intermed S.r.l. Milan, Italy), with children in light clothing, without shoes, and stood upright at the center of the platform of the mass scale. We calculated the age of the children from the birth date and subsequently rounded down values.

Table 1. Demographic and anthropometric information by sex. Numerosity following age: 8–9 y (1175 males, 1074 females), 9–10 y (1240 males, 1200 females), and 10–11 y (1275 males, 1353 females). All values are showed as mean ± DS.

Subjects	Numerosity	Age (y)	Height (cm)	Mass (kg)
Total	7317	9.4 ± 1	136.5 ± 8.5	33.8 ± 8.4
Males	3690	9.4 ± 1	136.4 ± 8.1	34.0 ± 8.2
Females	3627	9.4 ± 1	136.6 ± 8.9	33.7 ± 8.5

The explosive strength of the children was measured by the SBJ test (systematic error nearly to 0) [5], a practical, time-efficient, and low-cost field test widely adopted in school or gym contexts [7,11,16,28]. Every child jumped for distance from a standstill. During the performance of the jumps, the children were asked to bend their knees with their arms in front of them, parallel to the ground, then swing both arms, push off vigorously, and jump as far as possible. The test was performed three times, scored in centimeters, and the best value was recorded. The score was obtained by measuring the distance between the last heel mark and the take off line [29].

All tests were conducted by a team of three students of the sport science degree course during scheduled physical education classes in the morning. Previous training and calibration of the operators were performed to ensure the accuracy and repeatability of the procedure. The presence and collaboration of the curricular teachers were guaranteed at any time to meet the confidence of the students [30].

2.4. Statistical Analysis

The biological maturation (MO) was estimated through the somatic maturation method proposed by Werneck et al. [27].

This method estimates the MO from stature and chronological age using an algorithm, providing the result offset in years to peak height velocity (PHV). In particular, this easy approach was adopted because, briefly, involving only one anthropometric measure reduces operator-dependent errors, especially because it meets the full compliance of children and parents and avoids other maturity scales (i.e., Tanner; Marshall & Tanner 1969, 1970). In brief, the MO was determined using a specific formula for girls and boys:

Maturity offset for girls (years) = −7.709133 + (0.0042232 × (age × height))

Maturity offset for boys (years) = −7.999994 + (0.0036124 × (age × height))

Then, the age of PHV was determined by subtracting the maturity offset from the chronological age. Participants were classified as late, early, or on time through the one-SD method derived from the current sample.

The multiplicative model with allometric body size components of Body Mass (M) and Height (H) was used to identify the most appropriate body size and shape characteristics (Equation (1)) associated with, as well as detect any maturity (using MO) and categorical differences (e.g., sex, age) in, the physical performance variable (SBJ). The model is an extension of the one used to predict the physical performance variables of Greek children [23]:

$$Y = a \cdot M^{k_1} \cdot H^{k_2} \cdot \exp(c \cdot MO) \cdot \varepsilon \tag{1}$$

where k1 and k2 are the ontogenetic allometric coefficients; a, b, and c are allowed to vary randomly from child to child; and Log (ε), is assumed to have a constant error variance. The constant a is also allowed to vary for different populations, in this case the fixed factor: sex.

The model has the advantage of having proportional body size components and a multiplicative error that assumes they will increase proportionally with the physical performance variable Y (e.g., see Figure 1a,b).

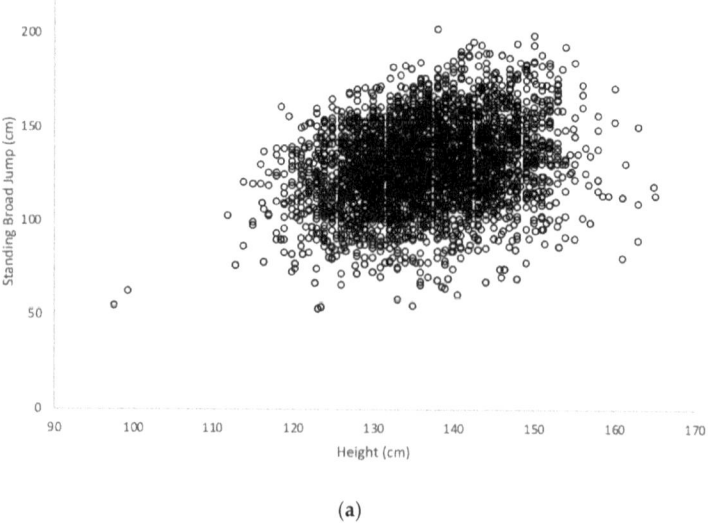

(a)

Figure 1. Cont.

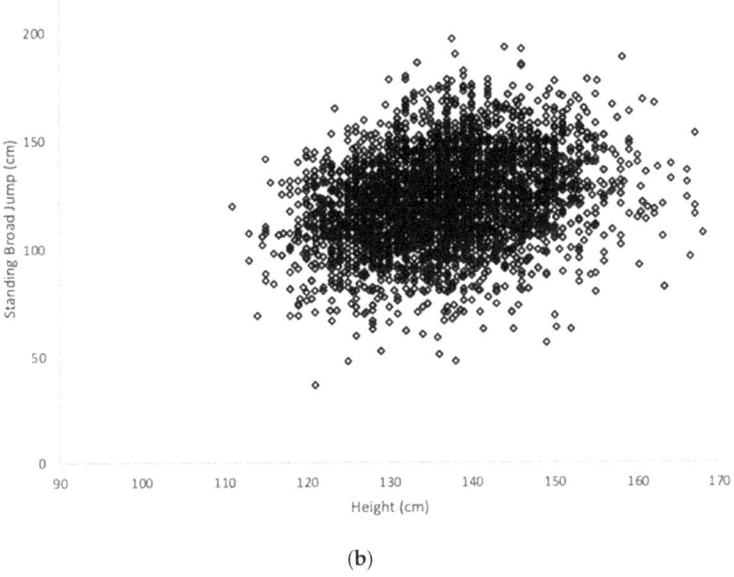

(b)

Figure 1. (a) The association between SBJ and height in 8–11-year-old male children, and (b) the association between SBJ and height in 8–11-year-old female children.

The model (Equation (1)) can be linearized with a log transformation (Equation (2)). A linear regression analysis or analysis of covariance (ANCOVA) on log(Y) can then be used to estimate the unknown parameters of the log-transformed model:

$$Log(Y) = \log(a) + k1 \cdot \log(M) + k2 \cdot \log(H) + c \cdot MO + \log(\varepsilon) \qquad (2)$$

Further categorical differences within the population (e.g., sex and age) can be explored by allowing the constant intercept parameter log(a) to vary for each group by introducing them as fixed factors (plus possible interactions) within an ANCOVA. The significance level was set at $p < 0.05$.

3. Results

The explosive strength expressed by the SBJ revealed a mean value (SD) of 128.29 cm (22.76) and 121.17 cm (21.49), while the MO was, on average, 3.36 y (0.72) and 6.35 y (0.44) for boys and girls, respectively. A significant difference between sex was found ($p < 0.001$). Figure 2 shows the results between sexes (with the covariates factored in), suggesting that females outperformed males in the SBJ; females had greater performances than males by up to 20 cm (on average). Furthermore, the parameter Log a that results from interaction between height, mass, MO, sex, and age was 0.973, 0.985, 0.982, and 0.995 for males and 1.199, 1.211, 1.208, and 1.211 for females, respectively, for 8, 9, 10, and 11-year-olds.

The estimated parameters from the multiplicative model relating the SBJ distance to the body size components in Equation (1), incorporating the MO, are given in Table 2.

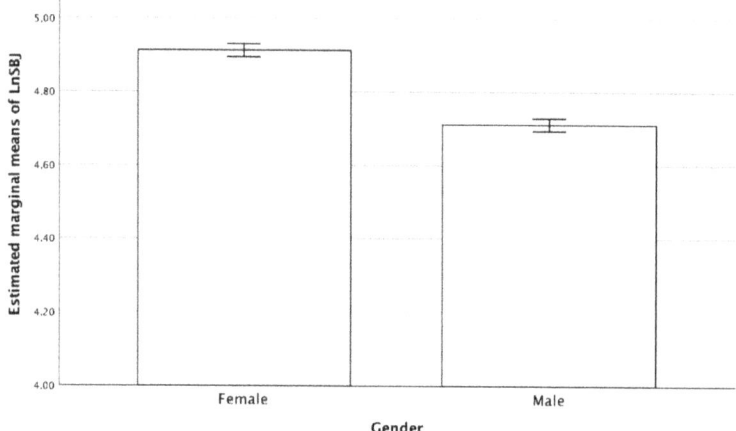

Figure 2. Estimated marginal means of SBJ by sex. Covariates appearing in the model are evaluated as follows: Ln Height = 4.9147, LN Mass = 3.4928, and MO = −4.8206.

Table 2. Parameters of Equation (1) about SBJ performance. The parameter Log a for males is 0.973, 0.985, 0.982, and 0.995, and 1.199, 1.211, 1.208, and 1.211 for females, respectively, for 8, 9, 10, and 11-year-olds. Note that the baseline group is the 11-year-old boys from which all other sex and age groups are compared.

Parameter	B	Std. Error	t	Sig.	95% Confidence Interval	
					Lower Bound	Upper Bound
Intercept Log(a)	0.995	0.327	3.043	0.002	0.354	1636
Log(M) (k1)	1.152	0.064	18.092	0.000	1027	1276
Log(H) (k2)	−0.435	0.015	−28.935	0.000	−0.465	−0.406
MO (c)	0.084	0.012	7.155	0.000	0.061	0.107
Sex (Female)	0.226	0.043	5.311	0.000	0.143	0.310
Age (8.00 y)	−0.022	0.019	−1.205	0.228	−0.059	0.014
Age (9.00 y)	−0.010	0.014	−0.704	0.482	−0.037	0.017
Age (10.00 y)	−0.013	0.009	−1.376	0.169	−0.032	0.006
Age (8.00) *Sex (Female)	−0.083	0.017	−4746	0.000	−0.117	−0.049
Age (9.00) *Sex (Female)	−0.065	0.014	−4631	0.000	−0.092	−0.037
Age (10.00) *Sex (Female)	−0.009	0.012	−0.785	0.432	−0.032	0.014

The model (Equation (1)) relating the SBJ distance to the body size components was

$$\text{SBJ distance (cm)} = a \cdot M^{-0.435} \cdot H^{1.152} \qquad (3)$$

With a positive height (H) and negative mass (M), the model suggested that the optimal body shape associated with the SBJ is to be taller, but lighter (less body mass).

Fittingly, the model (Equation (1)) revealed significant differences in the constant Log a parameter (Table 2) due to sex ($p < 0.001$) and age ($p < 0.001$), together with the interactions of age and sex ($p < 0.001$, Figure 3).

In particular, the parameter Log a appears in the footnote of Table 2. Note that the maturity offset (MO) made significant positive contributions to predicting the log-transformed SBJ distance ($p < 0.001$).

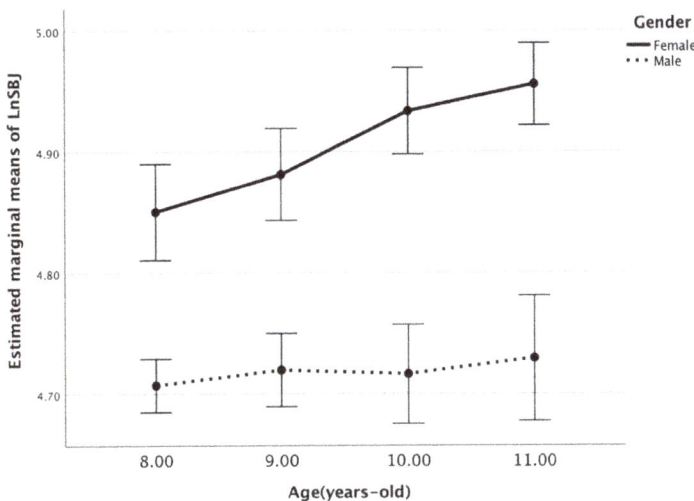

Figure 3. Estimated marginal means of the SBJ according to sex and age group. Covariates appearing in the model are evaluated as follows: LN height = 4.9147, LN weight = 3.4928, and MO = −4.8206.

4. Discussion

Since childhood, musculoskeletal fitness evaluation has been a crude indicator of both child performance and general health. To evaluate muscular power, the SBJ was included in all field test batteries. Researchers created reference values to characterize growth curves, not only in terms of anthropometrics (body mass and height) but also regarding physical performance. A close relation does exist, in fact, between the BMI and SBJ performance. In contrast, recent studies found that the BMI has limitations for measuring growth during childhood. From the age of seven to eight, body mass and height did not follow the same growth trends, making the BMI an improper predictor of SBJ performance [11,31]. In this light, this study aimed to investigate SBJ performance according to a robust scaling in which height and body mass are objectively valued, considering their actual trends owing to PHV assessment as a crucial individual factor of all physical performances. The data of this study confirmed the efficacy of the allometric approach to identify the most appropriate body size and shape characteristics associated with SBJ performance through the PHV. For boys and girls 8–11 years old, it is the ectomorph one (M = −0.435; H = 1.1152). In fact, in explosive strength, the MO contributed to predicting log-transformed SBJ distance since childhood. Without an allometric approach, consistent with other studies [13,14], child SBJ performance differs between boys and girls, with boys outperforming in a constant growth trend. Instead, the introduction of the size approach through allometric modeling to investigate SBJ performance with MO evaluation allowed us to refine the analysis, releasing different results. Males throughout the studied time frame (8–11 years) did not significantly augment their performances, whereas females showed a significant increase with a better SBJ performance (Figure 2). In line with other results [31,32], males did not outperform females in SBJ performance until reaching 11 years old. Furthermore, Newton's second law suggests that the force acting on a body is directly proportional to acceleration and shares its direction and orientation, with a proportionality constant given by the mass of the body. With that being said, Martin et al. [33] also showed that during maturation, female peak power is most likely to be determined by the quantitative properties of the muscle. Even in our study, the influence of body mass and related MO on strength performance in females was supported by the significant relationship that emerged between the SBJ and PHV offset. Moreover, Armstrong et al. [18] identified that, during the growth period, an index of lower limb power (assessed through the Wingate test) is strongly linked with both body mass and fat-free mass. This is probably explained by a lower body mass of the participants, which allows them to perform more efficiently. However, the possibility of a genuine comparison is hard due to the lack of data investigated with allometric approaches in the same age group. A small number of studies investigated such a performance during the early stages of maturity. Dos Santos et al. [34] suggested a better SBJ performance in 10–15-year-old boys controlled by body and shape with respect to their female peers. On the other hand, Meylan et al. [21] suggested that, when maturity was adjusted, the horizontal jump length results were slightly better ($p = 0.04$) for males than females.

Overall, the results of this study highlighted that females outperformed males in SBJ performance. A putative explanation may reside in the lower mass and higher coordination level of the females, with respect to males. Although our study did not investigate coordination, D'Hondt et al. [31] found an inverse correlation between motor coordination and lower mass in children of 5–10 years, and Stodden et al. [35] reported that children with a higher level of motor coordination exhibit greater performance (explosive strength). In this sense, sex differences in lower limb power performance have been related to the expression of significant differences in fat-free mass [36]. Subsequently, changes in force production at the age of 13–14 years have been attributed to the dramatic increase in steroid concentrations in males [37]. From a body shape view, the explosive strength in the lower limbs is facilitated through an ectomorphic body shape [23]. This is of relevance since these values are similar to those found by Lovecchio et al. [11] in middle school students (11–14 years old, $Log(M) = -0.357$, $Log(H) = 1.302$). Interestingly, in the two studies the trend was comparable, as though the explosive force paralleled the growth factors. Furthermore, the values of the a parameter for males and females (Table 2) are very practical, as they effectively complete the predictive equation for a field test widely used to evaluate physical fitness and, possibly, related general health beyond the performance extent by itself. Future studies may concern other field tests very commonly employed in children, such as speed and agility tests.

5. Conclusions

This study suggested some practical applications for young people in the early stages of maturation. First, coaches of young athletes must be aware of the sex differences because of maturity issues; therefore, females with lower body masses than males may be favored in lower limb performance. Second, coaches should be adopting tests and sample-specific scaling modeled after body mass, rather than using theoretical models based on the assumption of body dimension similarity. From this perspective, the use of the parameter a (Table 2) would be of meaningful assistance. Third, sex-specific training may also be needed, given the early PHV in girls. This should make coaches and physical education teachers aware that females can train strength earlier than males. Furthermore, this approach was aligned with the bio-banding rationale that employed a stratification per maturity offset, within a competitive context (and not only assessment procedure or in-training evaluation) [38,39]. Finally, age, maturity offset, body shape, and body mass should be carefully considered when interpreting children's lower limb performance, as they are relevant indicators to the growth curves.

Author Contributions: Conceptualization, N.L., M.G., and A.M.N.; methodology, R.C., G.C., and N.L.; validation, M.G., M.V., and A.M.N.; investigation, R.C. and M.V.; data curation, M.G. and M.V.; writing—original draft preparation, R.C. and G.C.; writing—review and editing, N.L. and M.G.; supervision, N.L. and A.M.N.; project administration, V.C.P., R.C., and M.V. All authors have read and agreed to the published version of the manuscript.

Funding: This research received no external funding.

Acknowledgments: The authors would like to acknowledge all the students, teachers, and staff of the schools, university students, and graduates. All authors disclose professional relationships with companies or manufacturers who will benefit from the results of the present study.

Conflicts of Interest: The authors declare no conflict of interest.

References

1. Rønnestad, B.R.; Kojedal, O.; Losnegard, T.; Kvamme, B.; Raastad, T. EVect of heavy strength training on muscle thickness, strength, jump performance, and endurance performance in well-trained Nordic Combined athletes. *Eur. J. Appl. Physiol.* **2012**, *112*, 2341–2352. [CrossRef] [PubMed]
2. Taipale, R.S.; Mikkola, J.; Vesterinen, V.; Nummela, A.; Häkkinen, K. Neuromuscular adaptations during combined strength and endurance training in endurance runners: Maximal versus explosive strength training or a mix of both. *Eur. J. Appl. Physiol.* **2013**, *113*, 325–335. [CrossRef] [PubMed]
3. Vicente-Rodriguez, G.; Jimenez-Ramirez, J.; Ara, I.; Serrano-Sanchez, J.A.; Dorado, C.; Calbet, J.A.L. Enhanced bone mass and physical fitness in prepubescent footballers. *Bone* **2003**, *33*, 853–859. [CrossRef] [PubMed]
4. Buehring, B.; Krueger, D.; Binkley, N. Jumping mechanography: A potential tool for sarcopenia evaluation in older individuals. *J. Clin. Densitom.* **2013**, *13*, 283–291. [CrossRef] [PubMed]
5. Ortega, F.B.; Ruiz, J.R.; Castillo, M.J.; Sjöström, M. Physical fitness in childhood and adolescence: A powerful marker of health. *Int. J. Obes.* **2008**, *32*, 1–11. [CrossRef] [PubMed]
6. Wilson, G.J.; Murphy, A.J. The use of isometric tests of muscular function in athletic assessment. *Sports Med.* **1996**, *22*, 19–37. [CrossRef]
7. Ruiz, J.R.; Castro-Piñero, J.; España-Romero, V.; Artero, E.G.; Ortega, F.B.; Cuenca, M.A.M.; Castillo, M.J. Field-based fitness assessment in young people: The ALPHA health-related fitness test battery for children and adolescents. *Br. J. Sports Med.* **2011**, *45*, 518–524. [CrossRef]
8. Castro-Piñero, J.; Artero, E.G.; Espana-Romero, V.; Ortega, F.B.; Sjöström, M.; Suni, J.; Ruiz, J.R. Criterion-related validity of field-based muscular fitness tests in youth. *Br. J. Sports Med.* **2010**, *44*, 934–943. [CrossRef]
9. Plowman, S.A.; Sterling, C.L.; Corbin, C.B.; Meredith, M.D.; Welk, G.J.; Morrow, J.R. The History of FITNESSGRAM®. *J. Phys. Act. Health* **2016**, *3*, S5–S20. [CrossRef]
10. Tomkinson, G.R.; Carver, K.D.; Atkinson, F.; Daniell, N.D.; Lewis, L.K.; Fitzgerald, J.S.; Ortega, F.B. European normative values for physical fitness in children and adolescents aged 9–17 years: Results from 2 779 165 Eurofit performances representing 30 countries. *Br. J. Sports Med.* **2018**, *52*, 1445–1456. [CrossRef]
11. Lovecchio, N.; Novak, D.; Sedlacek, J.; Hamar, P.; Milanovic, I.; Radisavljevic-Janic, S.; Zago, M. Physical fitness for sedentary students: A common trend from six European countries. *J. Sports Med. Phys. Fit.* **2019**, *59*, 1389–1396. [CrossRef] [PubMed]
12. Catley, M.J.; Tomkinson, G.R. Normative health-related fitness values for children: Analysis of 85347 test results on 9-17-year-old Australians since 1985. *Br. J. Sports Med.* **2013**, *47*, 98–108. [CrossRef] [PubMed]
13. Sauka, M.; Priedite, I.S.; Artjuhova, L.; Larins, V.; Selga, G.; Dahlström, Ö.; Timpka, T. Physical fitness in northern European youth: Reference values from the Latvian Physical Health in Youth Study. *Scand. J. Public Health* **2011**, *39*, 35–43. [CrossRef]
14. Halme, T.; Parkkisenniemi, S.; Kujala, U.M.; Nupponen, H. Relationships between standing broad jump, shuttle run and Body Mass Index in children aged three to ei. *J. Sports Med. Phys. Fit.* **2009**, *49*, 395–400. Available online: http://www.ncbi.nlm.nih.gov/pubmed/20087299 (accessed on 15 September 2020).
15. Giuriato, M.; Nevill, A.; Kawczynski, A.; Lovecchio, N. Body size and shape characteristics for Cooper's 12 minutes run test in 11–13 years old Caucasian children: An allometric approach. *J. Sports Med. Phys. Fit.* **2020**, *60*, 417–421. [CrossRef] [PubMed]
16. Lovecchio, N.; Zago, M. Fitness differences according to BMI categories: A new point of view. *J. Sports Med. Phys. Fit.* **2019**, *59*, 298–303. [CrossRef]
17. Cole, T.J.; Lobstein, T. Extended international (IOTF) body mass index cut-offs for thinness, overweight and obesity. *Pediatric Obes.* **2012**, *7*, 284–294. [CrossRef]
18. Armstrong, N.; Welsman, J. Sex-Specific Longitudinal Modeling of Short-Term Power in 11- to 18-Year-Olds. *Med. Sci. Sports Exerc.* **2019**, *51*, 1055–1063. [CrossRef]
19. Lovecchio, N.; Novak, D.; Eid, L.; Casolo, F.; Podnar, H. Urban and Rural Fitness Level: Comparison between Italian and Croatian Students. *Percept. Motor Skills* **2015**, *120*, 367–380. [CrossRef]
20. Van Praagh, E.; Doré, E. Short-term muscle power during growth and maturation. *Sports Med.* **2002**, *32*, 701–728. [CrossRef]
21. Meylan, C.M.P.; Cronin, J.B.; Oliver, J.L.; Rumpf, M.C. Sex-related differences in explosive actions during late childhood. *J. Strength Cond. Res.* **2014**, *28*, 2097–2104. [CrossRef] [PubMed]

22. Nevill, A.M.; Holder, R.L. Scaling, normalizing, and per ratio standards: An allometric modeling approach. *J. Appl. Physiol.* **1995**, *79*, 1027–1031. [CrossRef] [PubMed]
23. Nevill, A.; Tsiotra, G.; Tsimeas, P.; Koutedakis, Y. Allometric associations between body size, shape, and physical performance of Greek children. *Pediatric Exerc. Sci.* **2009**, *21*, 220–232. [CrossRef]
24. Murtagh, C.F.; Brownlee, T.E.; O'Boyle, A.; Morgans, R.; Drust, B.; Erskine, R.M. Importance of Speed and Power in Elite Youth Soccer Depends on Maturation Status. *J. Strength Cond. Res.* **2018**, *32*, 297–303. [CrossRef] [PubMed]
25. Beunen, G.; Malina, R.M. Growth and physical performance relative to the timing of the adolescent spurt. *Exerc. Sport Sci. Rev.* **1988**, *16*, 503–540. [CrossRef] [PubMed]
26. Mirwald, R.L.; Baxter-Jones, A.D.G.; Bailey, D.A.; Beunen, G.P. An assessment of maturity from anthropometric measurements. *Med. Sci. Sports Exerc.* **2002**, *34*, 689–694. [CrossRef]
27. Werneck, A.O.; Silva, D.R.; Oyeyemi, A.L.; Fernandes, R.A.; Romanzini, M.; Cyrino, E.S.; Ronque, E.R.V. Tracking of physical fitness in elementary school children: The role of changes in body fat. *Am. J. Hum. Biol.* **2019**, *31*, e23221. [CrossRef]
28. Artero, E.G.; España-Romero, V.; Castro-Piñero, J.; Ortega, F.B.; Suni, J.; Castillo-Garzon, M.J.; Ruiz, J.R. Reliability of Field-Based Fitness Tests in Youth. *Int. J. Sports Med.* **2011**, *32*, 159–169. [CrossRef]
29. Ortega, F.B.; Cadenas-Sánchez, C.; Sánchez-Delgado, G.; Mora-González, J.; Martínez-Téllez, B.; Artero, E.G.; Ruiz, J.R. Systematic Review and Proposal of a Field-Based Physical Fitness-Test Battery in Preschool Children: PREFIT Battery. *Sports Med.* **2015**, *45*, 533–555. [CrossRef]
30. Ceccarelli, G.; Bellato, M.; Zago, M.; Cusella, G.; Sforza, C.; Lovecchio, N. BMI and inverted BMI as predictors of fat mass in young people: A comparison across the ages. *Ann. Hum. Biol.* **2020**, *47*, 237–243. [CrossRef]
31. D'Hondt, E.; Deforche, B.; De Bourdeaudhuij, I.; Lenoir, M. Relationship between motor skill and body mass index in 5- to 10-year-old children. *Adapt. Phys. Act. Q.* **2009**, *26*, 21–37. [CrossRef]
32. Bustamante Valdivia, A.; Maia, J.; Nevill, A. Identifying the ideal body size and shape characteristics associated with children's physical performance tests in Peru. *Scand. J. Med. Sci. Sports* **2015**, *25*, e155–e165. [CrossRef] [PubMed]
33. Martin, R.J.F.; Dore, E.; Twisk, J.; van Praagh, E.; Hautier, C.A.; Bedu, M. Longitudinal changes of maximal short-term peak power in girls and boys during growth. *Med. Sci. Sports Exerc.* **2004**, *36*, 498–503. [CrossRef] [PubMed]
34. dos Santos, M.A.M.; Nevill, A.M.; Buranarugsa, R.; Pereira, S.; Gomes, T.N.Q.F.; Reyes, A.; Maia, J.A.R. Modeling children's development in gross motor coordination reveals key modifiable determinants. An allometric approach. *Scand. J. Med. Sci. Sports* **2018**, *28*, 1594–1603. [CrossRef]
35. Stodden, D.F.; Langendorfer, S.J.; Goodway, J.D.; Roberton, M.A.; Rudisill, M.E.; Garcia, C.; Garcia, L.E. A developmental perspective on the role of motor skill competence in physical activity: An emergent relationship. *Quest* **2008**, *60*, 290–306. [CrossRef]
36. Doré, E.; Bedu, M.; Van Praagh, E. Squat jump performance during growth in both sexes: Comparison with cycling power. *Res. Q. Exerc. Sport* **2008**, *79*, 517–524. [CrossRef] [PubMed]
37. Almuzaini, K.S. Muscle function in Saudi children and adolescents: Relationship to anthropometric characteristics during growth. *Pediatric Exerc. Sci.* **2007**, *19*, 319–333. [CrossRef] [PubMed]
38. Bradley, B.; Johnson, D.; Hill, M.; McGee, D.; Kana-ah, A.; Sharpin, C.; Malina, R.M. Bio-banding in academy football: Player's perceptions of a maturity matched tournament. *Ann. Hum. Biol.* **2019**, *46*, 400–408. [CrossRef]
39. Malina, R.M.; Cumming, S.P.; Rogol, A.D.; Coelho-e-Silva, M.J.; Figueiredo, A.J.; Konarski, J.M.; Kozieł, S.M. Bio-Banding in Youth Sports: Background, Concept, and Application. *Sports Med.* **2019**, *49*, 1671–1685. [CrossRef]

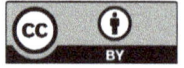

© 2020 by the authors. Licensee MDPI, Basel, Switzerland. This article is an open access article distributed under the terms and conditions of the Creative Commons Attribution (CC BY) license (http://creativecommons.org/licenses/by/4.0/).

Article

Contributions of Anthropometric and Strength Determinants to Estimate 2000 m Ergometer Performance in Traditional Rowing

Sergio Sebastia-Amat, Alfonso Penichet-Tomas *, Jose M. Jimenez-Olmedo and Basilio Pueo

Department of General and Specific Didactics, University of Alicante, 03690 Alicante, Spain; sergio.sebastia@ua.es (S.S.-A.); j.olmedo@ua.es (J.M.J.-O.); basilio@ua.es (B.P.)
* Correspondence: alfonso.penichet@ua.es

Received: 29 August 2020; Accepted: 18 September 2020; Published: 20 September 2020

Abstract: The purpose of this study was to analyze the contribution of anthropometric and strength determinants of 2000 m ergometer performance in traditional rowing. Nineteen rowers competing at national level participated in this study. Anthropometric characteristics, vertical jumps and bench pull tests were assessed to determine conditional factors, whereas the 2000 m test was used to set rowing performance. Pearson correlation coefficient, linear stepwise and allometric regression analyses were used to predict rowing performance ($R^2 > 50\%$). Height, body mass and body muscle correlated with rowing performance in male and female rowers. Similarly, power output for squat jump and countermovement jump power correlated with performance. Finally, mean propulsive velocity, mean power and maximum power in bench pull also correlated with the test. Stepwise multiple regression analysis identified body mass ($R^2 = 0.69$, $p < 0.001$) and mean propulsive velocity in bench pull ($R^2 = 0.76$, $p < 0.001$) for male rowers and body muscle ($R^2 = 0.89$, $p = 0.002$) and maximum power in bench pull ($R^2 = 0.62$, $p = 0.036$) for female rowers as the best predictors of rowing performance. These results determine the relevance of anthropometric characteristics and, in contrast to Olympic rowing, support the greatest importance of upper body power in traditional rowing training.

Keywords: bench pull; vertical jump; power; talent detection; training

1. Introduction

Rowing is a cyclic, strength-endurance sport that requires high levels of aerobic and anaerobic capacity to displace a boat through the water [1,2]. Rowers use the whole body to perform the rowing stroke for a distance that differs according to the modality [3]. There are two different rowing modalities, traditional—or fixed—rowing and Olympic rowing, with different performance indicators: distance, race time, mean force, total number of strokes and power per stroke and velocity of the boat [4]. Traditional rowing is a non-Olympic modality that demands high physical condition to carry out between 35–40 strokes per minute throughout a 19–20-min race, slightly longer than in Olympic rowing [4]. Traditional rowers show a 250–350 W average force applied for an optimal stroke length [4,5]. The power-capacity at each stroke has been identified as a key factor of rowing performance [4,6], together with other factors like large body size, relatively large limbs, high muscular strength, high muscular and cardiovascular endurance and proper balance [6–9].

Whereas approximately 46% of the power produced in Olympic modalities is generated by legs, the remaining is produced by trunk and arms [10]. In traditional rowing, the contribution of legs is slightly lower (40%) and the role of trunk and arms are slightly higher (60%) [11]. This fact may be due, among other factors, to the semi-flexed position of legs during the recovery of the traditional rowing cycle [12]. This position must be adopted as a consequence of the fixed seat, which entails an increase in the degree of body extension [13].

Traditional rowing is experiencing a significant increase in athletes worldwide and has attracted the attention of sports scientists in the same way was as in Olympic rowing. International research interest has enhanced due to physiological, performance and championships differences [4], the professionalization of this modality and the rise of worldwide championships in Europe (Spain, Italy, United Kingdom, etc.), America (Canada, USA, etc.) and other regions like Saudi Arabia [13]. Traditional rowing studies has increased in the field of sports profile [14], championships performance [13], supplementation [15], physiological factors [4] and different training characteristics and methodologies [4,16].

Most studies have mainly focused on describing performance factors in Olympic rowing [11], mainly those related with physiological and anthropometric variables and, to a lesser extent, in traditional rowing [4,13,16,17]. In the same way, research conducted to date relates the importance of some anthropometric characteristics like height, body mass, muscle mass or body fat in Olympic rowing performance [1]. Most of these studies have investigated the determinants of both Olympic and indoor rowing using correlation and linear regression techniques, assuming a linear relationship between rowing performance and determinants [8,18,19]. For curvilinear relationships between various measures of power output, a proportional allometric model can also be used [20,21]. However, the contribution of these determinants to rowing ergometer performance in traditional rowing has not been widely demonstrated. Several studies showed the relationship between 1500 m or 2000 m rowing ergometer performance in Olympic modality and lower body power obtained from different types of jump [8,22,23]. Similarly, a link has been shown between rowing ergometer performance and power produced by the upper body during different protocols of bench pull (BP) tests [4,24,25]. Even peak power output sustained during maximal incremental testing is an overall index of physiological rowing capacity and rowing efficiency and allows predicting rowing ergometer performance [26]. However, to the knowledge of the authors, there are no studies that relate the rowing ergometer performance in traditional rowing, considering that the contribution of the upper body is slightly higher in traditional rowing than in Olympic rowing [11,27]. Likewise, no available studies in the literature have considered the use of proportional allometric modeling to predict 2000 m ergometer rowing performance in traditional rowing.

Therefore, the purpose of this study was to analyze the contribution of anthropometric and strength determinants of rowing ergometer performance in traditional rowing. To that end, the relation of anthropometric characteristics and upper/lower body contribution with 2000 m rowing ergometer performance test was carried out using correlation, linear and allometric regression techniques.

2. Materials and Methods

2.1. Participants

Nineteen sweep (board) rowers competing at the national level participated in this study: 12 males (7 port and 5 starboard, 10 heavyweight and 2 lightweight, age: 24.6 ± 3.9 years, height: 178.4 ± 8.9 cm, body mass: 77.3 ± 7.9 kg) and 7 females (3 port and 4 starboard, 2 heavyweight and 5 lightweight, age: 25.7 ± 4.4 years, height: 166.3 ± 7.5 cm, body mass: 59.9 ± 8.3 kg). The requirement to participate was to have classified for the national championship, to train regularly a minimum of five days per week (> 12 h/week) for the last 3 years and not to have any musculoskeletal or neurological disorders, heart or respiratory failures, or any circulatory disturbance that may influence the results of the investigation. Rowers were requested to abstain from caffeine and alcohol consumption for 24 h and to avoid high-intensity training for 48 h before testing. All participants gave their written consent after project information, which was previously approved by the research ethics committee of the University of Alicante (IRB No. UA-2019-07-23).

2.2. Procedures

To determine the contribution of the different variables in rowing ergometer performance, the strength of lower/upper body and 2000 m rowing ergometer performance were tested. Data collection was conducted on three sessions carried out at the same time of the day in a controlled laboratory environment. Dynamic muscle strength and power tests appear to discriminate better between levels of rowing performance than isometric strength tests [28,29]; therefore, during the second session, rowers performed vertical jump tests and the bench pull test (BP). Finally, rowers completed a 2000 m test on a rowing ergometer in the third session. All athletes were familiarized with the testing protocols used in the present study. Pearson correlation statistical test and stepwise multiple linear regression calculations were used to establish strong common variances shared between predictors.

Anthropometric measurements were collected with an astra stadiometer with a mechanical scale to measure height (0.1 cm) and with a body composition analysis device for body mass (0.1 kg), body muscle (0.1 kg) and percentage of fat mass (0.1%) (TanitaBC-545N) [1], through the use of bioelectrical impedance analysis, which is based on the rate at which a weak electrical current travels through the body [30,31].

2.2.1. Vertical Jump Test

Three vertical jump types, squat jump (SJ), countermovement jump (CMJ) and repeat jump (RJ) [13], were used to evaluate the lower body power with a jump-mat system (Chronojump, Bosco-System, Barcelona, Spain), capturing 1000 samples per second. Each participant completed three trials of each type of jump with a rest period between actions of 2 min. The best performance was used for data analysis. In SJ, participants began from a flexed position with knees to 90 degrees and hold this position for 3 s before executing jump without any countermovement. The CMJ test started with the standing position, hands on hips and using the countermovement to jump as high as possible after descending to the half squat position. The RJ followed the same procedure that CMJ but with a continuous execution during 30 s. Elastic index (EI) was calculated from the difference between two jump types (SJ and CMJ), mechanical power (MchP) was calculated with Test time ($T = 30$ s), flight time (f_t) and the number of jumps (n) as MchP = $(g^2 \cdot T \cdot f_t)/[4n \cdot (T-f_t)]$. Finally, to calculate the resistance index (RI) to fast strength, the average height reached in RJ was related to CMJ height as RI = h_{RJ}/h_{CMJ} [13]. Power output prediction equations based on body mass, jump height in SJ (h_{SJ}) and CMJ (h_{CMJ}) were: predicted power SJ = $60.7 \cdot h_{SJ}$ + 45.3·body mass—2055 and predicted power CMJ = $51.9 \cdot h_{CMJ}$ + 48.9 · body mass—2007 [32].

2.2.2. Bench Pull Test

The bench pull test is a specific tool to assess the pulling strength of the upper torso in rowers owing to similar shoulder adduction that take place during rowing stroke [3,24]. BP data were recorded by an optoelectronic encoder (Velowin, Deportec, Murcia, Spain) capturing 500 samples per second from which a dedicated software calculated velocity, power and force output for each repetition. Mean and maximum values of velocity, power and force, both for the entire concentric action and for the propulsive phase during BP were recorded. In such a test, the rower is laying, face down on the bench, whose height from the floor is adjusted according to the length of the rower's arms so that both elbows are in full extension and the arms completely suspended. The barbell is held with hands apart at shoulder level or slightly wider [3,17]. A light load (30% from the 1RM) as the minimum load that can discriminate the different levels of traditional rowers [4], was used for this study. Although some studies did not find a relationship between BP test and rowing performance, it may be a consequence of having used too high intensity to perform BP. The test was cancelled when the rower was unable to flex the arms sufficiently to touch the underside of the bench phase [33].

2.2.3. 2000 m Rowing Ergometer Test

The performance test was carried out on a rowing ergometer (Model D; Concept 2, Inc., Morrisville, VT, USA) [11,24,34,35] with the aim of reducing external influences, such as wind, temperature and waves, that could influence the final result [36]. The control of these cofactors is advisable in traditional rowing, practiced in open waters or rough sea, and in Olympic rowing, which is practiced in flat waters, mainly rivers and lakes. Therefore, a rowing ergometer allows for individual testing in a controlled way, providing a valid proxy for rowing performance [4]. The rowers performed an all-out 2000 m test on a rowing ergometer, with the drag factor set to 130 for males and 110 for females [24]. The warm-up consisted of 10 min of moderate intensity (heart rate below 140 beats per minute and 18–20 strokes per minute). The rowers' coach was continuously motivating and giving feedback to the rowers so that they could carry out the test in the shortest time possible. The rowers could see all the power, stroke rate, distance and time information on the screen of the ergometer. Power output, stroke rate and time to complete 2000 m rowing ergometer performance test were recorded.

2.3. Statistical Analysis

The Statistical Package for Social Sciences (SPSS) v.24 program was used to compare the means of variables (IBM, Armonk, NY: IBM Corp). Descriptive statistics (mean ± SD) were used to report the characteristics of conditional factors. Shapiro–Wilk statistical test was used to determine whether the quantitative variables fulfil the criterion of normality. Pearson correlation coefficient (r) with 95% confidence intervals (CI) via bootstrapping was used to establish relationships between anthropometric characteristics, jump test, and bench pull test results with rowing performance. The magnitude of the correlation coefficient was interpreted with the following thresholds: 0.0–0.09 (trivial); 0.1–0.29 (small); 0.3–0.49 (moderate); 0.5–0.69 (strong); 0.7–0.89 (very strong); 0.9–0.99 (nearly perfect); and 1.0 (perfect) [37]. A stepwise multiple regression analysis was used to predict the 2000 m test performance. Additionally, a proportional curvilinear allometric scaling of 2000 m test performance was considered to identify key determinants of rowing performance [38,39]. For both regression techniques, predictors were iteratively adding and removing to the predictive model to find the subset of variables resulting in models which explained 50% or more of the variance of the data ($R^2 > 0.5$). The resulting best-fit equations for the best predictive models of rowing performance within the current population for male and female rowers were also shown, together with adjusted R^2 to account for non-significant predictors in the regression models. Statistical significance was set at $p < 0.05$.

3. Results

As shown in Table 1, height resulted in strong correlation with performance ($r = 0.68$, $p = 0.014$) in male rowers. Body mass ($r = 0.83$, $p < 0.001$) and body muscle ($r = 0.81$, $p < 0.001$) had a very strong correlation but percentage of body fat and Body Mass Index (BMI) were not correlated with performance test. Jump tests heights (h_{SJ}, h_{CMJ} and h_{RJ}), RI, EI and MP showed low correlation with performance test. Besides, the power output prediction equation based on body mass for SJ showed strong correlation with performance ($r = 0.58$, $p = 0.048$). Slightly higher correlations were found for CMJ ($r = 0.70$, $p = 0.012$). Mean velocity ($r = 0.84$, $p < 0.001$) and mean propulsive velocity ($r = 0.87$, $p < 0.001$) in BP test showed very strong correlation with performance. Likewise, mean power ($r = 0.85$, $p < 0.001$) resulted in very strong correlation and maximum power ($r = 0.73$, $p = 0.007$) showed very strong correlation with performance.

Table 1. Relationship of anthropometric and strength determinants with 2000 m rowing ergometer performance.

Conditional Factors	Male			Female		
	Mean ± SD	95% CI	2-km (r)	Mean ± SD	95% CI	2-km (r)
Anthropometry						
Height (cm)	178.4 ± 8.9	173.3–183.3	0.68 *	166.3 ± 7.5	161.3–171.9	0.67
Body mass (kg)	77.3 ± 7.9	72.8–82.0	0.83 †	59.9 ± 8.3	54.8–65.5	0.66
Body fat (%)	11.9 ± 3.8	9.9–13.9	−0.18	20.5 ± 4.1	17.8–23.4	0.24
BMI (kg/m^2)	24.3 ± 1.7	23.3–25.2	0.25	21.7 ± 2.6	20.0–23.6	0.28
Body muscle (kg)	64.5 ± 7.1	60.1–68.4	0.81 †	45.9 ± 4.8	42.9–49.0	0.94 †
Jump tests						
H$_{SJ}$ (cm)	35.6 ± 6.1	32.8–39.3	−0.17	25.2 ± 1.5	24.2–26.2	−0.72
W$_{SJ}$ (W)	3608.0 ± 404.8	3382.9–3834.0	0.58 *	2184.2 ± 314.9	1981.0–2399.8	0.57
H$_{CMJ}$ (cm)	38.0 ± 5.1	35.7–41.2	−0.23	26.4 ± 1.5	25.6–27.6	−0.60
W$_{CMJ}$ (W)	3744.1 ± 377.3	3519.7–3948.8	0.70 *	2303.8 ± 368.1	2087.6–2568.4	0.59
H$_{RJ}$ (cm)	29.4 ± 4.4	27.3–32.1	−0.14	18.5 ± 3.4	16.3–21.0	−0.58
RI	0.8 ± 0.1	0.7–0.8	0.13	0.7 ± 0.1	0.6–0.8	−0.50
EI	2.4 ± 2.8	0.8–3.6	−0.03	1.5 ± 1.2	0.7–2.4	0.14
MchP (W/kg)	19.5 ± 3.5	17.7–21.7	−0.06	13.4 ± 1.3	12.6–14.3	0.01
Bench Pull test						
MV (m·s^{-1})	1.8 ± 0.1	1.7–1.8	0.84 †	1.5 ± 0.1	1.4–1.5	0.63
MPV (m·s^{-1})	1.8 ± 0.1	1.8–1.9	0.87 †	1.5 ± 0.1	1.4–1.6	0.67
V$_{max}$ (m·s^{-1})	2.5 ± 0.2	2.4–2.6	0.79 †	2.0 ± 0.2	1.9–2.1	0.65
MF (N)	141.3 ± 1.8	140.4–124.3	0.34	91.6 ± 0.4	91.4–91.9	−0.39
MPF (N)	296.0 ± 32.6	278.3–313.8	0.58 *	158.1 ± 11.6	150.4–165.1	0.20
F$_{max}$ (N)	630.3 ± 85.6	583.4–677.8	0.60 *	350.7 ± 35.6	325.3–373.8	0.07
MP (W)	238.5 ± 16.2	230.1–248.0	0.85 †	126.8 ± 10.5	119.7–133.8	0.64
MPP (W)	445.8 ± 72.6	407.8–487.8	0.71 †	200.6 ± 24.5	185.4–218.6	0.55
P$_{max}$ (W)	626.7 ± 93.7	573.7–676.7	0.73 †	271.9 ± 33.9	250.2–295.2	0.79 *

BMI: Body Mass Index; H$_{SJ}$: squat jump height; W$_{SJ}$: squat jump power; H$_{CMJ}$: countermovement jump height; W$_{CMJ}$: countermovement jump power; H$_{RJ}$: repeat jump height; RI: resistance index; EI: elastic Index; MchP: mechanical power; MV: mean velocity; MPV: mean propulsive velocity; V$_{max}$: maximum velocity; MF: mean force; MPF: mean propulsive force; F$_{max}$: maximum force; MP: mean power; MPP: mean propulsive power; P$_{max}$: maximum power; * statistical significance $p < 0.05$; † statistical significance $p < 0.01$.

Female rowers showed strong to nearly perfect correlation between the same anthropometric variables than males with performance: height ($r = 0.67$, $p = 0.101$), body mass ($r = 0.66$, $p = 0.107$) and body muscle ($r = 0.94$, $p = 0.002$). Similarly to male rowers, the power output prediction equation based on body mass for SJ (W$_{SJ}$) showed strong correlation ($r = 0.57$, $p = 0.179$), and stronger correlation values were found for CMJ (W$_{CMJ}$) with performance ($r = 0.59$, $p = 0.159$). Finally, female rowers showed strong correlation in mean velocity ($r = 0.63$, $p = 0.126$), mean propulsive velocity ($r = 0.67$, $p = 0.102$) and mean power ($r = 0.64$, $p = 0.124$) in BP test with performance. Furthermore, very strong correlation in maximum power ($r = 0.79$, $p = 0.036$) were found.

The results of the stepwise multiple linear regression analysis in male rowers indicated that body mass is the only predictor variable for anthropometric characteristics explaining 69% ($R^2 = 0.69$, $p < 0.001$) of W$_{2000m}$. Similarly, the only predictor variable for BP test were the mean propulsive velocity that explained 76% of rowing performance ($R^2 = 0.76$, $p < 0.001$) (Table 2). The rest of the anthropometric and power variables in jump and BP tests did not contribute significantly and were excluded from the prediction equation. The best predictor of rowing performance among anthropometric characteristics for female rowers was body muscle, accounting for 89% of variance ($R^2 = 0.89$, $p = 0.002$) and maximum power for BP measures, explaining 62% of rowing performance ($R^2 = 0.62$, $p = 0.036$). As with the male linear regression models, the inclusion of the remaining variables resulted in models predicting less than 50% of the variance so they were excluded from the equations.

Table 2. Stepwise multiple regression analysis and proportional allometric scaling to predict rowing performance in male and female rowers according to anthropometric and power determinants.

Model	Sex	Equation	R^2	Adj. R^2	SEE	p
Linear	M	W_{2000m} (W) = 5.54 · Body mass (kg) − 154.97	0.69	0.66	30.96	$p < 0.001$
	M	W_{2000m} (W) = 384.10 · MPV (m·s^{-1}) − 431.99	0.76	0.73	27.30	$p < 0.001$
	F	W_{2000m} (W) = 4.28 · Body muscle (kg) − 30.02	0.89	0.86	8.00	$p = 0.002$
	F	W_{2000m} (W) = 0.50 · P_{max} (W) + 30.10	0.62	0.54	14.71	$p = 0.036$
Allometric	M	W_{2000m} (W) = 0.34 · [Body mass (kg)]$^{1.537}$	0.70	0.67	0.11	$p < 0.001$
	M	W_{2000m} (W) = 57.89 · [MPV (m·s^{-1})]$^{2.535}$	0.76	0.73	0.10	$p < 0.001$
	F	W_{2000m} (W) = 1.84 · [Body muscle (kg)]$^{1.177}$	0.88	0.85	0.00	$p = 0.002$
	F	W_{2000m} (W) = 1.72 · [P_{max} (W)]$^{0.815}$	0.60	0.52	0.10	$p = 0.040$

SEE: standard error of estimate; W: power; MPV: mean propulsive velocity in bench pull; P_{max}: maximum power in bench pull; M: Male; F: Female.

The proportional allometric model relationships between rowing performance (W_{2000m}) and determinants (anthropometric and BP) showed approximately linear associations, indicated by the exponent near unity. The only prediction equation showing power-function characteristics is the mean propulsive velocity for male rowers, which explained 76% of the variance. The proportional slopes of the rest of the predicting equations gave similar prediction power (R^2) but with lower estimate errors. The same variables that explain most of the variance in the stepwise linear regression were the remaining predictor variables making a significant contribution to the proportional allometric model. The remaining predicting variables lead to models explaining less than half the variance of rowing performance, so they were excluded from the equations.

4. Discussion

The main aim of the study was to analyze the relationship of anthropometric and strength determinants with 2000 m rowing ergometer performance in traditional rowing. According to several studies, high-performance rowers of both sexes are usually heavier and taller than low-performance counterparts [9,40,41]. Our results are in accordance with other studies in which height, body mass and body muscle correlated with better performance [34,42,43]. Furthermore, among all variables, body mass for male rowers and body muscle for female rowers were the best predictors of rowing performance. Akça [1] found taller and heavier Olympic male college rowers (185.8 cm and 80.2 kg) compared to traditional rowers of our study (178.4 cm and 77.3 kg). This difference can be due to traditional rowing requiring shorter and lighter rowers in some boat positions for hydrodynamic reasons, so the crew must be not homogeneous [11]. For that reason, some physical advantages of heavier and taller rowers in Olympic rowing could become a disadvantage in boat hydrodynamics and rowing technique in traditional rowing [4,11,27].

In line with our findings, Yoshiga and Higuchi [44] reported that rowing performance is highly influenced by body size, in such a way that large body size increased the rowing performance. However, these authors found that female rowers were slower than males when both groups were matched based on the body size, possibly due to the larger body fat of females which deteriorates the rowing performance. Nevertheless, the differences between sexes in rowing performance were reduced when the fat-free mass was taken into consideration. Therefore, the results support the idea that muscle mass and fat-free mass are key factors related to rowing performance [45], especially in female rowers [19].

High percentage of body fat negatively affects rowing performance because body fat contributes a metabolically non-productive load [46] and low body fat percentage was associated with higher aerobic capacity [47]. Nevertheless, it is difficult to combine high level of musculature with low percentage of body fat [9]. In this study, body fat showed a small correlation with rowing performance [1,34]. This finding was consistent with previous studies which showed significant differences between age categories, although the differences between elite and sub-elite categories were minimal [4,41].

Despite this fact, it seems accepted that rowers with low body fat percentage perform a shorter time in the 2000 m test [4,48].

In this study, traditional male rowers had a low percentage of body fat of 11.9%, which is in accordance with Majumdar et al. [34], who reported similar values (11.1%) in the combined group (light body mass and open category), although elite rowers showed lower percentage of body fat (7.8%). The same trend is observed when the female group (20.9%) were compared with female elite rowers (16.3%). The difference between sex showed higher body fat percentage in the female group compared with the male group ($\Delta 56.8\%$), usually accumulated around hips and thighs due to physiological and hormone characteristics [49]. Hence, rowers with high height and lean body mass values as well as low percentage of body fat seem to contribute to a greater power output stroke [9].

In the present study, there was a strong correlation in both sexes between power output in SJ (W_{SJ}) and CMJ (W_{CMJ}) with performance when body mass was considered. Greater muscle volume of the vastus lateralis could explain variance in rowing ergometer performance, sprint, and endurance capacity [50]. Battista et al. [8] did not find correlations between jump test and endurance test, probably since body mass, an important variable for rowing performance, has not been considered as an additional factor to assess vertical jump height [50]. To solve this problem, different authors proposed methods to estimate the lower limb power output during squat jump adding body mass variable to the equations [32,51]. Considering the contributions of these authors, the correlations between rowing performance test and jumps increased considerably. Comparing sex categories, our results showed a strong to very strong correlation between lower limb strength and rowing performance, although results were only significant in the male group. Similarly, Ingham et al. [20] reported a higher correlation between lower limb strength and rowing performance in male than female rowers, although these differences in correlation were considerably larger than our results.

The BP test, in contrast to Olympic rowing, showed higher correlations with rowing performance for all variables compared to jump tests. This fact can be due to the major contribution of the upper body in traditional rowing stroke. High correlation values between BP power average and rowing performance suggest that upper body power is one of the most important factors influencing the performance of traditional rowing, possibly due to the use of lower limbs in a flexed position and the greater degree of body extension compared to Olympic rowing [13]. In the same way, our results showed that mean propulsive velocity in BP was the best predictor of rowing performance for male rowers and maximum power in BP for female rowers, both for linear and proportional curvilinear (allometric) models, suggesting approximately linear associations between these determinants and rowing performance. The fact that seats are fixed in traditional rowing reduces legs freedom of movement and consequently their intervention in the stroke, although legs still have an important role in the first phase of paddling (isometric contraction). Comparing sex categories, male group showed higher correlation between BP power average and 2000 m test. These differences could be related to higher values of body muscle and less percentage of body fat of the male group since BP, 2000 m test is strongly correlated with the ratio between power and body mass [4]. Moreover, Attenborough, Smith, and Sinclair [52] studied the upper contribution to rowing performance of female rowers compared to male rowers and suggest to spend time to specific upper body conditioning as a key factor to improve rowing performance in the female category.

4.1. Limitations

In this study, the vertical jump test was performed to evaluate the power of the lower body by the similarity of the jumping movement gesture and the first phase of the leg drive. Further research could perform other measures, such as the Wingate test, to assess lower-body power, more specifically, peak power, mean power and fatigue index, and the possible relationship with traditional rowing performance.

Another limitation of this study is the small sample size and, therefore, the findings of the study should be interpreted with caution. Future studies are required to confirm our results in a larger population, including other traditional rowing modalities and nationalities to avoid a possible bias derived from an exclusively Spanish sample.

4.2. Practical Applications

The results of this study provide further insight regarding the influence of different determinants of anthropometry and strength on 2000 m rowing ergometer performance in traditional rowing. This study demonstrates that some anthropometric characteristics may influence rowing success and a higher correlation between the upper body and rowing performance than lower body. Therefore, coaches should consider it to perform effective talent identification programs for rowing and training planning.

5. Conclusions

In summary, the data presented within this investigation suggest that large values of height, body mass and body muscle were highly correlated with 2000 m rowing ergometer performance in traditional rowing. Furthermore, body mass for male rowers and body muscle for female rowers were found to be good predictors. The main results showed a strong correlation of W_{SJ} and W_{CMJ} with 2000 m rowing ergometer performance in traditional rowing. However, BP variables were those that most strongly correlated with performance, highlighting the relevant role of the upper trunk in traditional rowing. Mean propulsive velocity in BP in male rowers and maximum power in bench pull in female rowers were found to be good predictors of rowing performance.

Author Contributions: Conceptualization, S.S.-A., A.P.-T. and B.P.; Data curation, A.P.-T. and J.M.J.-O.; Formal analysis, S.S.-A., A.P.-T. and B.P.; Investigation, S.S.-A. and J.M.J.-O.; Methodology, A.P.-T., J.M.J.-O. and B.P.; Project administration, S.S.-A.; Resources, A.P.-T. and J.M.J.-O.; Software, S.S.-A. and B.P.; Supervision, B.P.; Validation, S.S.-A. and B.P.; Visualization, J.M.J.-O.; Writing—original draft, S.S.-A.; Writing—review and editing, S.S.-A., A.P.-T., J.M.J.-O. and B.P. All authors have read and agreed to the published version of the manuscript.

Funding: This study was supported by a pre-doctoral grant (ACIF/2018/209) from the Generalitat Valenciana, Spain, and vice-rectorate program of research and knowledge transfer for the promotion of R+D+I at the University of Alicante (Ref. GRE18-19).

Acknowledgments: The authors would like to express their gratitude to Jennifer Guerra, from the Department of Chemistry and Biochemistry, and to Elena Gandía García, from the Department of World Languages and Cultures, at the University of Nevada, Las Vegas, NV, USA, for providing assistance in preparing this manuscript.

Conflicts of Interest: The authors declare no conflict of interest.

References

1. Akça, F. Prediction of rowing ergometer performance from functional anaerobic power, strength and anthropometric components. *J. Hum. Kinet.* **2014**, *41*, 133–142. [CrossRef] [PubMed]
2. Gee, T.; Olsen, P.; Fritzdorf, S.; White, D.; Golby, J.; Thompson, K. Recovery of rowing sprint performance after high intensity strength training. *Int. J. Sport. Sci. Coach.* **2012**, *7*, 109–120. [CrossRef]
3. Maestu, J.; Jiirimae, J.; Jiirimae, T. Monitoring of performance and training in rowing. *Sport. Med.* **2005**, *35*, 597–618. [CrossRef] [PubMed]
4. Izquierdo-Gabarren, M.; González, R.; Sáez, E.; Izquierdo, M. Physiological factors to predict on traditional rowing performance. *Eur. J. Appl. Physiol.* **2010**, *108*, 83–92. [CrossRef]
5. Pollock, C.L.; Jones, I.C.; Jenkyn, T.R.; Ivanova, T.D.; Garland, S.J. Changes in kinematics and trunk electromyography during a 2000m race simulation in elite female rowers. *Scand. J. Med. Sci. Sport.* **2012**, *22*, 478–487. [CrossRef]
6. Lawton, T.W.; Cronin, J.B.; McGuigan, M.R. Strength testing and training of elite rowers. *Sport. Med.* **2011**, *41*, 413–432. [CrossRef]
7. Chimera, N.; Kremer, K. Sportsmetrics[TM] Training Improves Power and Landing in High School Rowers. *Int. J. Sports Phys. Ther.* **2016**, *11*, 44–53.
8. Battista, R.A.; Pivarnik, J.M.; Dummer, G.M.; Sauer, N.; Malina, R.M. Comparisons of physical characteristics and performances among female collegiate rowers. *J. Sports Sci.* **2007**, *25*, 651–657. [CrossRef]

9. Shephard, R.J. Science and medicine of rowing: A review. *J. Sports Sci.* **1998**, *16*, 603–620. [CrossRef]
10. Kleshnev, V. *The Biomechanics of Rowing*; Crowood Press: Malborough, UK, 2016.
11. González, J.M. Olympic rowing and traditional rowing: biomechanical, physiological and nutritional aspects. *Arch. Med. Deport.* **2014**, *31*, 51–59.
12. Mujika, I.; de Txabarri, R.G.; Maldonado-Martín, S.; Pyne, D.B. Warm-up intensity and duration's effect on traditional rowing time-trial performance. *Int. J. Sports Physiol. Perform.* **2012**, *7*, 186–188. [CrossRef] [PubMed]
13. Penichet-Tomás, A.; Pueo, B.; Jiménez-Olmedo, J. Physical performance indicators in traditional rowing championships. *J. Sports Med. Phys. Fit.* **2019**, *59*, 767–773. [CrossRef]
14. León-Guereño, P.; Urdampilleta, A.; Zourdos, M.C.; Mielgo-Ayuso, J. Anthropometric profile, body composition and somatotype in elite traditional rowers: A cross-sectional study. *Rev. Española Nutr. Diet.* **2018**, *2*, 279–286. [CrossRef]
15. Mielgo-Ayuso, J.; Calleja-González, J.; Urdampilleta, A.; León-Guereño, P.; Córdova, A.; Caballero-García, A.; Fernandez-Lázaro, D. Effects of vitamin D supplementation on haematological values and muscle recovery in elite male traditional rowers. *Nutrients* **2018**, *10*, 1968. [CrossRef] [PubMed]
16. Penichet-Tomas, A.; Pueo, B.; Jimenez-Olmedo, J.M. Relationship between experience and training characteristics with performance in non-Olympic rowing modalities. *J. Phys. Educ. Sport* **2016**, *16*, 1273–1277.
17. Izquierdo-Gabarren, M.; González, R.; García-Pallarés, J.; Sánchez-Medina, L.; Sáez, E.; Izquierdo, M. Concurrent endurance and strength training not to failure optimizes performance gains. *Med. Sci. Sports Exerc.* **2010**, *42*, 1191–1199. [CrossRef] [PubMed]
18. van der Zwaard, S.; Weide, G.; Levels, K.; Eikelboom, M.R.I.; Noordhof, D.A.; Hofmijster, M.J.; van der Laarse, W.J.; de Koning, J.J.; de Ruiter, C.J.; Jaspers, R.T. Muscle morphology of the vastus lateralis is strongly related to ergometer performance, sprint capacity and endurance capacity in Olympic rowers. *J. Sports Sci.* **2018**, *36*, 2111–2120. [CrossRef] [PubMed]
19. Riechman, S.E.; Zoeller, R.F.; Balasekaran, G.; Goss, F.L.; Robertson, R.J. Prediction of 2000 m indoor rowing performance using a 30 s sprint and maximal oxygen uptake. *J. Sports Sci.* **2002**, *20*, 681–687. [CrossRef]
20. Ingham, S.; Whyte, G.; Jones, K.; Nevill, A. Determinants of 2000 m rowing ergometer performance in elite rowers. *Eur. J. Appl. Physiol.* **2002**, *88*, 243–246. [CrossRef]
21. Nevill, A.M.; Allen, S.V.; Ingham, S.A. Modelling the determinants of 2000 m rowing ergometer performance: A proportional, curvilinear allometric approach. *Scand. J. Med. Sci. Sport* **2011**, *21*, 73–78. [CrossRef]
22. Chun-Jung, C.; Nesser, T.; Edwards, J. Strength and power determinants of rowing performance. *J. Exerc. Physiol. Online* **2010**, *13*, 52–57.
23. Perera, A.; Ariyasinghe, A.; Makuloluwa, P. Relationship of competitive success to the physique of Sri Lankan rowers. *Am. J. Sport. Sci. Med.* **2015**, *3*, 61–65. [CrossRef]
24. Lawton, T.W.; Cronin, J.B.; McGulgan, M.R. Does extensive on-water rowing increase muscular strength and endurance? *J. Sports Sci.* **2012**, *30*, 533–540. [CrossRef] [PubMed]
25. Giroux, C.; MacIejewski, H.; Ben-Abdessamie, A.; Chorin, F.; Lardy, J.; Ratel, S.; Rahmani, A. Relationship between force-velocity profiles and 1,500-m ergometer performance in young rowers. *Int. J. Sports Med.* **2017**, *38*, 992–1000. [CrossRef]
26. Bourdin, M.; Messonnier, L.; Hager, J.P.; Lacour, J.R. Peak power output predicts rowing ergometer performance in elite male rowers. *Int. J. Sports Med.* **2004**, *25*, 368–373. [CrossRef]
27. Baudouin, A.; Hawkins, D. A biomechanical review of factors affecting rowing performance. *Br. J. Sports Med.* **2002**, *36*, 396–402. [CrossRef]
28. Secher, N.H. Isometric rowing strength of experienced and inexperienced oarsmen. *Med. Sci. Sports Exerc.* **1975**, *7*, 280–283. [CrossRef]
29. Murphy, A.J. Poor correlations between isometric tests and dynamic performance: Relationship to muscle activation. *Eur. J. Appl. Physiol. Occup. Physiol.* **1996**, *73*, 353–357. [CrossRef]
30. Bera, T.K. Bioelectrical impedance methods for noninvasive health monitoring: A review. *J. Med. Eng.* **2014**, *2014*. [CrossRef]
31. Beaudart, C.; Bruyère, O.; Geerinck, A.; Hajaoui, M.; Scafoglieri, A.; Perkisas, S.; Bautmans, I.; Gielen, E.; Reginster, J.Y.; Buckinx, F. Equation models developed with bioelectric impedance analysis tools to assess muscle mass: A systematic review. *Clin. Nutr. ESPEN* **2020**, *35*, 47–62. [CrossRef]

32. Sayers, S.P.; Harackiewicz, D.V.; Harman, E.A.; Frykman, P.; Rosenstein, M.T. Cross-validation of three jump power equations. *Med. Sci. Sport. Exerc.* **1999**, *31*, 572–577. [CrossRef]
33. Sánchez-Medina, L.; González-Badillo, J.J.; Pérez, C.E.; Pallarés, J.G. Velocity- and power-load relationships of the bench pull vs Bench press exercises. *Int. J. Sports Med.* **2014**, *35*, 209–216. [CrossRef]
34. Majumdar, P.; Das, A.; Mandal, M. Physical and strength variables as a predictor of 2000m rowing ergometer performance in elite rowers. *J. Phys. Educ. Sport* **2017**, *17*, 2502–2507.
35. Mikulić, P.; Smoljanović, T.; Bojanić, I.; Hannafin, J.; Pedišić, Ž. Does 2000-m rowing ergometer performance time correlate with final rankings at the World Junior Rowing Championship? A case study of 398 elite junior rowers. *J. Sports Sci.* **2009**, *27*, 361–366. [CrossRef] [PubMed]
36. Smith, T.B.; Hopkins, W.G. Measures of rowing performance. *Sport. Med.* **2012**, *42*, 343–358. [CrossRef] [PubMed]
37. Hopkins, W.G. A Scale of Magnitudes for Effect Statistics—A new view of statistics. Available online: www.sportsci.org/resource/stats/effectmag.html (accessed on 1 March 2020).
38. Nevill, A.M.; Jobson, S.A.; Davison, R.C.R.; Jeukendrup, A.E. Optimal power-to-mass ratios when predicting flat and hill-climbing time-trial cycling. *Eur. J. Appl. Physiol.* **2006**, *97*, 424–431. [CrossRef] [PubMed]
39. Ingham, S.A.; Whyte, G.P.; Pedlar, C.; Bailey, D.M.; Dunman, N.; Nevill, A.M. Determinants of 800-m and 1500-m running performance using allometric models. *Med. Sci. Sports Exerc.* **2008**, *40*, 345–350. [CrossRef] [PubMed]
40. Malina, R.M. Physical activity and training: Effects on stature and the adolescent growth spurt. *Med. Sci. Sports Exerc.* **1994**, *26*, 759–766. [CrossRef]
41. Mikulić, P. Anthropometric and physiological profiles. *Hum. Perform.* **2008**, *40*, 80–88. [CrossRef]
42. Mikulic, P. Anthropometric and metabolic determinants of 6,000-m rowing ergometer performance in internationally competitive rowers. *J. Strength Cond. Res.* **2009**, *23*, 1851–1857. [CrossRef]
43. Kerr, D.A.; Ross, W.D.; Norton, K.; Hume, P.; Kagawa, M.; Ackland, T.R. Olympic lightweight and open-class rowers possess distinctive physical and proportionality characteristics. *J. Sports Sci.* **2007**, *25*, 43–53. [CrossRef] [PubMed]
44. Yoshiga, C.C.; Higuchi, M. Rowing performance of female and male rowers. *Scand. J. Med. Sci. Sports* **2003**, *13*, 317–321. [CrossRef]
45. Tachibana, K.; Yashiro, K.; Miyazaki, J.; Ikegami, Y.; Higuchi, M. Muscle cross-sectional areas and performance power of limbs and trunk in the rowing motion. *Sport. Biomech.* **2007**, *6*, 44–58. [CrossRef] [PubMed]
46. Olds, T. Body composition and sports performance. In *The Olympic Textbook of Science in Sports*; Maughan, R., Ed.; Blackwell Science: London, UK, 2009; pp. 131–145. ISBN 9781405156387.
47. Yoshiga, C.C.; Higuchi, M. Oxygen uptake and ventilation during rowing and running in females and males. *Scand. J. Med. Sci. Sport.* **2003**, *13*, 359–363. [CrossRef]
48. Drarnitsyn, O.; Ivanova, A.; Sazonov, V. The relationship between the dynamics of cardiorespiratory variables and rowing ergometer performance. *Hum. Physiol.* **2009**, *35*, 325–331. [CrossRef]
49. Bredella, M.A. Sex differences in body composition. In *Sex and Gender Factors Affecting Metabolic Homeostasis, Diabetes and Obesity. Advances in Experimental Medicine and Biology*; Springer: Cham, Switzerland, 2017; Volume 1043, pp. 9–29. ISBN 978-3-319-70177-6.
50. Maciejewski, H.; Rahmani, A.; Chorin, F.; Lardy, J.; Samozino, P.; Ratel, S. Methodological considerations on the relationship between the 1500-m rowing ergometer performance and vertical jump in national-level adolescent rowers. *J. Strength Cond. Res.* **2018**. [CrossRef]
51. Samozino, P.; Morin, J.B.; Hintzy, F.; Belli, A. A simple method for measuring force, velocity and power output during squat jump. *J. Biomech.* **2008**, *41*, 2940–2945. [CrossRef]
52. Attenborough, A.S.; Smith, R.M.; Sinclair, P.J. Effect of gender and stroke rate on joint power characteristics of the upper extremity during simulated rowing. *J. Sports Sci.* **2012**, *30*, 449–458. [CrossRef]

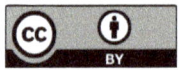

© 2020 by the authors. Licensee MDPI, Basel, Switzerland. This article is an open access article distributed under the terms and conditions of the Creative Commons Attribution (CC BY) license (http://creativecommons.org/licenses/by/4.0/).

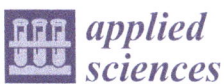

Article

Effects of Achilles Tendon Moment Arm Length on Insertional Achilles Tendinopathy

Takuma Miyamoto [1], Yasushi Shinohara [2,*], Tomohiro Matsui [3], Hiroaki Kurokawa [1], Akira Taniguchi [1], Tsukasa Kumai [4] and Yasuhito Tanaka [1]

[1] Orthopaedic Surgery, Nara Medical University, Nara 634-8521, Japan; k166136@naramed-u.ac.jp (T.M.); blackandriver@hotmail.co.jp (H.K.); a-tani@naramed-u.ac.jp (A.T.); yatanaka@naramed-u.ac.jp (Y.T.)
[2] College of Sport and Health Science, Ritsumeikan University, Shiga 525-8577, Japan
[3] Orthopaedic Surgery, Saiseikai Nara Hospital, Nara 630-8145, Japan; t.matsui19810671@live.jp
[4] Faculty of Sport Sciences, Waseda University, Tokyo 169-8050, Japan; kumakumat@waseda.jp
* Correspondence: ysr15159@fc.ritsumei.ac.jp; Tel.: +81-77-561-2617

Received: 21 August 2020; Accepted: 22 September 2020; Published: 23 September 2020

Abstract: Insertional Achilles tendinopathy (IAT) is caused by traction force of the tendon. The effectiveness of the suture bridge technique in correcting it is unknown. We examined the moment arm in patients with IAT before and after surgery using the suture bridge technique, in comparison to that of healthy individuals. We hypothesized that the suture bridge method influences the moment arm length. An IAT group comprising 10 feet belonging to 8 patients requiring surgical treatment for IAT were followed up postoperatively and compared with a control group comprising 15 feet of 15 healthy individuals with no ankle complaints or history of trauma or surgery. The ratio of the moment arm (MA) length/foot length was found to be statistically significant between the control group, the IAT group preoperatively and the IAT group postoperatively ($p < 0.01$). Despite no significant difference in the force between the control and preoperative IAT groups, a significantly higher force to the Achilles tendon was observed in the IAT group postoperatively compared to the other groups ($p < 0.05$). This study demonstrates that a long moment arm may be one of the causes of IAT, and the suture bridge technique may reduce the Achilles tendon moment arm.

Keywords: insertional Achilles tendinopathy; Achilles tendon moment arm; suture bridge method

1. Introduction

The Achilles tendon, attached to the posterior process of the calcaneus, is the largest and strongest tendon in the body. It is composed of the gastrocnemius muscle, originating from the condyle of the femur, and the soleus muscle, originating from the upper tibia. The gastrocnemius and soleus muscles, collectively known as the triceps surae, flex the ankle joint during gait. In the gait cycle, balance is maintained against gravity during the stance phase, and flexing the ankle joint during the toe-off phase provides a forward propulsive force [1].

The contraction of the triceps surae is exerted as a rotational force (torque) around the ankle axis, which can be calculated theoretically as the product of the muscle cross-section and the moment arm (MA) (Figure 1) [2–4].

In general, the length of the MA is known to change depending on the angles of plantarflexion and dorsiflexion of the ankle joint, which is different in each individual [2–4]. However, the length of the MA of the triceps surae has been reported to change depending on the angle of plantar- and dorsiflexion of the ankle joint [5–7]. Yet, it has also been reported that motion does not cause any change in the length of the MA [8,9], and that the plantarflexion moment length, from the plantarflexion region to the dorsiflexion region, is different in each individual, with little change caused by motion [2–4]. Thus, the changes in the length of the MA in motion has attracted great attention. Moreover, the shape of the foot has been shown to influence the Achilles tendon MA [10]. However, these studies examined the length of the MA only in healthy individuals and it has not been investigated in patients with Achilles tendon disorders.

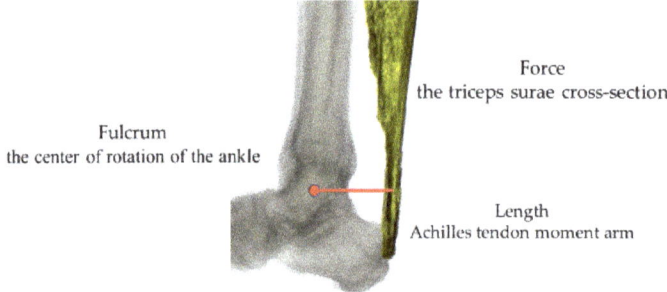

Figure 1. The contraction of the triceps surae can be calculated theoretically as the product of the triceps surae muscle cross-section area and the Achilles tendon moment arm using the lever rule.

The center of rotation (COR) and tendon excursion (TE) methods are mainly used for the measurement of the lever arm of Achilles tendon [5], with MRI and ultrasound generally used for these methods, respectively. Manja et al. [10] proposed a new method using a weight-bearing X-ray. The method allowed the evaluation of the morphology and anatomical position of the bone and soft tissue. Therefore, we are now able to investigate in various patients with Achilles tendon disorders.

Insertional Achilles tendinopathy (IAT), an Achilles tendon disorder, is caused by the traction force of the Achilles tendon [11,12]. This traction force is influenced by the rotational torque of the ankle joint, and the moment arm length is proportional to the plantar flexion torque of the ankle joint [13]. Therefore, when force is applied to the ankle joint, the Achilles tendon moment arm length is inversely proportional to the traction force applied to the insertion of the Achilles tendon. On the other hand, with a short moment arm, the circular arc associated with ankle rotation is thought to shorten, reducing the length displacement of the muscle-tendon complex, and further reducing the consumption of elastic energy of the Achilles tendon [13,14]. Thus, the moment arm of the ankle joint is expected to influence the traction force applied to the insertion of the Achilles tendon, the length displacement of the muscle-tendon complex, and the elastic energy.

Surgical treatments for IAT include para-tendon excision, adhesion detachment, intra-tendon degeneration excision, and calcaneal wedge osteotomy [15,16]. Of these, we preferred surgical treatment of insertional Achilles tendinosis with reattachment of the Achilles tendon using the suture bridge technique (Figure 2). This method firmly fixes the enthesis by pressing the tendon with the surface, and good outcomes have been reported with this method [17].

However, due to the lack of basic research on this surgical technique, its effectiveness remains unknown. This study aimed to examine the moment arm length as an anatomical feature in patients with IAT. We hypothesized that the suture bridge method for IAT influences the moment arm length.

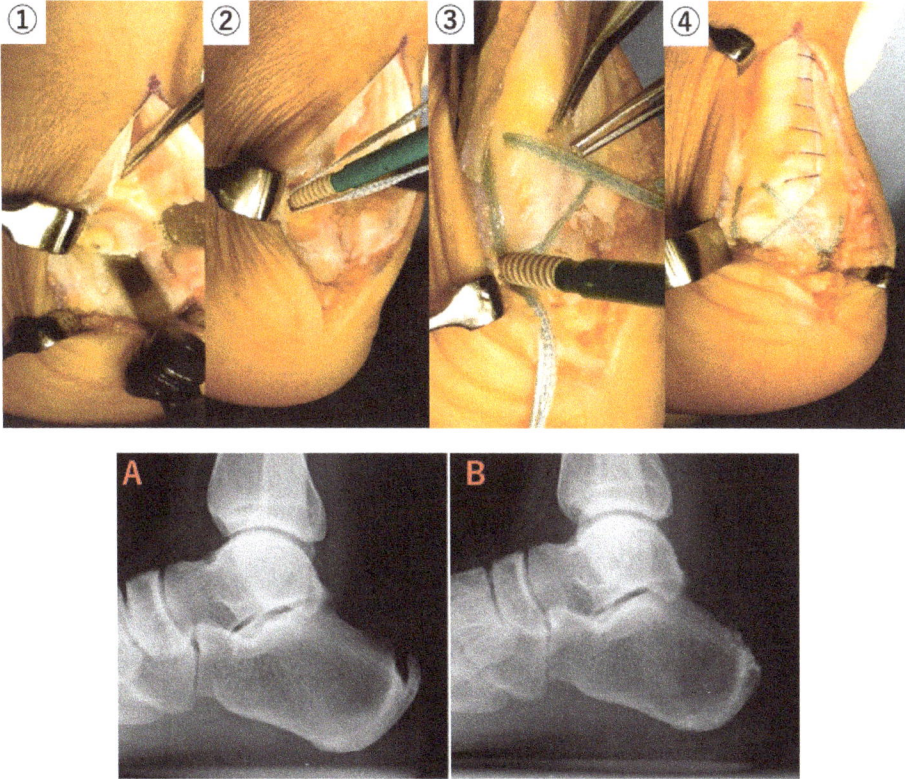

Figure 2. We performed a reconstruction of the Achilles tendon with a suture bridge technique. ①: Bone spurs, calcifications in the tendon, and Haglund's prominence is removed. ②: Two Swive Locks with Fiber Tape inserted in the proximal hole. ③: Fiber Tape is passed through the Achilles tendon and inserted into the prepared distal hole using Swive Lock. ④: The tails on the distal row flushed to the anchor. (**A**): Preoperative X-ray. (**B**): Postoperative X-ray for the same case.

2. Materials and Methods

This is a retrospective study. Fourteen individuals (16 feet) who required surgical treatment for IAT at our hospital between 2014 and 2019 were included in the IAT group. Those with a history of collagen diseases or trauma other than Achilles tendon injuries, and those who could not be followed up for more than one year after surgery were excluded from the study. As a result, 8 individuals (10 feet; IAT group) were examined in this study. Fifteen healthy individuals (with no complaints of ankle joint injuries nor history of surgical trauma) were included for examination in the control group.

The reconstruction in all IAT cases was performed using the Achilles SpeedBridge system (Arthrex, FL, USA). After extending the Achilles tendon in the midline and partly separating it from the insertion, the osteophytes, intra-tendinous degeneration site, and posterior superior calcaneus at the enthesis were excised. Subsequently, fiber tape was used to fix the Achilles tendon to the calcaneus using four knotless anchors. We analyzed a clinical evaluation by the American Orthopedic Foot and Ankle Society ankle/hindfoot scale (AOFAS scale) and visual analog pain scale (VAS) 1 year after the surgery.

At 6 months to 1 year after the surgery, 1.5T MRI (Vantage Titan Ver3.0, Canon, Tokyo, Japan) images were taken to evaluate the morphology of the Achilles tendon insertion area and abnormal signal in the tendon before and after surgery.

Plain X-ray images were used to measure the lever arm. The images of the affected side were taken for patients in the IAT group, while those of the healthy side were taken for patients in the control group. As described by Manja et al. [10], who used plain X-ray images of the feet during weight-bearing, the weight-bearing plane was taken as the plantar axis from the lateral image; a straight line perpendicular to this plantar axis, passing through the center of the Achilles tendon, was set as the central axis of the Achilles tendon. The shortest distance from the central axis of the Achilles tendon to the center of the first metatarsal head parallel to the plantar axis was defined as the length of the sole. A perfect circle was drawn to fit the pulley surface of the talus, and the center point was used as the center of motion. The shortest distance from the center of motion to the central axis of the Achilles tendon was defined as the MA length. In addition, the angle between the Achilles tendon moment arm and the line from the center of the ankle joint movement to the insertion of the Achilles tendon was defined as the α angle (Figure 3). The central axis of the Achilles tendon at the time of postoperative measurement was the midpoint from the most dorsal surface to the bottom of the insertion (Figure 4). Also, the ratio of the MA length/foot length was used to standardize the difference in foot size. Furthermore, in order to take the influence of body weight into account, the force applied to the Achilles tendon at the time of heel raise can be calculated as the rotational force around the ankle joint axis. Then, the force applied to the Achilles tendon, F, can be estimated by:

$$F = w \times (L - MA)/MA$$

where w is the body weight, MA is the Achilles tendon moment arm length, and L is the length of the sole [14,18,19] (Figure 5). In the present study, this formula was used to calculate the force applied to the Achilles tendon, and the average value of three measurements performed by one examiner was used.

Both the control group and the IAT group were examined, and all measurements were taken pre- and post-operatively. Statistical tests were performed using Microsoft Excel. Data were tested using unpaired student t-tests, and effects were considered significant at 95% CI and $p < 0.05$. All subjects gave their informed consent for inclusion before they participated in the study. The study was conducted in accordance with the Declaration of Helsinki, and the protocol was approved by the Ethics Committee of Nara Medical University (Approval number: 2740).

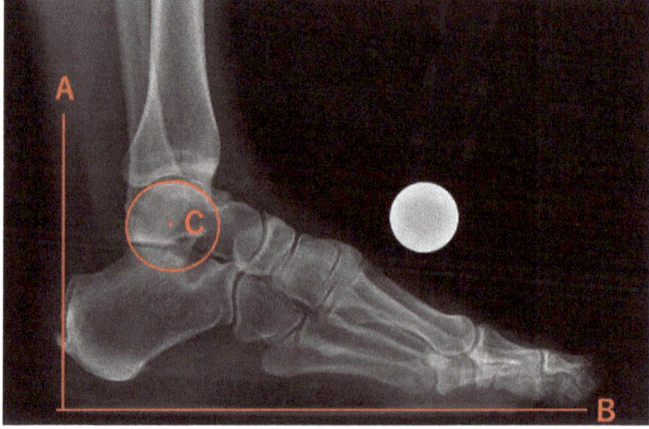

Figure 3. *Cont.*

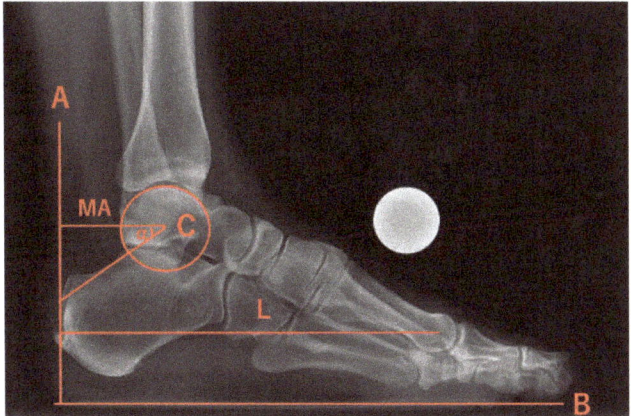

Figure 3. The measurement of the lateral weightbearing radiograph were (A) the centerline of the Achilles tendon insertion, (B) plantar axis, (C) the center of rotation of the ankle, (L) the length of the sole, (MA) the Achilles tendon moment arm (α). The angle between the Achilles tendon moment arm and the line connecting the insertion point and the center of rotation.

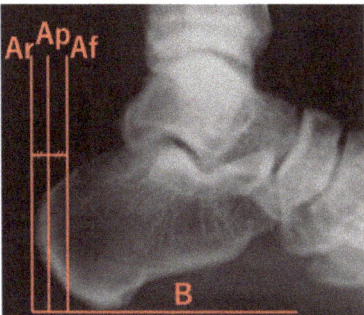

Figure 4. B: Plantar axis. Af: Front edge of the Achilles tendon insertion. Ar: Rear edge of the Achilles tendon insertion. The central axis of Ar and Af was defined as Ap (the central axis of post-operated Achilles tendon insertion).

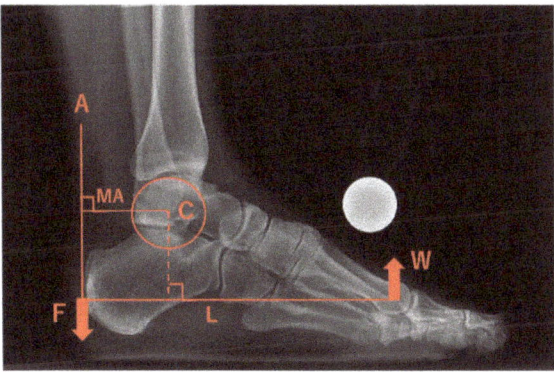

Figure 5. (A) The centerline of the Achilles tendon insertion, (C) the center of rotation of the ankle, (L) the length of the sole, and (MA) the Achilles tendon moment arm. (F) Traction force of the Achilles tendon. (W) Reaction force by body weight. We calculated F using principle of lever.

3. Results

The average height of subjects in the healthy group was 163 ± 7.4 cm, with average body weight and BMI of 64.5 ± 12.1 kg and 24.3 ± 4.8 kg/m², respectively. The average height of subjects in the IAT groups was 163.6 ±13.3 cm, with average body weight and BMI of 73.5 ± 11.0 kg and 27.7 ± 4.5 kg/m², respectively. Thus, there was no significant difference between the groups for these items (Table 1).

Table 1. Patient Characteristics.

	IAT	Control	p Value
n	10 feet (8 people)	15 feet (15 people)	
Sex	Male: 4 Female: 4	Male: 8 Female: 7	
Age, y	55.5 ± 14.4	37.4 ± 16.2	
Height, cm	164 ± 13.3	163 ± 7.44	>0.05
Body weight, kg	73.5 ± 11.0	64.5 ± 12.1	>0.05
BMI, kg/m²	27.7 ± 4.58	24.3 ± 4.83	>0.05

Abbreviations: IAT, insertional Achilles tendinopathy. BMI, body mass index. Values are given as mean ± standard deviation (SD).

The AOFAS scale and VAS improved in all cases (AOFAS scale: Preoperative averaged 71.7, postoperative averaged 92.3; VAS: Preoperative averaged 5.0, postoperative averaged 0.83).

MRI assessment after surgery for IAT revealed Achilles tendon insertion running from the proximal knotless anchor insert to the distal knotless anchor insert via the suture bridge technique in all cases (Figure 6). Also, MRI findings showed the disappearance of abnormal signals in the Achilles tendon in all cases.

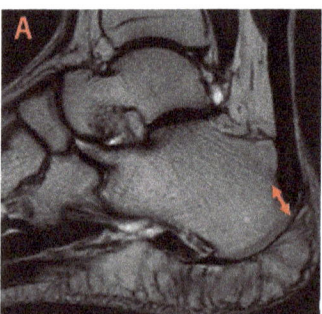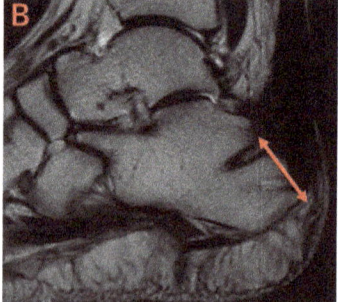

Figure 6. The MRI images of T2-weighted images of the same patient. ↔: Length of Achilles tendon insertion. (A): Pre-operation of the Achilles tendon insertion. (B): Post-operation of the Achilles tendon insertion. We can see the postoperative Achilles tendon insertion presence from the proximal knotless anchor insert to the distal knotless anchor insert.

There was no significant difference in the α angle between the control and IAT groups. The ratio of MA length/foot length was $0.30 ± 0.9 \times 10^{-3}$, in the control group, $0.31 ± 1.0 \times 10^{-2}$, in the IAT group preoperatively, and $0.27 ± 0.2 \times 10^{-1}$ in the IAT group postoperatively, showing significant differences between these groups ($p < 0.05$). The force applied to the Achilles tendon was 148.5 ± 24.9 kg in the control group, 166.2 ± 23.0 kg in the IAT group preoperatively, and 200.8 ± 25.4 kg in the IAT group postoperatively. Despite no significant difference in the force between the control and preoperative IAT groups, a significantly higher force to the Achilles tendon was observed in the IAT group postoperatively, compared to the other groups ($p < 0.05$) (Figure 7).

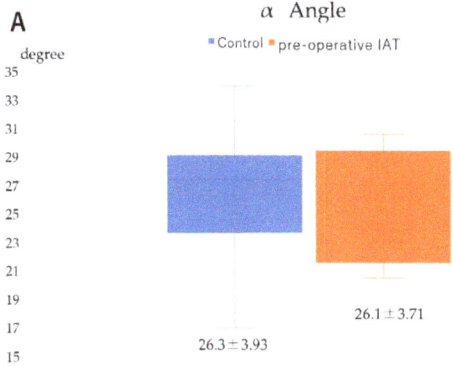
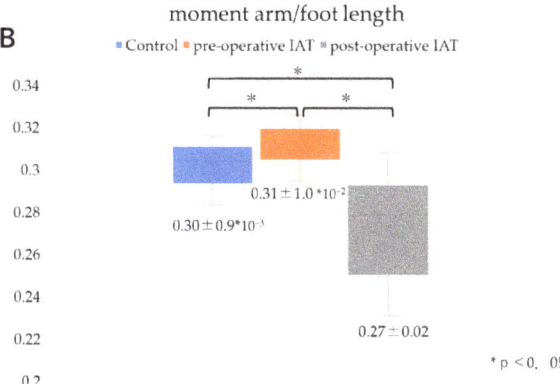
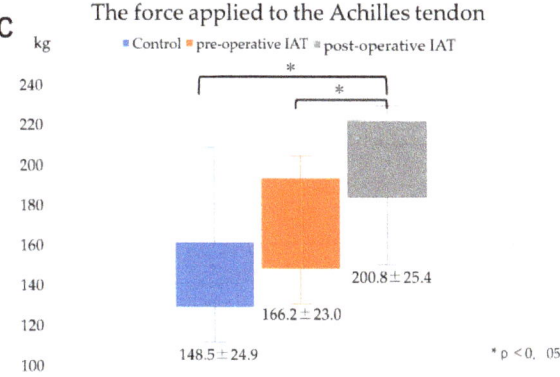

Figure 7. Radiographic Measurement. (**A**): Comparison of the α angle between the control and pre-operative IAT groups. (**B**): Comparison of the ratio of MA length/foot length between the control group, the preoperative IAT group, and the postoperative IAT group, showing significant differences between these groups ($p < 0.05$). (**C**): Comparison of the force applied to the Achilles tendon between the control group, the preoperative IAT group, and the postoperative IAT group, showing that a significantly higher force to the Achilles tendon was observed in the IAT group postoperatively, compared to the other groups ($p < 0.05$). Values are given as mean ± SD.

4. Discussion

COR method and TE methods are mainly used for the measurement of the lever arm of Achilles tendon [5]. It has been reported that the TE method shows a shorter moment arm than the COR method [5]. However, it has also been reported that there is no difference in measurements between the two methods [20]. Thus, there is no unified view on this issue. Furthermore, the Achilles tendon moment arm has been shown to be influenced by weight-bearing [21], and an evaluation method using weight-bearing X-ray has been developed for taking images during weight-bearing [10]. It is also feasible to use radiographs to measure the Achilles tendon moment arm [10]. In the present study, we examined the group of patients with IAT before and after surgery, in comparison to a control group of healthy individuals. In order to measure the moment arm and evaluation of the morphology of the bone during weight-bearing in each group, we decided to use a weight-bearing X-ray for evaluation. Also, the usage of an X-ray is a simple method and allows us to perform anatomical calculations easily. Therefore, we determined that it was a good method in our study.

A study using this measurement method reported a moment arm length of 64.3 mm [10]. In the present study, the average moment arm lengths of the healthy and IAT groups were 51.7 mm and 53.7 mm, respectively, both of which were shorter than the previously reported value. However, the length of the sole of subjects in the previous report was 185.7 mm, in contrast to 171 mm and 170.1 mm in healthy and IAT groups, respectively, in the present study. This suggests that the moment arm length may be influenced by the difference in the physical constitution.

In addition, Manja et al. [10] showed that the moment arm length and α angle are influenced by the difference in the shape of the foot, such as flat and concave feet. In the present study, no significant difference in α angle between the control and experimental groups was observed, indicating that the results are not influenced by the difference in the shape of the subject's foot, even in flat and concave feet.

To date, there have been no reports comparing the Achilles tendon moment lengths between healthy individuals and patients with IAT, but many factors are known to influence the pathophysiology of IAT. Lyman et al. [22] stated that it is caused by the traction force of the Achilles tendon during ankle movement. In the present study, those with IAT had a significantly longer Achilles tendon moment arm than healthy individuals. However, there was no significant difference in the force applied to the Achilles tendon between two groups. This indicates that the traction force of the Achilles tendon, which is the cause of IAT, is not influenced simply by the force applied to the Achilles tendon.

It has been shown that the Achilles tendon exerts approximately 4 to 6 times its weight during running [23,24], stretching approximately 8% of the total length of the Achilles tendon [25]. It has also been shown that, despite the smaller force applied during walking than in running, approximately 7% of the total length of the Achilles tendon is stretched during walking [26]. This indicates that the insertion of the Achilles tendon is influenced not only by simple tension but also by the elastic energy due to the stretching of the Achilles tendon [27]. In fact, triceps surae eccentric exercise has been recommended as a conservative therapy for IAT [28,29], and the extension of the Achilles tendon is a major cause of IAT. Our data revealed that individuals with IAT had a longer moment arm length than healthy individuals. This suggests that, with a long moment arm, the arc length associated with the ankle rotation lengthens, increasing the length displacement of the muscle-tendon complex, and further increasing the elastic energy consumption of the Achilles tendon [13,14]. Therefore, the elasticity of the Achilles tendon is shown to be greatly responsible for the development of IAT.

In addition, any measurements of the moment arm length before and after surgery using the suture bridge technique have not been reported to date. As a surgical treatment for IAT, the calcaneal wedge osteotomy takes the influence of the moment arm into account and aims to reduce stress on the insertion of the Achilles tendon by shortening the calcaneus length and slightly lifting the insertion of the Achilles tendon [30]. The suture bridge technique used in the present study has also been reported to have good long-term outcomes [17,31]. This method can treat various pathological conditions that influence IAT with minimal invasion [31]. Furthermore, by comparing the preoperative and postoperative data in this study, the postoperative Achilles tendon moment arm was found to be shortened. On the other hand, the force applied to the Achilles tendon was significantly increased in individuals with IAT compared to healthy individuals. This indicates that this method may not reduce the force applied to the Achilles tendon. Rather, it may reduce the length displacement of the Achilles tendon by reducing the Achilles tendon moment arm, thereby reducing the energy applied to the Achilles tendon.

There are three limitations to this study. First, the number of cases was small. The study needs to proceed with an increased number of cases, and proper statistical analysis needs to be performed. Secondly, the Achilles tendon insertion is an area, but for the sake of simplicity, it was considered to be a point. Performing 3D analyses allows more precise analyses, and we will need to investigate the area of the Achilles tendon insertion. Third, the moment arm measurement method used in this study was the static evaluation. An X-ray or MRI scan is required to measure the Achilles tendon moment arm after the reconstruction of Achilles tendon insertion using the suture bridge technique. However, it is difficult to measure the dynamic change of the moment arm before and after surgery with the measurement methods reported to date. Therefore, a new measurement method needs to be developed for measuring a dynamic moment arm using X-ray or ultrasonic waves in the future.

5. Conclusions

In this study, we examined the moment arm in patients with IAT before and after undergoing the suture bridge technique compared to that of healthy individuals. The Achilles tendon moment arm was significantly longer in patients with IAT. We hypothesized that the suture bridge technique for IAT influences the moment arm length. To test this, we examined the changes in the moment arm length of patients with IAT before and after the surgery by analyzing the X-ray images of the lateral side of their feet during under weight-bearing. This study demonstrates that a long moment arm may be one of the causes of IAT, and the suture bridge technique may reduce the Achilles tendon moment arm. These findings suggest that it is important to consider the influence of the Achilles tendon moment arm in the treatment of IAT.

Author Contributions: Conceptualization, Y.S.; methodology, Y.S. and T.M. (Takuma Miyamoto); software, T.M. (Takuma Miyamoto); validation, T.M. (Takuma Miyamoto), Y.S. and Y.T.; formal analysis, T.M. (Takuma Miyamoto); investigation, T.M. (Takuma Miyamoto); resources, Y.T., T.K., A.T., H.K. and T.M. (Tomohiro Matsui); data curation, Y.T., T.K., A.T., H.K. and T.M. (Tomohiro Matsui); writing—original draft preparation, T.M. (Takuma Miyamoto); writing—review and editing, Y.S. and Y.T.; visualization, T.M. (Takuma Miyamoto); supervision, Y.S. and Y.T.; project administration, Y.S. All authors have read and agreed to the published version of the manuscript.

Funding: This research received no external funding.

Conflicts of Interest: The authors declare no conflict of interest.

References

1. Dayton, P. Anatomic, Vascular, and Mechanical Overview of the Achilles Tendon. *Clin. Podiatr. Med. Surg.* **2017**, *34*, 107–113. [CrossRef]
2. Carbone, V.; Fluit, R.; Pelilaan, P.; van der Krogt, M.M.; Janssen, D.; Damsgaard, M.; Vigneron, L.; Feilkas, T.; Koopman, H.F.J.M.; Verdonschot, N. TLEM 2.0-A comprehensive musculoskeletal geometry dataset for subject-specific modeling of the lower extremity. *J. Biomech.* **2015**, *48*, 734–774. [CrossRef]
3. Klein Horsman, M.D.; Koopman, H.F.J.M.; van der Helm, F.C.T.; Poliacu Prose, L.; Veeger, H.E.J. Morphological muscle and joint parameters for musculoskeletal modeling of the lower extremity. *Clin. Biomech.* **2007**, *22*, 239–247. [CrossRef]
4. Klein, P.; Mattys, S.; Rooze, M. Moment arm length variations of selected muscles acting on talocrural and subtalar joints during movement: An in vitro study. *J. Biomech.* **1996**, *29*, 21–30. [CrossRef]
5. Fath, F.; Blazevich, A.J.; Waugh, C.M.; Miller, S.C.; Korff, T. Direct comparison of in vivo Achilles tendon moment arms obtained from ultrasound and MR scans. *J. Appl. Physiol.* **2010**, *109*, 1644–1652. [CrossRef] [PubMed]

6. Maganaris, C.N. Imaging-based estimates of moment arm length in intact human muscle-tendons. *Eur. J. Appl. Phsyol.* **2004**, *91*, 130–139. [CrossRef] [PubMed]
7. Olzewski, K.; Dick, T.J.; Wakeling, J.M. Achilles tendon moment arms: The importance of measuring at constant tendon load when using the tendon excursion method. *J. Biomech.* **2015**, *48*, 1206–1209. [CrossRef] [PubMed]
8. Csapo, R.; Hodgson, J.; Kinugasa, R.; Edgerton, V.R.; Sinha, S.; Edgerton, V.R.; Sinha, S. Ankle morphology amplifies calcaneus movement relative to triceps surae muscle shortening. *J. Appl. Physiol.* **2013**, *115*, 468–473. [CrossRef]
9. Manal, K.; Cowder, J.D.; Buchanan, T.S. Subject-specific measures of Achilles tendon moment arm using ultrasound and video-based motion capture. *Physiol. Rep.* **2013**, *1*, e00139. [CrossRef]
10. Manja, D.; Zwicky, L.; Horn, T.; Hintermann, B. The effect of foot type on the Achilles tendon moment arm and biomechanics. *Foot* **2019**, *38*, 91–94. [CrossRef]
11. Rufai, A.; Ralphs, J.R.; Benjamin, M. Structure and histopathology of the insertional region of the human Achilles tendon. *J. Orthop. Res.* **1995**, *13*, 585–593. [CrossRef] [PubMed]
12. Benjamin, M.; Kumai, T.; Milz, S.; Boszczyk, B.M.; Boszczyk, A.A.; Ralphs, J.R. The skeletal attachment of tendons-tendon 'entheses'. *Comp. Biochem. Physiol. A Mol. Integr. Physiol.* **2002**, *133*, 931–945. [CrossRef]
13. Baxter, J.R.; Piazza, S.J. Plantar flexor moment arm and muscle volume predict torque-generating capacity in young men. *J. Appl. Physio.* **2014**, *116*, 538–544. [CrossRef]
14. Kunimasa, Y.; Sano, K.; Oda, T.; Nicol, C.; Komi, P.V.; Locatelli, E.; Ito, A.; Ishikawa, M. Specific muscle-tendon architecture in elite Kenyan distance runners. *Scand. J. Med. Sci. Sports* **2014**, *24*, e269–e274. [CrossRef]
15. Irwin, T.A. Current concepts review: Insertional Achilles tendinopathy. *Foot Ankle Int.* **2010**, *31*, 933–939. [CrossRef] [PubMed]
16. Chimenti, R.L.; Cychosz, C.C.; Hall, M.M.; Phisitkul, P. Current concepts review Update: Insertional Achilles tendinopathy. *Foot Ankle Int.* **2017**, *38*, 1160–1169. [CrossRef]
17. McGravey, W.C.; Palumbo, R.C.; Baxter, D.E.; Leibman, B.D. Insertional Achilles Tendinosis: Surgical Treatment through a Central Tendon Splitting Approach. *Foot Ankle Int.* **2002**, *23*, 19–25. [CrossRef]
18. Blazevich, A.J.; Coleman, D.R.; Horne, S.; Cannavan, D. Anatomical predictors of maximum isometric and concentric knee extensor moment. *Eur. J. Appl. Physiol.* **2009**, *105*, 869–878. [CrossRef]
19. Carrier, D.R.; Heglund, N.C.; Earls, K.D. Variable Gearing During Locomotion in the Human Musculoskeletal System. *Science* **1994**, *265*, 651–653. [CrossRef]
20. Magnaris, C.N.; Balizopolos, V.; Sargeant, A.J. In vivo measurement-based estimations of the human Achilles tendon moment arm. *Eur. J. Appl. Physiol.* **2000**, *83*, 363–369. [CrossRef]
21. Rasske, K.; Thelen, D.G.; Prahz, J.R. Variation in the human Achilles tendon moment arm during walking. *Comput. Method Biomech. Biomed. Engin.* **2017**, *20*, 201–205. [CrossRef] [PubMed]
22. Lyman, J.; Weinhold, P.S.; Almekinders, L.C. Strain behavior of the distal Achilles tendon: Implications for insertional Achilles tendinopathy. *Am. J. Sports Med.* **2004**, *32*, 457–461. [CrossRef] [PubMed]
23. Andrew, G.; Jonathan, S. Comparison of Achilles tendon loading between male and female recreational runners. *J. Hum. Kinet.* **2014**, *44*, 155–159. [CrossRef] [PubMed]
24. Willy, R.W.; Halsey, L.; Hayek, A.; Johnson, H.; Willson, J.D. Patellofemoral joint and Achilles tendon loads during overground and treadmill running. *J. Orthop. Sports Phys. Ther.* **2016**, *46*, 664–672. [CrossRef]
25. Farris, D.J.; Buckeridge, E.; Trewartha, G.; McGuigan, M.P. The effects of orthotic heel lifts on Achilles tendon force and strain during running. *J. Appl. Biomech.* **2012**, *28*, 511–519. [CrossRef]
26. Franz, J.R.; Slane, L.C.; Rasske, K.; Thelen, D.G. Non-uniform in vivo deformations of the human Achilles tendon during walking. *Gait Posture* **2015**, *41*, 192–197. [CrossRef]
27. Frankewycz, B.; Penz, A.; Weber, J.; da Silva, N.P.; Freimoser, F.; Bell, R.; Nerlich, M.; Jung, E.M.; Docheva, D.; Pfeifer, C.G. Achilles tendon elastic properties remain decreased in long term after rupture. *Knee Surg. Sports Traumatol. Arthrosc.* **2018**, *26*, 2080–2087. [CrossRef]
28. Fahlstrom, M.; Jonsson, P.; Lorentzon, R.; Alfredson, H. Chronic Achilles tendon pain treated with eccentric calf-muscle training. *Knee Surg. Sports Traumatol. Arthrosc.* **2003**, *11*, 327–333. [CrossRef]
29. Rompe, J.D.; Furia, J.; Maffuli, N. Eccentric loading versus eccentric loading plus shock-wave treatment for midportion Achilles tendinopathy: A randomized controlled trial. *Am. J. Sports Med.* **2009**, *37*, 463–470. [CrossRef]

30. Perlman, M.D. Enlargement of the entire posterior aspect of the calcaneus: Treatment with the Keck and Kelly calcaneal osteotomy. *J. Foot Surg.* **1992**, *31*, 424–433.
31. Greenhagen, R.M.; Shinabarger, A.B.; Pearson, K.T.; Burns, P.R. Intermediate and long-term outcomes of the suture bridge technique for the management of insertional Achilles tendinopathy. *Foot Ankle Spec.* **2013**, *6*, 185–190. [CrossRef] [PubMed]

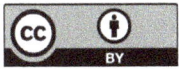

© 2020 by the authors. Licensee MDPI, Basel, Switzerland. This article is an open access article distributed under the terms and conditions of the Creative Commons Attribution (CC BY) license (http://creativecommons.org/licenses/by/4.0/).

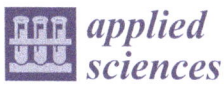

Article

Immediate Effects of an Inverted Body Position on Energy Expenditure and Blood Lactate Removal after Intense Running

Moo Sung Kim [1] and Jihong Park [2,*]

[1] Athletic Training Laboratory, Department of Physical Education, Graduate School, Kyung Hee University, Yongin 17104, Korea; kms_ss@khu.ac.kr
[2] Athletic Training Laboratory, Department of Sports Medicine, Kyung Hee University, Yongin 17104, Korea
* Correspondence: jihong.park@khu.ac.kr; Tel.: +82-31-201-2721

Received: 5 September 2020; Accepted: 21 September 2020; Published: 23 September 2020

Abstract: We compared the immediate effects of a cool-down strategy including an inverted body position (IBP: continuous 30-s alternations of supine and IBP) after a short period of an intense treadmill run with active (walking) and passive (seated) methods. Fifteen healthy subjects (22 years, 172 cm, 67 kg) completed three cool-down conditions (in a counterbalanced order) followed by a 5-min static stretch on three separate days. Heart rate, energy expenditure, blood lactate concentration, fatigue perception, and circumference of thighs and calves were recorded at pre- and post-run at 0, 5, 10, 20, and 30 min. At 5 min post-run, subjects performing the IBP condition showed (1) a 22% slower heart rate ($p < 0.0001$, ES = 2.52) and 14% lower energy expenditure ($p = 0.01$, ES = 0.48) than in the active condition, and (2) a 23% lower blood lactate than in the passive condition ($p = 0.001$, ES = 0.82). Fatigue perception and circumferences of thighs and calves did not differ between the conditions at any time point ($F_{10,238} < 0.96$, $p < 0.99$ for all tests). IBP appears to produce an effect similar to that of an active cool-down in blood lactate removal with less energy expenditure. This cool-down strategy is recommended for tournament sporting events with short breaks between matches, such as Taekwondo, Judo, and wrestling.

Keywords: cool-down strategy; heart rate; fatigue perception

1. Introduction

Progressive overload is an essential principle in developing physical fitness, and it often requires fatigue-inducing training [1]. Fatigue is defined as a physiological (and psychological) constraint that results in failure to maintain a certain amount or intensity of voluntary muscle contractions [2]. By overloading exercise-induced fatigue, athletes may experience a temporary (e.g., a few days) performance reduction, referred to as functional overreaching [3]. Nonfunctional overreaching is also considered as the normal process of training adaptation, although it may take a longer time (e.g., a few weeks) to restore function [4]. Overtraining results in performance decrease with persistent physical and/or psychological fatigue for an extended period of time (e.g., a few months) [5]. While athletes and coaches seek optimal training adaptations, inadequate physiological (and psychological) recovery between training sessions can lead to overtraining [6]. Therefore, cool-down strategies to balance training stimulation and physical recovery are just as important as the training program.

Since "active recovery", defined as submaximal exercise or movement immediately following a training session, was first introduced in 1975 [7], its relative superiority over passive recovery has been reported in many studies [8–11]. Specifically, faster decreases of blood lactate [9], intramuscular pH level (due to reduced H+) [12], and oxyhemoglobin [13] as well as faster phosphocreatine resynthesis [14] are known advantages although the most effective working intensity remains controversial [9,15].

Enhancement of oxidation due to a higher rate or volume of blood flow to the working muscles [15] enhances the lactic acid removal [16] and prevents H+ release [17], which allows faster recovery from exercise-induced fatigue. Because of the increase in blood flow, practicing active recovery is preferred, especially when multiple exercise bouts are performed.

If the rate or volume of blood flow is an important causal factor, an inverted body position (IBP) might expedite the recovery process. This gravity-independent position (elevation of the lower body) decreases vascular hydrostatic pressure, resulting in increased venous return and lymphatic drainage [18]. According to the Frank–Starling mechanism [19], an increased venous return increases myocardial stretch (preload), which results in increased stroke volume and cardiac output [20]. Therefore, IBP activity could increase peripheral circulation in the lower extremities and enhance the process of physiological recovery. Previously, a position of head-down tilt at 15° was shown to increase stroke volume, mean arterial pressure, and cutaneous vascular conductance [21,22]. Another study [23] used the same position for 5 min and reported a 36% increase in tibial microvascular flow. Although an acute increase of cardiovascular function from holding a head-down tilt position is evident [21–23], changes of blood lactate removal and fatigue perception have not been evaluated.

Hence, the primary purpose of this study was to examine how a 10-min cool-down protocol containing IBP affects physiological and psychological recovery after intense running compared to the same duration of active (walking) and passive (seated) cool-down strategies. Since the effects of increasing blood flow were achieved on the 15° head-down tilt [21–23], our IBP protocol had a maximal inclination (up to 90°) in expectation of the greatest effects of circulation of blood and body fluids [18]. Considering results from previous head-down tilt studies [21–23], the effects of elevation [18], and the Frank–Starling mechanism theory [19], we hypothesized that the lactate removal rate at the end of IBP would be greater than that of passive recovery at the same time point. Due to more voluntary muscle contractions and movements, we further expected higher values of heart rate and energy expenditure in the active recovery condition than in the IBP and passive recovery conditions.

2. Materials and Methods

2.1. Experimental Design

We used a three (condition) × six (time) single-blinded cross-over design with repeated measures of time. To objectively increase exercise-induced blood lactate, a treadmill run was implemented. In this approach, we assumed that heart rate increase by exercise correlates linearly with the amount of blood lactate. To test the condition effect, dependent measurements among the conditions were compared at each time point. Each condition had a 10-min cool-down activity that consisted of 5 min of IBP, walking on the treadmill or sitting on a chair, and another 5 min of static stretching (same activity for each condition). Therefore, the post-run 5-min time point reflected the acute effect of the IBP whereas the post-run 20- and 30-min time points corresponded to the combined effect of IBP and stretching. The temperature and relative humidity in the laboratory were maintained at 25 °C and 50% during the data collection period. One researcher guided the treadmill run and conducted the measurements while being blinded to the cool-down condition by leaving the laboratory while another researcher conducted the cool-down protocol. The study was approved by the Institutional Review Board and was conducted in accordance with the Declaration of Helsinki.

2.2. Subjects

Fifteen healthy active adults (5 females: 20.4 ± 0.6 years, 161.4 ± 3.3 cm, 57.8 ± 4.2 kg; 10 males: 22.9 ± 0.9 years, 176.5 ± 1.9 cm, 72.1 ± 0.7 kg) who were participating in club sports (>240 min/week) were recruited for this study. Subjects had no history of lower-extremity surgery and were free from musculoskeletal injury within the last six months. Subjects with current lower-extremity musculoskeletal pain, anemia, diabetes, or cardiovascular disease were excluded. Prior to participation, all subjects gave informed consent, as approved by the University's Institutional Review Board.

2.3. Procedures

Each subject visited the laboratory three times (with a week wash-out period) on separate days at the same time of day (Figure 1).

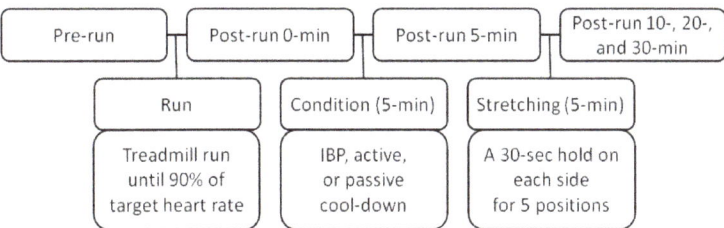

Figure 1. Testing procedures, IBP: inverted body position. Heart rate, energy expenditure, fatigue perception, circumference of lower-extremity, and blood lactate were recorded at each measurement time.

Upon arrival at the laboratory for the first time, subjects read and signed the informed consent form. At each visit, subjects were fitted with a heart rate monitor, and asked to lie down on a treatment table for a 10-min rest to achieve cardiovascular stability before measuring their resting heart rate.

Pre-run measurements were recorded in the order of heart rate, energy expenditure, fatigue perception, circumference of the thighs and calves, and blood lactate (measurements were recorded in the same order at all other time points). Subjects then performed an exercise protocol on the treadmill (Jog Forma, Technogym S.p.A, Gambettola, Italy) where the run began at 4 km/h without treadmill inclination and the speed and inclination increased by 1 km/h and 0.5% every minute. The exercise protocol was ended when the subjects reached the target heart rate (90% of the maximal heart rate calculated using the Karvonen formula) [24]. The post-run 0-min measurements were recorded immediately. After a set of measurements, the researcher left the laboratory and a different researcher came into the laboratory to guide the cool-down conditions.

Subjects executed the three cool-down conditions (IBP, active, and passive) in a counterbalanced order. For the IBP condition, subjects performed five sets of continuous alternating positions on the inversion table. Each set was defined as a position change from A to B for 30 s (Figure 2A,B) followed by a position change from B to A (Figure 2A,B). The duration of inversion was determined to prevent discomfort due to increased intracranial pressure [25]. To change positions, the researcher asked a subject to press a button on the inversion table. For the active condition, subjects walked on the treadmill at speeds of 5 and 6 km/h for females and males, respectively, for 5 min. The walking treadmill speed was determined in our pilot study where we wanted it to be neither too fast (to avoid additional fatigue) nor too slow (no effect on active recovery). For the passive condition, subjects remained seated on a chair for 5 min. After the next set of measurements (post-run 5 min), a 5-min static stretch of the hip adductors, extensors, abductors, and flexors, and knee extensors with a 30-s hold on each side (the same protocol was applied for each condition) was performed. After completion of the static stretch, the post-run 10-, 20-, and 30-min measurements were recorded.

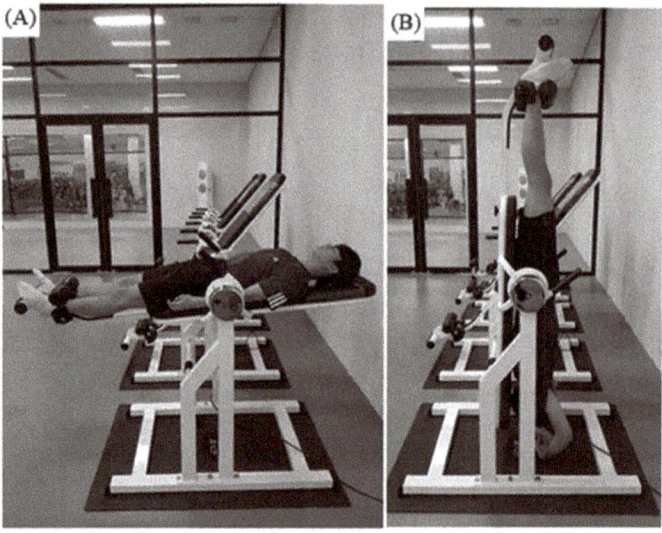

Figure 2. The inverted body position, once subjects moved from (**A**) a supine position to (**B**) the IBP, 30 s were counted and then they were returned to the starting position (**A**). It took 17 s to move from position A to B or vice versa. Subjects then spent about 13 s in the IBP (**B**) before returning to position (**A**).

2.4. Measurements

The total running time, average treadmill speed, and inclination were recorded for each subject during each treadmill run.

For the blood lactate measurements, a finger-pricking lancet needle (26 G, Lancets, Moa, Korea) was administered to collect 0.7 µL blood samples on lactate test strips (Lactate Plus Lactate Test Strips, Nova Biomedical, Waltham, MA, USA). The strips were then inserted into a lactate meter (Lactate Plus, Nova Biomedical, USA) for analysis. The blood lactate analysis using this device was previously validated [26].

To measure heart rate and energy expenditure, the subjects wore a heart rate monitor consisting of a Polar M400 GPS watch on their wrist and a Polar H7 strap on their chests throughout the experiment (Polar Electro Oy, Kempele, Finland). After the device was wirelessly connected to the mobile application (Polar Beat), the subject's age, sex, height, and mass were entered. All data recorded throughout the experiment were downloaded from a website (http://flow.polar.com).

The perception of subjective fatigue level was quantified using a modified 10-cm visual analogue scale [27,28] with the terms "unfatigued" and "fatigued" at each end. Subjects were asked to mark their fatigue level at each measurement time.

Using a tape measure, the circumferences of the thighs and calves were recorded (to the nearest 0.1 cm) at the midpoint between the anterior superior iliac spine and the superior pole of the patella and the thickest circumference on the triceps surae, respectively. Both sides were recorded each time (left side first).

2.5. Statistical Analyses

Our sample size was calculated based on a pilot study conducted in our laboratory. We expected a mean difference in blood lactate concentration of 3 mmol/L with a standard deviation of 3.5 mmol/L (an effect size of 0.86). These calculations estimated that 14 individuals would be necessary in each condition (an alpha of 0.05 and a beta of 0.2). This calculation was supported by a similar previous study ($n = 14$) that reported a difference of 3.17 mmol/L [10].

Descriptive data (means and 95% confidence intervals) were calculated and checked for normality using the Shapiro–Wilk test. To test condition effects over time, a mixed model analysis of variance (random variable: subjects; fixed variables: condition and time) and Tukey's test were performed on each dependent measurement. To determine practical significance, Cohen's d effect size [29] was also calculated when statistical significance was found. To test for a correlation between the blood lactate concentration and fatigue perception, Pearson's correlation coefficient was calculated. SAS software (SAS 9.3, Institute Inc., Cary, NC, USA) was used for all tests ($p < 0.05$).

3. Results

The mean ± 95% confidence interval total running time was 7 min and 39 s ± 46 s at a treadmill speed of 7.3 ± 0.4 km/h and an inclination of 1.7 ± 0.2%. The mean treadmill speed and inclination at the end of each run were 11.1 ± 0.8 km/h and 3.6 ± 0.4%, respectively.

The blood lactate concentration was different among the three conditions at post-run 5 and 10 min (condition × time interaction: $F_{10,238} = 3.04$, $p = 0.001$; condition effect: $F_{2,238} = 12.38$, $p < 0.0001$; Table 1). Specifically, the IBP condition (6.7 mmol/L, 23%, $p = 0.001$, ES = 0.82) and the active condition (6.9 mmol/L, 20%, $p = 0.01$, ES = 0.75) showed lower blood lactate values than the passive condition (8.6 mmol/L) at post-run 5 min. At post-run 10 min, the active condition showed lower blood lactate values than the passive condition (4.4 vs. 6.0 mmol/L, 27%, $p = 0.02$, ES = 0.90). Regardless of the condition (time effect: $F_{5,238} = 314.95$, $p < 0.0001$), the blood lactate values decreased gradually after running and they did not return to the pre-run level (1.3 mmol/L) at the end of the experiment (post-run 30-min: 3.1 mmol/L, $p < 0.0001$, ES = 2.41; Figure 3A).

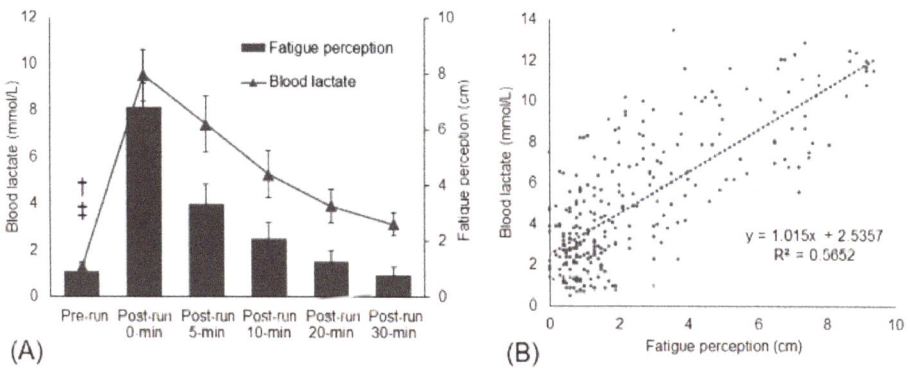

Figure 3. (**A**) Changes in blood lactate and fatigue perception regardless of conditions. Error bars are upper and lower limits of 95% confidence intervals. † Different from other time points in blood lactate ($p < 0.0001$). ‡ Different from post-run 0, 5, and 10 min in fatigue perception ($p < 0.0001$). (**B**) Correlation between blood lactate and fatigue perception. There is a high correlation ($r = 0.75$) between blood lactate and fatigue perception.

The heart rate values differed between the conditions at each time point (condition × time interaction: $F_{10,238} = 8.39$, $p < 0.0001$; condition effect: $F_{2,238} = 17.61$, $p < 0.0001$; time effect: $F_{5,238} = 1243.89$, $p < 0.0001$; Table 1). The IBP condition (96 bpm, 22%, $p < 0.0001$, ES = 2.52) and the passive condition (103 bpm, 17%, $p = 0.002$, ES = 1.92) resulted in lower heart rate values than the active condition (123 bpm) at post-run 5 min.

Energy expenditure among the three cool-down conditions at each time point did not differ (no condition × time interaction: $F_{10,238} = 1.65$, $p = 0.09$; time effect: $F_{5,238} = 224.40$, $p < 0.0001$; Table 1).

However, the total energy expenditure between the conditions was different (condition effect: $F_{2,238} = 4.81$, $p = 0.01$) in that subjects in the active condition had a 14% higher total energy expenditure compared to the IBP condition (219 vs. 189 kcal, $p = 0.01$, ES = 0.48; Figure 4).

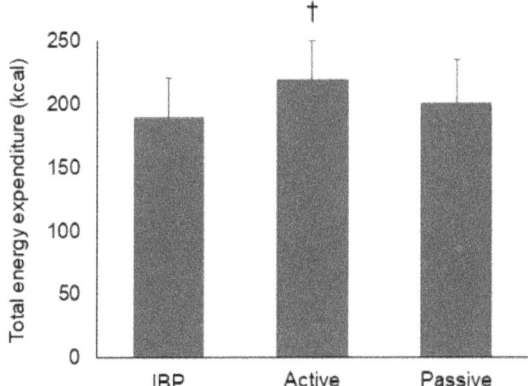

Figure 4. Changes in total energy expenditure regardless of time, IBP: inverted body position; Error bars are upper limits of 95% confidence intervals, † Condition effect ($F_{2238} = 4.81$, $p = 0.01$): Active was recorded at higher total energy expenditure values compared with the IBP (219 vs. 189 kcal, 14%, $p = 0.01$, ES = 0.48).

Table 1. Changes in heart rate, energy expenditure, blood lactate, and fatigue perception.

Mean (95% CIs)	Condition	Pre-Run	Post-Run 0 Min	Post-Run 5 Min	Post-Run 10 Min	Post-Run 20 Min	Post-Run 30 Min
Blood lactate (mmol/L) ICC: 0.75	IBP	1.3 (0.2)	9.8 (1.1)	6.7 (1.2)	5.4 (1.1)	4.2 (0.8)	3.3 (0.5)
	Active	1.3 (0.2)	9.4 (1.0)	6.9 (1.1)	4.4 (0.8)	3.3 (0.6)	2.7 (0.4)
	Passive	1.3 (0.3)	9.3 (1.2)	8.6 † (1.2)	6.0 ‡ (0.9)	4.3 (0.7)	3.5 (0.5)
Heart rate (bpm) ICC: 0.91	IBP	72.3 (6.2)	185.0 (2.0)	95.9 (5.7)	110.2 (7.6)	95.3 (6.9)	90.1 (5.1)
	Active	73.8 (5.2)	184.9 (1.5)	123.3 # (5.3)	117.9 (8.2)	96.3 (4.8)	91.1 (5.0)
	Passive	72.8 (5.8)	185.5 (1.1)	102.9 (5.5)	114.0 (7.3)	94.2 (5.4)	90.9 (4.9)
Energy expenditure (kcal) ICC: N/A	IBP	-	74.5 (10.9)	20.5 (4.6)	29.9 (7.1)	33.2 (7.9)	30.6 (6.8)
	Active	-	76.3 (12.5)	38.8 (5.1)	34.1 (6.2)	37.3 (8.1)	31.9 (7.1)
	Passive	-	75.7 (12.0)	24.7 (5.5)	31.9 (6.5)	36.0 (8.0)	31.9 (7.3)
Fatigue perception (cm) ICC: 0.76	IBP	1.1 (0.4)	6.8 (0.8)	3.4 (0.9)	2.1 (0.5)	1.3 (0.4)	0.8 (0.2)
	Active	0.7 (0.2)	6.6 (0.9)	3.3 (0.7)	1.9 (0.5)	1.2 (0.4)	0.7 (0.2)
	Passive	0.9 (0.3)	7.0 (0.9)	3.3 (0.6)	2.2 (0.8)	1.2 (0.4)	0.8 (0.4)

IBP: inverted body position; ICC: intraclass correlation coefficient, † Different from the IBP (23%, $p = 0.001$, ES = 0.82) and active (20%, $p = 0.01$, ES = 0.75) conditions at post-run 5 min; ‡ Different from the active condition (27%, $p = 0.02$, ES = 0.90) at post-run 10 min; # Different from the IBP (22%, $p < 0.0001$, ES 2.52) and passive (17%, $p = 0.002$, ES = 1.92) conditions at post-run 5 min.

Fatigue perception did not differ among the three cool-down conditions at each time point (no condition × time interaction: $F_{10,238} = 0.13$, $p = 0.99$; no condition effect: $F_{2,238} = 0.87$, $p = 0.42$; time effect: $F_{5,238} = 245.80$, $p < 0.0001$; Table 1). Regardless of the condition, fatigue perception was 87% higher after running (6.8 cm, $p < 0.0001$, ES = 4.63) and returned to the pre-run level (0.9 cm) at post-run 20 min (1.2 cm, $p = 0.55$; Figure 3A).

The circumference of the left (no condition × time interaction: $F_{10,238} = 0.28$, $p = 0.99$; condition effect: $F_{2,238} = 3.72$, $p = 0.03$; time effect: $F_{5,238} = 3.88$, $p = 0.002$; Table 2) and right (no condition × time interaction: $F_{10,238} = 0.25$, $p = 0.99$; no condition effect: $F_{2,238} = 1.26$, $p = 0.29$; time effect: $F_{5,238} = 6.66$, $p < 0.0001$; Table 2) thighs, and left (no condition × time interaction: $F_{10,238} = 0.96$, $p = 0.48$; condition effect: $F_{2,238} = 22.32$, $p < 0.0001$; time effect: $F_{5,238} = 41.33$, $p < 0.0001$) and right (no condition × time interaction: $F_{10,238} = 0.79$, $p = 0.64$; condition effect: $F_{2,238} = 12.13$, $p < 0.0001$; time effect: $F_{5,238} = 44.57$, $p < 0.0001$) calves did not differ between the conditions at each time point.

Blood lactate was highly correlated with fatigue perception ($r = 0.75$, $p < 0.0001$; Figure 3B).

Good to excellent measurement consistency (ICC values from 0.75 to 0.99; Tables 1 and 2) was calculated for all measurements [30].

Table 2. Changes in circumference of lower-extremities.

Mean (95% CIs)	Condition	Pre-Run	Post-Run 0 Min	Post-Run 5 Min	Post-Run 10 Min	Post-Run 20 Min	Post-Run 30 Min
Left thigh (cm) ICC: 0.99	IBP	54.4 (1.2)	54.7 (1.2)	54.5 (1.2)	54.4 (1.2)	54.4 (1.2)	54.4 (1.2)
	Active	54.2 (1.4)	54.6 (1.4)	54.4 (1.4)	54.3 (1.4)	54.3 (1.4)	54.3 (1.4)
	Passive	54.4 (1.4)	54.7 (1.4)	54.7 (1.5)	54.5 (1.4)	54.4 (1.4)	54.4 (1.4)
Right thigh (cm) ICC: 0.99	IBP	54.6 (1.1)	54.9 (1.2)	54.6 (1.2)	54.6 (1.2)	54.6 (1.1)	54.5 (1.1)
	Active	54.4 (1.3)	55.0 (1.4)	54.7 (1.2)	54.6 (1.3)	54.5 (1.3)	54.5 (1.3)
	Passive	54.5 (1.3)	54.9 (1.3)	54.8 (1.3)	54.8 (1.3)	54.7 (1.3)	54.6 (1.3)
Left calf (cm) ICC: 0.99	IBP	36.3 (0.9)	36.9 (1.0)	36.6 (0.9)	36.5 (0.9)	36.4 (0.9)	36.4 (0.9)
	Active	36.4 (1.1)	37.0 (1.1)	36.9 (1.1)	36.7 (1.1)	36.6 (1.1)	36.6 (1.1)
	Passive	36.4 (1.0)	37.0 (1.0)	36.9 (1.0)	36.7 (1.0)	36.7 (1.0)	36.6 (1.0)
Right calf (cm) ICC: 0.99	IBP	36.5 (0.9)	37.2 (0.9)	36.9 (0.9)	36.7 (0.9)	36.6 (0.9)	36.6 (0.9)
	Active	36.5 (1.0)	37.2 (1.0)	37.0 (1.0)	36.8 (1.0)	36.7 (1.0)	36.7 (1.0)
	Passive	36.6 (0.9)	37.2 (1.0)	37.1 (1.0)	36.9 (1.0)	36.9 (1.0)	36.8 (1.0)

IBP: inverted body position; ICC: intraclass correlation coefficient, No condition × time interactions in circumference of left ($F_{10,238} = 0.28$, $p = 0.99$) and right ($F_{10,238} = 0.25$, $p = 0.99$) thigh, and circumference of left ($F_{10,238} = 0.96$, $p = 0.48$) and right ($F_{10,238} = 0.79$, $p = 0.64$) calf.

4. Discussion

The purpose of this study was to examine how the IBP condition consisting of continuous alternation between 30-s IBP and a supine position for 5 min would help physiological and psychological recovery after intense running relative to active (walking) and passive (sitting) recovery methods. While walking is a commonly recommended method [10,31] and sitting is considered as a control, we were interested in comparing these existing and frequently practiced methods to a recovery condition containing IBP. During the initial 5 min of the recovery period, the IBP was effective in reducing the blood lactate and heart rate to levels similar to the active and passive conditions. In other words, the IBP condition produced an effect similar to that of the active condition in blood lactate with less energy expenditure. This observation suggests that the recovery condition including IBP could be an alternative recovery strategy after a short bout of intense exercise. Since blood lactate removal is dependent on the amount of blood flow to working muscles, and the process is facilitated by muscle contraction [17], performing IBP could be beneficial for individuals who need a fast recovery while minimizing energy consumption.

The IBP and active (walking at a speed of 5 to 6 km/h) strategies in this study reduced blood lactate by 32% (9.8 to 6.7 mmol/L) and 27% (9.4 to 6.9 mmol/L), respectively, at 5 min postexercise (post-run 0 min). The effects of recovery strategies with active movements [10,31,32], electrotherapy [33], and massage [31] were previously reported. Comparable corresponding values at similar time points in other studies included a 19% (14.9 to 12.0 mmol/L) reduction with a 5-min treadmill run (at 50% of maximal speed) [32] and a 49% (3.9 to 2.0 mmol/L) reduction with 6 min of motor level electrotherapy (at 9, 8, and 7 Hz for 2 min each via 8 electrodes) [33]. At 10 min postexercise (after subjects had finished a 5-min static stretch in our study), blood lactate was reduced by 45% (9.8 to 5.4 mmol/L) and 53% (9.4 to 4.4 mmol/L) in the IBP and active conditions, respectively. Other studies reported reductions of 40% (14.9 to 8.9 mmol/L) with a 10-min treadmill run (at 50% of the maximal speed) [32], 51% (11.7 to 5.7 mmol/L) with a 10-min free style swim (at 65% of each individual's best 200-m front crawl swim velocity) [31], and 39% (11.6 to 7.1 mmol/L) with a 10-min massage (using the effleurage, petrissage, tapotement, and compression techniques) [31]. As indicated by these indirect comparisons at 5 and 10 min postexercise, our IBP condition (a combination of the 5-min IBP and static stretch) appears to be as effective as other recovery activities. Although not directly measured, we believe that the effect of the IBP could have been attributed to hemodynamic changes similar to those of using compression garments [34,35]. According to men's and women's Taekwondo Kyorugi schedules at the Olympic Games in Rio in 2016, the rests between matches ranged from 360 min to less than 60 min. In the Asian Games in Jakarta–Palembang in 2018, the rest times in the men's fencing épée ranged from 80 min to 175 min. During such short time periods, a recovery activity enhancing a rapid blood lactate removal with minimal energy expenditure would contribute to the performance in the subsequent match. Because all of the comparable recovery strategies reported require an electrical device [33], massage personnel [31], or to expend more energy [31,32], our method with IBP could be the best option. Although the blood lactate values in the three conditions in our study became similar at 20 min postexercise, IBP is still beneficial because it resulted in a longer time to rest with a low blood lactate level.

Fatigue perception did not differ among the three recovery conditions at each time point. Previously, electrotherapy (motor level stimulation via 8 electrodes) and the passive (sitting on a chair) recovery method reduced perceived exertion by 46% and 38% compared with active recovery, respectively [33]. Another study [32] reported 18% less perceived exertion with passive (sitting on a chair) recovery than with active (treadmill run at 50% maximal speed) recovery [32]. Although the results of the Borg scales (0 to 10 points: [33]; 6–20 points: [32]) are comparable to our fatigue perception because both are measures of subjective physical condition, the differences of the measurement characteristics could explain why there was no difference across the conditions in our study. The Borg scale matches a numeric scale with descriptions of exertion, asking subjects to indicate their exertion level, whereas our measurement simply asked subjects to place themselves between "unfatigued" and "fatigued" on a visual analogue scale. Measurements were also taken during exercise using the Borg scale and after exercise in our study. Since subjects in previous studies felt less exertion in the passive condition than those in the active condition [32,33], providing different descriptions (e.g., fresh or recovered) or using a more detailed numeric scale may have produced a different result. Interestingly, blood lactate and fatigue perception values had a strong correlation in our study ($r = 0.75$, $r^2 = 0.57$). Thus, at least 57% of an individual's perceived fatigue can be explained by blood lactate and vice versa. However, fatigue perception returned to the pre-run level at 20 min postexercise (post-run 20 min) whereas blood lactate levels did not. This observation has several practical implications. First, people may feel complete recovery although their bodies are still in the process of physiological recovery. Second, a complete physiological recovery may be unnecessary for psychological (perceptual) recovery. Third, in addition to blood lactate, there could be other factors which contribute to the level of fatigue perception. A future study should examine the relationships between psychological, physiological, and athletic performance.

Similarly, there were no changes in the circumferences of lower extremities at any time point. Given that a tape measure was used to obtain circumferences in many previous studies [34–37], the measurement reproducibility in our study was strong (ICC value of 0.99 for between-session reliability in all measurements), measurement technique or errors were unlikely to contribute to the results. In fact, we did not even observe a circumference change at the post-run measurements, which could be explained by the exercise duration and mode (specific energy system). Previously reported postexercise extremity circumference was induced by resistance [34,35] or endurance exercise [36,37]. Therefore, an approximately 7-min all-out treadmill run may not have been sufficient to increase leg swelling. Exercise-induced transient hypertrophy, also known as "the pump", is thought to be caused by the accumulation of intracellular fluid from reactive hyperemia [38] or osmolytic activity [39]. In endurance activities, the expansion of extracellular volume [37] due to increased plasma volume and sodium retention [40] is thought to be responsible for oedematous swelling. While we assumed that our intense treadmill run mostly used the combined energy system of anaerobic glycolysis, it produced neither of the physiological mechanisms, resulting in no circumference change. Because body fluid removal is an important facet of physical recovery, a future investigation should examine how the IBP strategy affects the increased circumference caused by either resistance or prolonged endurance exercise. Appendicular body composition analysis along with skinfold thickness would provide better accuracy in the assessment of exercise-induced anthropometric changes.

There are several limitations and assumptions in our study that may benefit future research. Although good criterion-related validity and high reliability in the estimation of energy expenditure using the same heart rate monitoring device were established [41], the major contributing factors such as the physical activity and sedentary levels [42], and percentage of body fat [43] were not reflected. Additionally, a lower heart rate recorded during the IBP might have underestimated the whole-body metabolism and energy consumption. Therefore, we acknowledge the level of accuracy in estimating energy expenditure as a limitation. While accepted, our hypothesis was based on increased blood flow for a body position with 15° head-down tilt [21–23] and the lack of direct measures on blood flow parameters limit us to explain and interpret the observed benefits. As an elevated blood pressure during and after exercise is typical, performing IBP immediately after exercise may be harmful by applying additional pressure to blood vessels. When comparing the inversion duration (90° for 2 min) in previous reports [44,45] to ours (90° for 13 s: Figure 2), we assume that the possibility of additional blood pressure was minimal. Additionally, our subjects' heart rate at the last minute of the treadmill run and the beginning of IBP were 183 and 121 bpm, respectively. A 2-min interval for the post-run measurements resulted in a 34% reduction in heart rate (183 to 121 bpm). Considering that both heart rate and blood pressure are linearly related to exercise intensity [46], a reduced heart rate value indirectly supports the idea that our subjects performing IBP were not in a deleterious situation. However, future studies should attempt to compare the change of blood flow volume and pressure during the recovery period to resolve our limitations. Lastly, the contraindications of IBP should be addressed since the IBP may be unsafe for pregnant individuals or those with abnormal blood pressure or other cardiovascular diseases, eye or ear injuries, or herniated discs.

According to our data, a 10-min recovery strategy consisting of 5 min of IBP and a 5-min static stretch was the most effective of the tested protocols in removing blood lactate and minimizing energy expenditure during the acute recovery period (the first 30 min, postexercise). Therefore, the recovery condition including our IBP protocol is an appropriate strategy to enhance physical and psychological recovery. We particularly recommend this IBP protocol for athletes who complete several matches (events) within a few hours on a single day (e.g., tournaments for Taekwondo, Judo, weightlifting, fencing, wrestling, sprint cycling, and swimming). In the final stage of matches (e.g., after quarterfinals), the fatigue level would be high. In this situation, physical fitness and stamina can play bigger roles than technical and tactical strategies. Therefore, we recommend practicing our IBP method between matches. If an IBP device is unavailable, peer-assisted IBP or a supine position with legs elevated against a wall could be used instead.

Author Contributions: Conceptualization, M.S.K. and J.P. Methodology, J.P. Formal analysis, M.S.K. and J.P. Investigation, J.P. Data curation, M.S.K. Writing—original draft preparation, M.S.K. and J.P. Writing—review and editing, J.P. Supervision, J.P. Project administration, J.P. All authors have read and agreed to the published version of the manuscript.

Funding: This research received no external funding.

Acknowledgments: This study received no specific grant from any funding agency. We thank Chae Rin Kim, Chaerin Yeom, and Gihum Kown for their data collection and reduction.

Conflicts of Interest: The authors declare no conflict of interest.

References

1. Ramírez-Campillo, R.; Henríquez-Olguín, C.; Burgos, C.; Andrade, D.C. Effect of progressive volume-based overload during plyometric training on explosive and endurance performance in young soccer players. *J. Strength Cond. Res.* **2015**, *29*, 1884–1893. [CrossRef]
2. Fry, A.; Mullinger, K.J.; O'Neill, G.C.; Mullinger, K.J.; Brookers, M.J. The effect of physical fatigue on oscillatory dynamics of the sensorimotor cortex. *Acta Physiol.* **2017**, *220*, 370–381. [CrossRef] [PubMed]
3. Meeusen, R.; Duclos, M.; Gleespn, M.; Foster, C.; Fry, A.; Gleeson, M.; Nieman, D.; Raglin, J.; Rietjens, G.; Steinacker, J.; et al. Prevention, diagnosis and treatment of the overtraining syndrome. *Eur. J. Appl. Physiol.* **2006**, *6*, 1–14. [CrossRef]
4. Halson, S.; Jeukendrup, A.E. Does overtraining exist? An analysis of overreaching and overtraining research. *Sports Med.* **2004**, *34*, 967–981. [CrossRef] [PubMed]
5. Thiel, C.; Vogt, L.; Bürklein, M.; Rosenhagen, A. Functional overreaching during preparation training of elite tennis professionals. *J. Hum. Kinet.* **2011**, *28*, 79–89. [CrossRef] [PubMed]
6. Hausswirth, C.; Mujika, I. *Recovery for Performance in Sport*; Human Kinetics: Champain, France, 2012.
7. Belcastro, A.N.; Bonen, A. Lactic acid removal rates during controlled and uncontrolled recovery exercise. *J. Appl. Physiol.* **1975**, *39*, 932–936. [CrossRef]
8. Dupont, G.; Moalla, W.; Guinhouya, C.; Ahmadi, S. Passive versus active recovery during high-intensity intermittent exercises. *Med. Sci. Sports Exerc.* **2004**, *36*, 302–308. [CrossRef]
9. Menzies, P.; Menzies, C.; McIntyre, L.; Paterson, P. Blood lactate clearance during active recovery after an intense running bout depends on the intensity of the active recovery. *J. Sports Sci.* **2010**, *28*, 975–982. [CrossRef]
10. Mota, M.R.; Dantas, R.A.E.; Oliveira-Silva, I.; Mahalhaes Sales, M.; da Costa Sotero, R.; Espiodola Mota Venancio, P.; Teixeira Junior, J.; Nobre Chaves, S.; de Lima, F.D. Effect of self-paced active recovery and passive recovery on blood lactate removal following a 200 m freestyle swimming trial. *Open Access J. Sports Med.* **2017**, *8*, 155–160. [CrossRef]
11. Soares, A.H.; Oliveira, T.P.; Cavalcante, B.R.; Farah, B.Q.; Lima, A.; Cucato, G.G.; Cardoso, C.G.; Ritti-Dias, R.M. Effects of active recovery on autonomic and haemodynamic responses after aerobic exercise. *Clin. Physiol. Funct. Imaging* **2017**, *37*, 62–67. [CrossRef]
12. Fairchild, T.J.; Armstrong, A.A.; Rao, A.; Hawk, L. Glycogen synthesis in muscle fibers during active recovery from intense exercise. *Med. Sci. Sports Exerc.* **2003**, *35*, 595–602. [CrossRef] [PubMed]
13. Baquet, G.; Dupont, G.; Gamelin, F.-X.; Aucountier, J.; Berthoin, S. Active versus passive recovery in high-intensity intermittent exercises in children: An exploratory study. *Pediatr. Exerc. Sci.* **2019**, *31*, 248–253. [CrossRef] [PubMed]
14. Toubekis, A.G.; Douda, H.T.; Tokmakidis, S.P. Influence of different rest intervals during active or passive recovery on repeated sprint swimming performance. *Eur. J. Appl. Physiol.* **2005**, *93*, 694–700. [CrossRef]

15. Monedero, J.; Donne, B. Effect of recovery interventions on lactate removal and subsequent performance. *Int. J. Sports Med.* **2000**, *21*, 593–597. [CrossRef]
16. Draper, N.; Bird, E.L.; Coleman, I.; Hodgson, C. Effects of active recovery on lactate concentration, heart rate and RPE in climbing. *J. Sports Sci. Med.* **2006**, *5*, 97–105. [PubMed]
17. Gladden, L.B. Muscle as a consumer of lactate. *Med. Sci. Sport Exer.* **2000**, *32*, 764–771. [CrossRef] [PubMed]
18. Starkey, C. *Therapeutic Modalities*; FA Davis Company: Philadelphia, PA, USA, 2013.
19. Maestrini, D. Genesis of the so-called insufficient contractions of the heart in decompensation. *Policlin. Prat.* **1951**, *58*, 257–268.
20. Brooks, G.A.; Fahey, T.D.; Baldwin, K.M. *Exercise Physiology: Human Bioenergenetics and Its Applications*; McGraw Hill: New York, NY, USA, 2005; pp. 293–308.
21. McInnis, N.H.; Journeay, W.S.; Jay, O.; Lelair, E.; Kenny, G.P. 15° Head-down tilt attenuates the postexercise reduction in cutaneous vascular conductance and sweating and decreases esophageal temperature recovery time. *J. Appl. Physiol.* **2006**, *101*, 840–847. [CrossRef]
22. Journeay, W.S.; Jay, O.; McInnis, N.H.; Lelair, E.; Kenny, G.P. Postexercise heat loss and hemodynamic responses during head-down tilt are similar between genders. *Med. Sci. Sports Exerc.* **2007**, *39*, 1308–1804. [CrossRef]
23. Siamwala, J.H.; Lee, P.C.; Macias, B.R.; Hargens, A.R. Lower-body negative pressure restores leg bone microvascular flow to supine levels during head-down tilt. *J. Appl. Physiol.* **2015**, *119*, 101–109. [CrossRef]
24. Karvonen, J.; Vuorimaa, T. Heart rate and exercise intensity during sports activities. *Sports Med.* **1988**, *5*, 303–311. [CrossRef] [PubMed]
25. Smith, D.M.; McAuliffe, J.; Johnson, M.J.; Button, D.C. Seated inversion adversely affects vigilance tasks and suppresses heart rate and blood pressure. *Occup. Ergon.* **2013**, *11*, 153–163. [CrossRef]
26. Hart, S.; Drevets, K.; Alford, M.; Salacinski, A.; Hunt, B.E. A method-comparison study regarding the validity and reliability of the Lactate Plus analyzer. *BMJ Open* **2013**, *3*, e001899. [CrossRef]
27. Shahid, A.; Wilkinson, K.; Marcu, S.; Shapiro, C.M. Visual analogue scale to evaluate fatigue severity (VAS-F.). In *STOP, THAT and One Hundred Other Sleep Scales*; Spinger: New York, NY, USA, 2011; pp. 399–402.
28. Wolfe, F. Fatigue assessments in rheumatoid arthritis: Comparative performance of visual analog scales and longer fatigue questionnaires in 7760 patients. *J. Rheumatol.* **2004**, *31*, 1896–1902. [PubMed]
29. Cohen, J. A power primer. *Psychol. Bull.* **1992**, *112*, 155. [CrossRef]
30. Koo, T.K.; Li, M.Y. A guideline of seletcing and reporting intraclass correlation coefficients for reliability research. *J. Chripract. Med.* **2016**, *15*, 155–163.
31. Ali Rasooli, S.; Koushkie Jahromi, M.; Asadmanesh, A.; Salesi, M. Influence of massage, active and passive recovery on swimming performance and blood lactate. *J. Sport Med. Phys. Fit.* **2012**, *52*, 122–127.
32. Ouergui, I.; Hammouda, O.; Chtourou, H.; Gmada, N.; Franchini, E. Effects of recovery type after a kickboxing match on blood lactate and performance in anaerobic tests. *Asian J. Sports Med.* **2014**, *5*, 99–107.
33. Warren, C.D.; Szymanski, D.J.; Landers, M.R. Effects of three recovery protocols on range of motion, heart rate, rating of perceived exertion, and blood lactate in baseball pitchers during a simulated game. *J. Strength Cond. Res.* **2015**, *29*, 3016–3025. [CrossRef]
34. Goto, K.; Morishima, T. Compression garment promotes muscular strength recovery after resistance exercise. *Med. Sci. Sports Exerc.* **2014**, *46*, 2265–2270. [CrossRef]
35. Kraemer, W.J.; Flanagan, S.D.; Comstock, B.A.; Fragala, M.; Earp, J.; Dunn-Lewis, C.; Ho, J.; Thomas, G.; Solomon-Hill, G.; Penwell, Z.; et al. Effects of a whole body compression garment on markers of recovery after a heavy resistance workout in men and women. *J. Strength Cond. Res.* **2010**, *24*, 804–814. [CrossRef]
36. Dawson, L.G.; Dawson, K.A.; Tiidus, P.M. Evaluating the influence of massage on leg strength, swelling, and pain following a half-marathon. *J. Sport Scimed.* **2004**, *3*, 37–43.
37. Knechtle, B.; Vinzent, T.; Kirby, S.; Knechtle, P. The recovery phase following a triple iron triathlon. *J. Hum. Kinet.* **2009**, *21*, 65–74. [CrossRef]
38. Schoenfeld, B.J.; Contreras, B. The pump: Potential mechanisms and applications for enhancing hypertrophic adaptations. *Strength Cond. J.* **2014**, *36*, 21–25. [CrossRef]
39. Schoenfeld, B.J. The mecahnisms of muscle hypertrophy and their application to resistance training. *J. Strength Cond. Res.* **2010**, *24*, 2857–2872. [CrossRef]

40. Fellmann, N.; Bedu, M.; Giry, J.; Pharmakis-amadieu, M.; Bezou, M.; Barlet, J.; Coudert, J. Hormonal, fluid, and electrolyte changes during a 72-h recovery from a 24-h endurance run. *Int. J. Sports Med.* **1989**, *10*, 406–412. [CrossRef]
41. Engström, E.; Ottosson, E.; Wohlfart, B.; Grundstorm, N.; Wisen, A. Comparison of heart rate measured by Polar RS400 and ECG, validity and repeatability. *Adv. Physiother.* **2012**, *14*, 115–122. [CrossRef]
42. Besson, H.; Brage, S.; Jakes, R.W.; Ekelund, U.; Wareham, N. Estimating physical activity energy expenditure, sedentary time, and physical activity intensity by self-report in adults. *Am. J. Clin. Nutr.* **2010**, *91*, 106–114. [CrossRef]
43. Irwin, M.L.; Ainsworth, B.E.; Conway, J.M. Estimation of energy expenditure from physical activity measures: Determinants of accuracy. *Obes. Res.* **2001**, *9*, 517–525. [CrossRef]
44. Haskvitz, E.M.; Hanten, W.P. Blood pressure response to inversion traction. *Phys. Ther.* **1986**, *66*, 1361–1364. [CrossRef]
45. LeMarr, J.D.; Golding, L.A.; Crehan, K.D. Cardiorespiratory responses to inversion. *Physician Sportsmed.* **1983**, *11*, 51–57. [CrossRef]
46. Cornelissen, V.A.; Verheyden, B.; Aubert, A.E.; Fagard, R.H. Effects of aerobic training intensity on resting, exercise and post-exercise blood pressure, heart rate and heart-rate variability. *J. Hum. Hypertens.* **2010**, *24*, 175–182. [CrossRef]

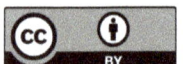

© 2020 by the authors. Licensee MDPI, Basel, Switzerland. This article is an open access article distributed under the terms and conditions of the Creative Commons Attribution (CC BY) license (http://creativecommons.org/licenses/by/4.0/).

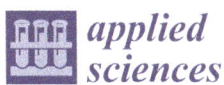

Article

Ultrasound-Guided Percutaneous Needle Electrolysis and Rehab and Reconditioning Program for Rectus Femoris Muscle Injuries: A Cohort Study with Professional Soccer Players and a 20-Week Follow-Up

Fermín Valera-Garrido [1,2,3,*], Sergio Jiménez-Rubio [4,5], Francisco Minaya-Muñoz [1,2,6], José Luis Estévez-Rodríguez [5,7] and Archit Navandar [8]

1. MVClinic Institute, 28600 Madrid, Spain
2. CEU San Pablo University, 28925 Alcorcón, Madrid, Spain
3. Invasive Physiotherapy Department, Getafe C.F., 28903 Getafe, Madrid, Spain
4. Reconditioning & Performance Department, Getafe C.F., 28903 Getafe, Madrid, Spain; sjimenezrubio@yahoo.es
5. Train Movements Center, 28923 Alcorcón, Madrid, Spain
6. Invasive Physiotherapy Department, A.D. Alcorcón, 28922 Alcorcón, Madrid, Spain; franminaya@mvclinic.es
7. Reconditioning & Performance Department, C.F. Fuenlabrada, 28942 Fuenlabrada, Madrid, Spain; joselu.estevez@gmail.com
8. Faculty of Sport Science, Universidad Europea de Madrid, 28670 Villaviciosa de Odón, Madrid, Spain; archit.navandar@universidadeuropea.es
* Correspondence: ferminvalera@mvclinic.es

Received: 4 September 2020; Accepted: 3 November 2020; Published: 8 November 2020

Abstract: Rectus femoris muscle strains are one of the most common injuries occurring in sports such as soccer. The purpose of this study was to describe the safety and feasibility of a combination of percutaneous needle electrolysis (PNE) and a specific rehab and reconditioning program (RRP) following an injury to the rectus femoris in professional soccer players. Thirteen professional soccer players received PNE treatment 48 h after a grade II rectus femoris muscle injury, followed by a the RRP 24 h later. Assessment of recovery from injury was done by registering the days taken to return to train (RTT), return to play (RTP), and structural and functional progress of the injured muscle was registered through ultrasound imaging and match-GPS parameters. Also, adverse events and reinjuries were recorded in the follow up period of twenty weeks. The RTT registered was 15.62 ± 1.80 days and RTP was 20.15 + 2.79 days. After fourteen days, the ultrasound image showed optimal repair. Match-GPS parameters were similar before and after injury. There were no relapses nor were any serious adverse effects reported during the 20-week follow-up after the RTP. A combination of PNE and a specific RRP facilitated a faster RTP in previously injured professional soccer players enabling them to sustain performance and avoid reinjuries.

Keywords: muscle strain; quadriceps; football; invasive physiotherapy; post-injury performance; reinjury; return to play

---

1. Introduction

Professional soccer players face significant mechanical, metabolic, and physiological demands as a result of their participation in the sport [1]. Regarding to these demands, scientific evidence shows, for example, that elite soccer players cover total distances of 11,173 ± 524 m [2], with 600–831 m ran at speeds exceeding 7 m·s^{-1} [3] and over 160 accelerations between 1.5–2 m·s^{-2} [4]. Given these demands, soccer has a high risk of injury [5,6]; in fact, at the elite level, up to two injuries per player per season occur [7]. Muscle strains are among the most frequent non-contact injuries [8], and 81–92% of all muscle injuries in professional soccer affect four muscle groups: the hamstrings, the adductors, the quadriceps, and the calf muscles, with the quadriceps being the most affected after the hamstrings and the adductors [9,10]. The biggest muscle among the quadriceps, the rectus femoris, is the anatomical area that is most affected during a tear in the quadriceps [10,11], representing 19% of all non-contact muscle injuries [10,12]. Among all rectus femoris injuries, 46.1% are grade I injuries (representing an edema during MRI evaluation), 37.3% are grade II (representing a partial tear during MRI evaluation) and 4.9% are grade III (representing a complete tear during MRI evaluation) [10].

The rectus femoris is composed of fast-twitch type II fibers [13] and is vulnerable to an injury because of its biarticular nature spanning over the hip and knee joint [12]. It has an important relationship with the iliopsoas helping in the flexion of the hip [14,15], and previous research has shown that a weak or an under-active psoas can result in the rectus femoris generating a greater hip flexion force, resulting in a rectus femoris strain [14–16]. It is mainly injured during kicking or sprinting [15]. In kicking, the rectus femoris plays an important role where it is subjected to changes in muscular length during the reduction of moment of inertia at the knee in the leg cocking phase (when the hip and knee both flex) to the subsequent increase in knee extension velocity in the leg acceleration phase [15,17]. Similarly, in sprinting, specifically during acceleration and deceleration, the quadriceps absorb a large amount of energy [15,17] when they are activated eccentrically as knee extensors while the hip flexes simultaneously. In such a scenario, the adoption of a correct posture is key in order to maintain stability and facilitate force transmission across the lower-limb joints, thereby avoiding compensation generated by an absence of coordination of the lumbopelvic complex [14,15,17].

Moreover, its high recurrence rate in the weeks following return to play (RTP) is a cause of concern in professional soccer [18–20]. Its recurrence rate is between 5% and 6.4% in the short-term (the first week following RTP) [21,22], between 50% and 77% in the medium-term (between the first and second month after RTP), and 15% in the long term (between 5–6 months after RTP) [22]. For these reasons, a successful management of these injuries constitutes a challenge for clinicians in order to define specific protocols of treatment that integrate biological stimulus [23–25] and reconditioning programs adapted for elite competition [17].

Ultrasound (US)-guided percutaneous needle electrolysis (PNE) is a minimally invasive technique that consists of the application of a galvanic current through an acupuncture needle under direct ultrasound visualization [26]. PNE stimulates a local inflammatory response leading to increased cellular activity and repair of the affected area [27]. It has proven to be effective in injuries such as tendinosis (for example, in patellar tendonitis [28], lateral epicondylitis [29], subacromial pain syndrome [30], etc.), and plantar heel pain [31]. The histological and functional evidence observed in an animal model of muscle lesion [32,33] demonstrates that the application of PNE during muscle regeneration induces a decrease in pro-inflammatory mediators (TNF-α and IL-1β), and an increase in the expression of anti-inflammatory proteins (PPAR-γ) and vascular endothelial growth factor (VEGF). The recovery time of the damaged muscle tissue is also reduced. However, such studies in humans are limited to case studies analyzing acute muscle injury [34,35]. Previous studies [36] have used different strength programs in participants with previous injuries to the rectus femoris in order to assess the effectiveness of the program. A review on the rectus femoris injuries has stressed the need to propose interventions through criteria-based reconditioning programs for this injury in order to ensure an optimal RTP scenario to sustain performance and prevent reinjuries [37]. Such criteria-based reconditioning interventions have been shown to be successful in the case of hamstring injuries [38,39].

The identification of elimination of potential risk factors for an injury can be aided by following a cohort of players in a single center over a large span of time. If the same rehabilitation program is applied to all players of the cohort, this also allows the evaluation of a particular program and helps look at the medium to large term development of the players. This has been seen in the case of hamstring injuries, where following a cohort of professional and youth players helped discarding isokinetic strength (of the hamstrings and quadriceps) [40] and flexibility [41] as weak indicators for a potential hamstring injury. In terms of medium to long-term evaluation of the program, the application of a criteria based reconditioning program showed the absence of reinjuries in a span of twenty-four weeks following injury [38] and the players actually managed to improve their performance as a result of individualized training they underwent [39]. However, to the best of the authors' knowledge, such programs following an injury to rectus femoris have not been described in the literature.

Hence, the aim of this study was to assess the safety and feasibility of a combination of percutaneous needle electrolysis and a specific rehab and reconditioning program (RRP) in professional soccer players with an acute muscle injury to the rectus femoris. A secondary aim of the study was to analyze possible reinjuries following RTP in the short, medium and long term. Based on previous research, the hypothesis was that the PNE and RRP program would reduce the layoff time, but the players' physical performance at RTP would be at a lower level as compared to the pre-injury levels.

2. Methods

2.1. Study Design

A single exposure cohort study design was used where a single group of players was followed over the course of three seasons. In case of sustaining an injury to the rectus femoris, their rehabilitation and performance was monitored in the short, medium, and long term.

2.2. Participants

Players from a single club playing in the top professional soccer division of the Spanish soccer league system, commonly known as *LaLiga* were followed over three seasons, i.e., the 2017–2018, 2018–2019, and 2019–2020 seasons. To be eligible for the study, participants were required to meet the inclusion criteria of being professional male soccer players, over 18 years of age and having suffered the acute onset of anterior thigh pain, confirmed via ultrasound imaging [42–45] as a grade II [46] injury to the rectus femoris muscle located at the myotendinous junction. The sports medicine physician confirmed the diagnosis 48 h after the injury incidence. Additional eligibility criteria are described in Table 1.

Table 1. Inclusion and exclusion criteria.

Inclusion Criteria	Exclusion Criteria
- Professional soccer players. - Age >18 years. - Acute onset of anterior thigh pain. - Indirect muscle injury. - Ultrasound imaging within 48 h from injury. - Rectus femoris injury at the myotendinous junction. - Available for follow-up.	- Reinjury or chronic rectus femoris injury - Concurrent other injury inhibiting rehabilitation & reconditioning. - Needle phobia (belonephobia). - Overlying skin infection. - History of diabetes, gout, or rheumatoid arthritis may all be predisposing factors for muscle tears. - Immunocompromised state.

Thirteen soccer players (age = 27.92 ± 3.17 years; height = 180.92 ± 3.42 cm; mass = 74.07 ± 3.42 Kg; 61.5% of whom were injured while kicking) (Table 2) were finally included in the cohort and volunteered to participate in the study. All participants provided written informed consent, and procedures were conducted under the guidance of the technical and medical staff of the team, always adhering to the ethical principles for medical research involving human subjects under the Declaration of Helsinki.

Table 2. Profile of professional soccer players.

Players (n)	Player Position	Age (Years)	Mass (Kg)	Height (cm)	Injury Mechanism	Dominant Leg	Phenotype
1	Full-Back	32	74	179	Kicking	D	Caucasian
2	Midfielder	28	77	184	Sprint	D	Caucasian
3	Midfielder	31	76	181	CoD *	ND	Caucasian
4	Central Defender	28	70	177	Kicking	D	Black
5	Winger	24	74	180	Kicking	D	Caucasian
6	Full-Back	25	75	181	Kicking	D	Caucasian
7	Stricker	27	73	179	Sprint	D	Caucasian
8	Stricker	26	69	176	Sprint	ND	Caucasian
9	Winger	27	70	180	Kicking	D	Caucasian
10	Winger	32	72	181	Kicking	D	Caucasian
11	Central Defender	31	81	189	CoD	D	Caucasian
12	Midfielder	30	78	185	Kicking	D	Caucasian
13	Midfielder	22	74	180	Kicking	D	Caucasian

* CoD: change of direction; D: dominant; ND: non-dominant; Kg: kilogram; cm: centimeter.

3. Intervention Protocol

3.1. US-Guided Percutaneous Needle Electrolysis (PNE)

The PNE technique was performed under ultrasound guidance on the muscle injury using an intensity of 1.5–2 mA during 3 s, five times (1.5–2:3:5), according to the protocol by Valera-Garrido and Minaya-Muñoz [47], 48 h after the injury because electromyographic recovery of endplate noise in muscles treated percutaneously with galvanic current is relatively quick (72 h), coinciding with the inflammatory reaction [47]. A specifically developed medically certified device (Physio Invasiva®, PRIM Physio, Spain) was used (Figure 1). The device produced a continuous galvanic current through the cathode (modified electrosurgical scalpel with the needle) while the patient held the anode (handheld electrode). A GE® LOGIQ™ E9 ultrasound machine with a ML6–15 linear transducer (GE Healthcare®, Wisconsin, USA) was used. During the PNE technique, the player was placed in the supine position on a reclining bed at an elevation of 45 degrees with both legs flat resting on the bed. Prior to inserting a needle, the underlying skin was cleaned with isopropyl alcohol and chlorhexidine (Lainco® 2%). The transducer, enclosed in a non-sterile rolled latex covered over non-sterile ultrasound gel, was placed on the target area. Subsequently, an acupuncture needle 0.30 mm × 30 mm (Physio Invasiva® needles, PRIM Physio, Spain; uncoated steel needle with rigid metal handle with guide, Korean type) was inserted using a short-axis approach at a 80-degree angle with skin and advanced toward the muscle injury according to the technique described by Valera-Garrido and Minaya-Muñoz [47] (Figure 2). A physiotherapist with more than 10 years of experience in ultrasound evaluation and over fifteen years of experience in invasive therapy applied the PNE technique. Oral paracetamol was used when necessary for the purpose of pain relief in the first 24 h after PNE intervention.

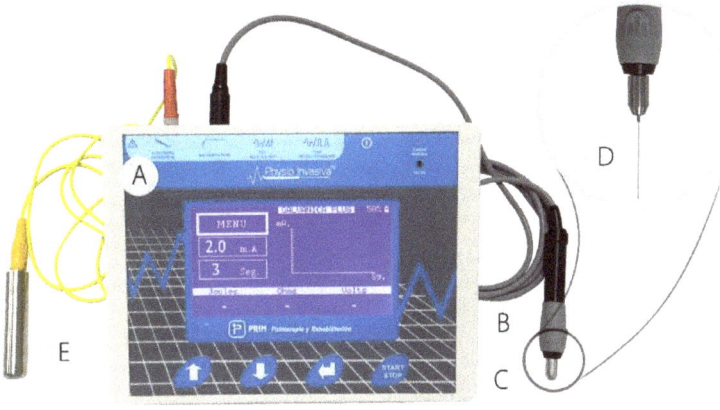

Figure 1. Medically certified device (Physio Invasiva®, PRIM Physio, Spain). (**A**) Device; (**B**) cathode (modified electrosurgical scalpel with the needle); (**C**) needle holder; (**D**) needle; (**E**) anode (handheld electrode).

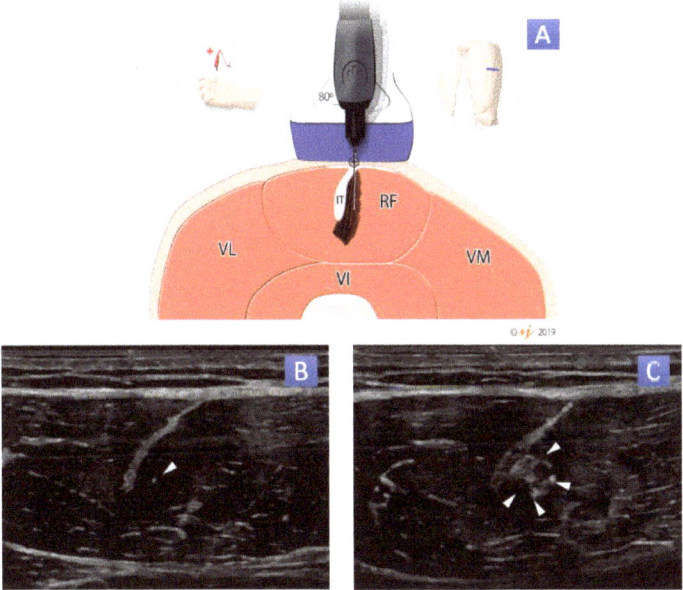

Figure 2. Percutaneous needle electrolysis (PNE) technique for rectus femoris muscle injury. (**A**) Graphic scheme in transverse plane. Short-axis approach at an 80-degree angle into the area of muscle injury (dark red part). (**B**) B-mode ultrasound image of PNE technique in which arrowhead represents the tip of the needle in a short-axis approach in area of muscle injury. (**C**) B-mode ultrasound image of PNE technique in which the white area represents the hydrogen gas released during the electrolysis. RF: rectus femoris; VM: vastus medialis; VL: vastus lateralis; VI: vastus intermedius; IT: intramuscular tendon of RF muscle.

3.2. Rehab and Reconditioning Program (RRP)

The rehab and reconditioning program was divided into two parts: an indoor rehab (IR) program and an on-field reconditioning (OFR) program. The IR program, focused on restoring the athlete's neuromuscular function [48], had a duration of approximately 8–9 days post-PNE. This program was further divided into two phases. The initial phase (Phase 1, Table 3) was based on the optimization of range of motion (ROM) and strength. Progressive muscular tensions at different ROMs and movement velocities [49] were prescribed to protect it against future demands and promote connective tissue repair (48 h, 72 h & 96 h post-PNE-Table 3). Hip, pelvic and thoracic spine mobility, single leg strength training, and dynamic tasks that combined isometric activation with stretch-shortening cycle of the lower limb muscles were included in this initial phase. The second phase (Phase 2, Table 4) began 5–7 days post-PNE and focused on tasks based on the absorption and production of force in different planes. This acted as a link toward the progression of movement skills in order to optimize lineal and multidirectional movements [38,39,50]. Players were instructed to perform the included exercises within a pain score of 2 on a numerical rating scale from 0 to 10, where 0 represented no pain and 10 was the most extreme pain possible. Players were encouraged to increase the load with minor pain corresponding to 2 of 10; that is, if pain was ≤ 1 of 10, they were encouraged to increase the load, and if pain was ≥ 3 of 10, the load was reduced [51].

The OFR program (Phase 3, Table 5) focused on an optimal reconditioning to prepare the player for the competition demands through technical and coordination drills (OF-1, OF-2, OF-3, and OF-4), which were increased in terms of complexity and demands of decision making [38,52]. In addition, global positioning system (GPS) and accelerometer data were used to training load monitoring during the OFR program. When the player successfully completed all item of the RRP and progression criteria, they were declared fit to train with the team.

Table 3. Indoor rehab program—Phase 1.

Indoor Phase	Date	Description	Volume (Time)
Phase 1 (ROM & Strength)	24 h-Post PNE	**Pelvic Assessment** - Assessment of the Pelvis architecture: Anterior-Posterior Pelvic Tilt. - Reestablish and identify deficits in ROM of Hip-Thoracic spine. - Activation synergists muscles + Inhibition over-actives muscles.	40′
	48 h-Post PNE	**24 h Post PNE + Strength Training Eccentric-quasi-isometric (EQI)** - Single leg Deadlift 2 × 6; Hip Thrust 2 × 8 × 4″; Step-Down on Box (45 cm) 4 × 4″ iso. - Lunge-position 4 × 7″ isom; Med Ball Lunge-position Isometric chest throw (×8) (3–5 Kg.) (Back position leg injured). - Med Ball Lunge-position Isometric overhead hold (4 × 12″) (3–5 Kg.) (Back position leg injured).	40′
	72 h-Post PNE	**48 h Post PNE + Strength Training (ISO + SSC) + Absorption/Landings (Frontal Plane)** - Single leg Squat Bulgarian 1—2 × 8″ + 2 SSC slow Motion; Lunge-position 2 × 6″ isom. + 2 Split Jumps in each cycle. - *Absorption/Landings* (*Single leg*): Lateral Bound and stick (×4); Single leg depth bound and stick (45 cm) (×4); Box Lateral Bound (25 cm) (1:1) (×4).	45′
	96 h-Post PNE	**72 h Post PNE + Strength Training + Absorption (Multiplane)** - Lunge-position iso. 3″ + Switch Jump Lunges (×6); Reverse Lunges on step + Med ball Overhead hold (×6 × 4″). - 2 Switch Jump Lunges + Step-up to Box (×5); Lunge-position (Front Leg on Box 25 cm—Back Leg Injured on Box 45 cm) + Reverse Step ×4 (5 Kg.). - Switch Jump Lunges + Med ball Chest Throw (×6); Switch Jump Lunges + Med ball Overhead Throw (×6). - *Absorption/Landings*: Drop Split Squat (×4); Single leg Squat Bulgarian + Med ball (2 Kg.) Overhead Throw + Reverse Step (×6).	50′

Exit Criteria
- Overcome items of phase 1 (with minor pair. corresponding to 2 of 10).
- No resting pain (DOMS accepted).
- Full pain free ROM of lower-velocity tasks.
- Pain free contractile function/strength in mid-, inner and outer range (with minor pain corresponding to 2 of 10).
- Absorption force pain free.
- Ultrasound imaging confirmed a correct alignment of muscle fibers without evidence of edema.

ROM: range of motion; EQI: eccentric-quasi-isometric; ISO: isometric tension; SSC: stretch-shortening cycle; DOMS: delayed onset muscle soreness; PNE: percutaneous needle electrolysis.

Table 4. Indoor rehab program—Phase 2.

Indoor Phase	Date	Description	Volume (Time)
Phase 2 (Development of movement skills)	Days 5–7 Post PNE	**Linear Running Performance + Rate of moment production and absorption (Multi-Plane-Plyos) (18–20 contacts)** - Reverse Sled Drag (2 × 12 + 15 m) (80–100%); Prowler march (2 × 12 + 15 m) (90–100% BW). - Running Drills (Mini-Medium Hurdles Running Training drill) (6 hurdles) (Slow Motion) (×4). - Switch Jump Lunges (Back position leg injured) + Lateral hop box and Stick (×4); Single leg Lateral Depth + Horizontal Jump (1:2) (×4). - Switch Jump Lunges on two boxes (45 cm) (×6); Bench between Leg-Jump (CMJ) 2:1 (45 cm) (Frontal Plane) (×4) (Injured leg).	50′
		Multidirectional performance + Rate of moment production and absorption (Multi-Plane-Plyos) (18–20 contacts) + Movement Skills - Shuffle resisted (×6); Band assisted Deceleration + Landings Single Leg (×6). - Split Step to Hip Turn (×6); Accel (5–7 steps) + Deceleration Mechanism (×4). - Single leg Depth Jump + Accel (3–4 Steps) (×4); Single leg Depth Jump + Cutting + Accel (3–4 Steps) (Frontal Plane) (×4). **Return to Running** - March, Skipping, Bounds (4 × 12–15 m). - Treadmill Running (14 Km·h^{-1}) (6 × 45″/45″).	60′

Exit Criteria
- Running movement performed pain free (45% maximum speed).
- Multidirectional movements performed pain free (low and medium speed).
- Optimize rate of moment production and absorption in multiplane motion.
- Ultrasound imaging confirmed a correct alignment of muscle fibers without evidence of edema.

CMJ: countermovement jump; BW: body weight.

Table 5. On-field reconditioning program—Phase 3.

On Field Phase	Date	Description	Volume (Time)
Phase 3	Day 9–10 Post PNE (OF-1)	- Change of directions drills in closed skills. - Sport-Specific technical skills with ball.	25'
	Day 11 Post PNE (OF-2)	- Analytics RSA (Linear / Curve Sprint). - Uphill submaximal sprint (14 m) (3 × 2) density 1:1. - Deceleration and re-acceleration patterns in closed skills. - Agility and coordination drills (with and without a ball in the same action) in closed skill.	35'
	Day 12 Post PNE	- Recovery Session: Mobility + Self-Myofascial release.	20'
	Day 13–14 Post PNE (OF-3)	- On-Field session 1. - Reeducation kicking drills. - Sport-specific RSA with agility and coordination drills closed/open skills. - Back pedal drill + 45° CoD in open skill (Inverted Y cone drill).	40'
	Day 15 Post PNE (OF-4)	- On-Field session 2. - Specific drills, including change of direction with uncertainty and RSA. - Tactical Skills with ball repeated efforts. - Specific kicking drill, including RSA (3 × 2 kicking) in open skill.	50'

Exit Criteria
- Overcome items of phase 3 in absence pain (with minor pain corresponding to 2 of 10).
- Individual sport-specific drills.
- Return to multidirectional skills, sprint speed, acceleration and deceleration velocities (High speed-RSA-open skills).
- Kicking in absence pain.
- Training load monitoring with GPS (>70% Game Load) (Running >90% Max. Speed, HSR, Sprints accumulated to RTT demands).
- Ultrasound imaging confirmed an optimal muscle repair.

OF-1: on-field 1 (days 9–10 post PNE); OF-2: day 11 post PNE; OF-3: days 13–14 post PNE; OF-4: day 15 post PNE; RSA: repeated sprint ability; CoD: change of direction; PNE: percutaneous needle electrolysis.

4. Variables and Data Analysis

4.1. Return to Training and Return to Play

The number of days between the injury and the return to training (RTT), return to play (RTP 1), and following match (RTP 2) were counted.

4.2. Ultrasound

Ultrasound scanning of the injured area was performed every three days with the help of Compare Assistant LOGIQ™ software (GE Healthcare®, Milwaukee, WI, USA) to compare prior examinations with the current one for confidence.

4.3. GPS Match Variables

GPS data (WIMU PRO™, Real Track Systems®, Almeria, Spain) was collected for all players from all matches in which they participated before (PRE: PRE 1 and PRE 2) and after (RTP: RTP 1 and RTP 2) injury. This pre-injury data would serve as a control group for this cohort, as it would permit the comparison with the aim of evaluating the effects of the intervention, on the performance of the injured player. This could only be registered on 10 players, since three players were injured in the preseason, and there were no data from official competitions prior to the injury.

The variables used to compare the performance represented actions where the quadriceps are known to be the most active: in accelerations, high intensity runs, and sub-maximal and maximal sprints [53]. The variables measured were (a) total distance covered in m (as a reference value); (b) distance covered at high intensities (between 18.1–21.0 Km·h^{-1}) in m; (c) distance covered at very high intensities (21.1–24.0 Km·h^{-1}) in m; (d) distance covered at sprint velocities (above 24.0 Km·h^{-1}) in m; (e) the peak speed registered in Km·h^{-1}; (f) the peak acceleration registered in m·s^{-2}; and (g) the explosive distance (i.e., the distance covered when the acceleration exceeded 1.2 m·s^{-2}) in m·min^{-1}.

4.4. Statistical Analysis

The GPS data recorded were compared, pre-injury vs. post-injury values, using a repeated measures ANOVA. Post-hoc corrections were made with Bonferroni corrections considering the following analyses only: PRE 2 vs. RTP 1, PRE 2 vs. RTP 2, PRE 1 vs. RTP 1, and PRE 1 vs. RTP 2. All calculations were carried out with Jamovi 1.2.17 (version 1.2) with $\alpha = 0.05$.

4.5. Adverse Events

The soccer players were asked to report any adverse events that they experienced during or after the PNE technique and RRP. Adverse events can be defined as sequelae of medium to long term in duration, with moderate to severe symptoms, perceived as distressing and unacceptable and requiring further treatment [54].

4.6. Follow-Up

After RTP, the players were followed up in the short term (1 week), medium term (8 weeks) and long term (20 weeks) to assess a possible re-injury and adverse effects.

5. Results

Participants returned to full team training (RTT) in 15.62 ± 1.80 days and returned to play (RTP 1) in 20.15 ± 2.79 days and played a total of 94.6 ± 1.20 min. The following match (RTP 2) was in 29.62 ± 3.95 days following the index injury with a match time 95.1 ± 1.14 min.

5.1. Ultrasound

Initially, all players presented images showing a fibrillar defect in the myotendinous junction of rectus femoris muscle with surrounding edema, without fluid collection/hematoma drainable, consistent with a grade II strain injury (Figure 3A). In 92.3% of the cases, the ultrasound examination in the day 7 post-PNE showed a significant change in the extent of edema and fiber disruption (Figure 3B). One player needed one additional session of PNE (7 days post-PNE-1). Ultrasound follow-up at 14 days showed an almost complete disappearance of the injury pattern of the muscle in all players in the ultrasound image (Figure 3C).

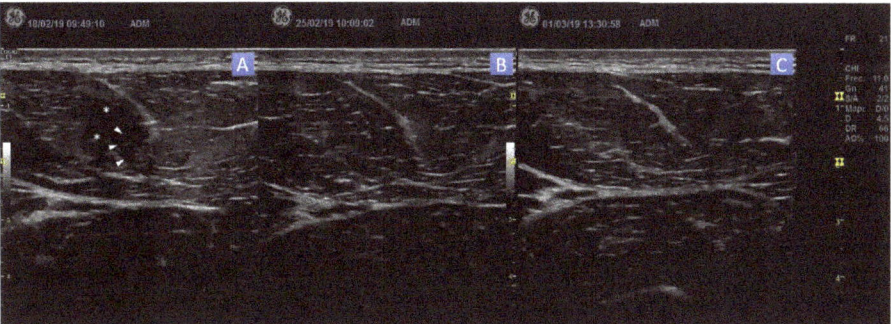

Figure 3. Transverse B-Mode ultrasound images of the evolution of the injured muscle. (**A**) Initial. 48 h post-injury. Ultrasound imaging shows muscle fiber discontinuity at the level of tear (arrowhead), with surrounding echogenic muscle edema (asterisk). (**B**) Ultrasound imaging at seven days post-PNE. (**C**) Ultrasound imaging at 14 days post-PNE.

5.2. GPS Parameters

On comparing the data from the GPS data (Figure 4), there were significant differences between the GPS recorded distances at high intensities (F (3,27) = 4.67, p = 0.009, η^2 = 0.087) and distances covered at sprint speeds (F (3,27) = 2.98, p = 0.049, η^2 = 0.108) but no significant differences for distances covered at very high intensities (F (3,27) = 0.699, p = 0.561, η^2 = 0.010). Post-hoc comparisons showed a significant decrease between PRE-1 and RTP 1 in distances covered at high intensities (p = 0.007). All other post-hoc comparisons between PRE and RTP data showed no significant differences between data registered at PRE and POST. A comparison of the total distance run showed significant differences between the matches, with the distances run during RTP 2 being significantly higher than PRE-2 (p < 0.001) and PRE-1 (p < 0.001); and the distance run at RTP 1 was higher than that at PRE-2 (p = 0.007).

The variation in peak speed (Figure 5) was not significant between the different instances (F (3,27) = 2.49, p = 0.136, η^2 = 0.126). However, a significant difference was observed for the peak acceleration registered (F (3,27) = 4.74, p = 0.009, η^2 = 0.257), although post-hoc comparisons showed no significant differences between the different instances. The explosive distance showed significant differences between the instances (F (3,27) = 13.4, p < 0.001, η^2 = 0.481), and post-hoc comparisons showed significantly higher values for RTP 2 compared to PRE-2 (p < 0.001) and PRE-1 compared to RTP 1 (p < 0.001).

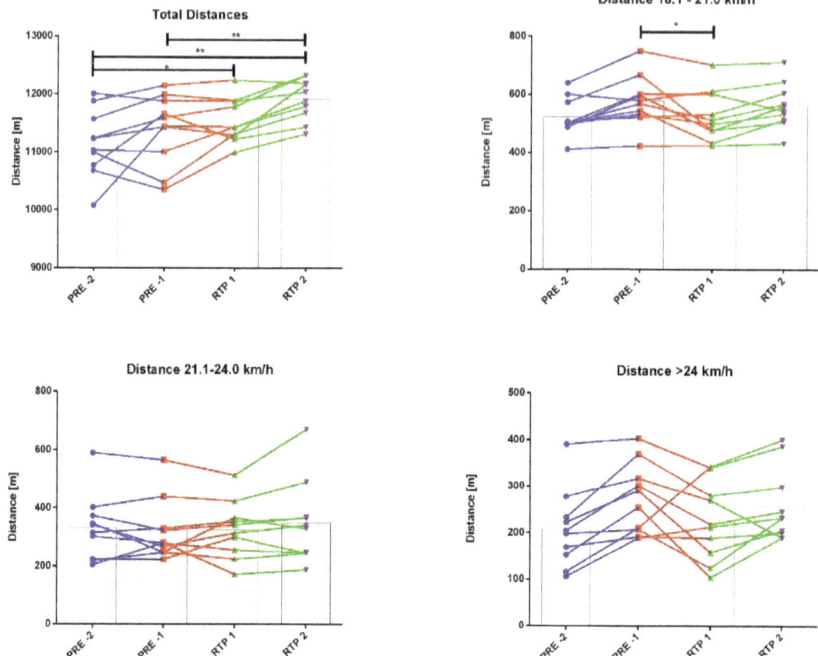

Figure 4. Absolute total distance and absolute distances run in different velocity ranges by the participants in matches before (PRE) and after (POST) a rectus femoris injury. * indicates a significant difference between instances at $p < 0.05$. ** indicates a significant difference between instances at $p < 0.001$.

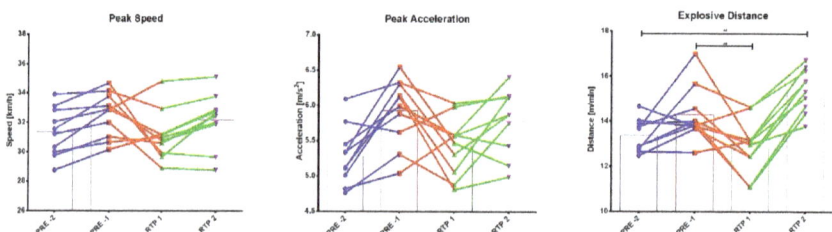

Figure 5. Peak speed, peak acceleration, and explosive distance covered by the participants in matches before (PRE) and after (POST) a rectus femoris injury. ** indicates a significant difference between instances at $p < 0.001$.

5.3. Adverse Events

There were no serious adverse events reported, whereas minor adverse events were common. It included pain during PNE (100%) and local soreness after treatment (23.1%) that resolved spontaneously within 24–48 h without any intervention.

5.4. Follow-Up

No player suffered a reinjury 20 weeks following RTP. Also, there were no dropouts during the development of the study.

6. Discussions

This study describes the intervention of percutaneous needle electrolysis treatment along with a rehab and reconditioning program following an injury to the rectus femoris in professional soccer players. Ultrasound images during the reconditioning and performance parameters after return to play were registered to assess the effectiveness of the intervention. A short-term, medium-term, and long-term follow-up was also carried out, and the results showed that the injured muscle recovered completely and were no reinjuries or adverse effects reported in the 20 weeks following the index injury.

The apparent success of the program was highlighted by the relatively short times for RTT and RTP and similar physical performance parameters before and after injury. The duration for RTT (mean: 15.62 days, median: 14 days) and RTP (mean: 20.15 days, median: 19 days) was lower than previous studies, which reported a mean layoff duration of 33 (median: 22 days) [10] to 46.8 days [55] for a grade II rectus femoris injuries, although these results must be taken with caution, given the lack of a control group in the study. When comparing physical match parameters before and after injury, the distances covered at the different speed thresholds were similar, and so were the peak values of speed and acceleration registered, suggesting that the participant not only recovered from the previous injury but also did not suffer a substantial loss in terms of their conditioning. Moreover, the gradual improvements in the variable of explosive distance suggests an optimal evolution in the ability to continue competing without a risk of reinjury. Given that the match schedule and opponents were not under the control of the researchers, nor the fact whether the player would go on to play the full 90 min, the similarity in values indicate a successful short-term recovery of the participant. Such a type of follow-up with GPS data has been previously reported to indicate the success of the rehabilitation applied [56]. This positive progress of the players appears to have been facilitated by the structural and functional changes noted during the injury reconditioning process.

Considering the structural data, important changes in terms of the extent of edema and fiber disruption were noted in all cases presented in this study early in the muscle healing process. Different authors [32,33] have evaluated the effect of the application of PNE such as on a model of muscle injury in animal tissue such as the rat, reproducing a physiological environment very similar to that in humans. They concluded that the application of PNE in an animal model of muscle injury reduces the recovery time of the damaged muscle tissue because of the galvanic current facilitates the inflammatory reaction and muscle irrigation, thereby, helping muscular regeneration and, simultaneously, improving the recovery of the injured muscle tissue at an earlier time (from 72 h to seven days post-PNE). The PNE protocol applied was similar in this study, and the results obtained are comparable and evident from the ultrasound scans. This regeneration of injured muscle is a crucial feature enabling the progression on to the functional tasks described in the RRP.

The RRP was designed in such a manner that it followed and complemented the PNE applied 48 h earlier. The early start of the RRP (Table 2) showed a promising advantage when compared other interventions [55], where the rehabilitation and reconditioning program for rectus femoris consisted initially of absolute rest for the first week with the application of ice, compression and non-steroidal anti-inflammatory medication. Furthermore, in this study, the progression criteria were defined based on previous research that has stated the importance of reestablishment neuromuscular function from the initial phases to reduce the layoff period and the risk of re-injury, and thereby, avoiding the loss of training capacity [48,57]. Mobility, core stability, and strength training exercises were prescribed from the first days after PNE for this reason. Due to the biarticular function of the rectus femoris, eccentric-quasi-isometric (EQI) strength training for the muscle at different ranges of movement and movement speeds were used to stimulate damaged fibers, thereby obtaining different ranges of muscular tension in the muscle healing process [49]. In the final phase of the indoor rehab program, the rate of force development and the improvement of movement skills in different planes were key, specifically in acceleration and deceleration patterns where the rectus femoris is highly involved [37]. Previous research has shown that such tasks help restore coordinated movement patterns that are essential for athletic success in the future [58].

During the on-field reconditioning program, drills with repeated sprints [59], multidirectional drills, and soccer-specific technical skills were included, with special emphasis in kicking drills [37]. The load and decision-making progressively increased in order to optimize the functions of the rectus femoris and reconditioning the players in order to prepare them for the demands of competition and training [38,52]. The constant monitoring of the evolution of the repair of injured tissue through ultrasound, provided the researchers with important progression criteria to be taken into account in the progress of the RRP.

An important part of the study was that the participants did not suffer any re-injury or serious adverse effects in 20 weeks following RTP. Epidemiological research has reported that the recurrence rate of a reinjury to the rectus femoris in the weeks following the RTP varied between 5% [21] and 6.4% [22]. As in previous studies, only post-needling soreness was reported, which is a frequent effect after PNE, usually lasting less than 48 h [60]. These results reinforce the medium and long-term success of the PNE + RRP, the progression of which is based on criteria and not time, and this in turn not only might reduce the reinjury risk, but also prepare the athletes for what they would be exposed to during the season.

However, given the small sample size, the results of this study, although promising, must be taken with caution. The absence of a control group is one of the main limitations of the present study. But it is important to highlight that in an elite professional environment is very difficult establish control or placebo group. The reason of choosing a single exposure cohort [61] was to reflect the practical realities in an elite, professional environment where all injured players were exposed to the same PNE and RRP program as per the decision taken by the club's medical and technical staff team. Nevertheless, in this paper, the results were compared to those obtained in the few previous studies that reported on rectus femoris injuries and showed faster mean and median recovery times.

Another limitation to this study was the use of a combination of qualitative and quantitative criteria to determine progress, although this is, to the authors' knowledge, the first study to detail progression criteria in scientific literature on rectus femoris injuries. There was an absence of a purely objective, biomechanical test that could measure the functional capacity of the rectus femoris during or after the rehabilitation and reconditioning process. On such an occasion, tests such as electromyographic evaluation could not be conducted due to decisions beyond the control of the researchers when working with elite athletes. Incorporating such testing could probably help reinforce the complete rehabilitation of the rectus femoris muscle. Although ultrasound was used for injury diagnosis and is a valid tool for the evaluation and monitoring of muscle injury in future studies, it was used qualitatively, and decisions were made based on the operator's experience. Objective quantification of these images could be carried out in future studies, and this could be complemented with the information provided by magnetic resonance imaging. Also, such a study could be implemented in the case of non-elite participants, where the possibility of a randomized clinical study could explain the findings of this study with more detail.

7. Conclusions

An early intervention with PNE and RRP in soccer players with injuries to rectus femoris appeared to allow a safe return to training and to competition without re-injuries in the short, medium, and long term. Assessment of the evolution of the injured tissue through a combination of ultrasound imaging and functional criteria give the impression that they were crucial to make better decisions during the process. In addition, the use of GPS provided information about the athlete's performance after the injury, where the injured player reached similar values when compared to those pre-injury, which possibly indicated the importance of the intervention.

Author Contributions: Conceptualization, F.V.-G., F.M.-M., S.J.-R., J.L.E.-R.; Methodology, F.V.-G., F.M.-M., S.J.-R., J.L.E.-R., A.N.; Validation, A.N.; Formal Analysis, A.N.; Investigation, F.V.-G. and S.J.-R.; Writing—Original Draft Preparation, F.V.-G., F.M.-M., S.J.-R., J.L.E.-R., A.N.; Writing—Review & Editing, F.V.-G., F.M.-M., S.J.-R., J.L.E.-R., A.N. All authors have read and agreed to the published version of the manuscript.

Funding: This research received no external funding.

Acknowledgments: Our thanks to the players who participated in the study. The authors also wish to express their gratitude to Javier Vidal Deltell for his involvement, dedication and active participation in the process of returning players to competition. Without him the results would not have been the same.

Conflicts of Interest: The authors declare no conflict of interest.

References

1. Rivilla-García, J.; Calvo, L.C.; Jiménez-Rubio, S.; Paredes-Hernández, V.; Muñoz, A.; Van den Tillaar, R.; Navandar, A. Characteristics of very high intensity runs of soccer players in relation to their playing position and playing half in the 2013-14 Spanish La Liga Season. *J. Hum. Kinet.* **2019**, *66*, 213–222. [CrossRef]
2. Dellal, A.; Chamari, K.; Wong, D.P.; Ahmaidi, S.; Keller, D.; Barros, R.; Bisciotti, G.N.; Carling, C. Comparison of physical and technical performance in European soccer match-play: FA Premier League and La Liga. *Eur. J. Sport Sci.* **2011**, *11*, 51–59. [CrossRef]
3. Taylor, J.B.; Wright, A.A.; Dischiavi, S.L.; Townsend, M.A.; Marmon, A.R. Activity demands during multi-directional team sports: A systematic review. *Sports Med.* **2017**, *47*, 2533–2551. [CrossRef]
4. Mallo, J.; Mena, E.; Nevado, F.; Paredes, V. Physical Demands of Top-Class Soccer Friendly Matches in Relation to a Playing Position Using Global Positioning System Technology. *J. Hum. Kinet.* **2015**, *47*, 179–188. [CrossRef] [PubMed]
5. Hägglund, M.; Waldén, M.; Ekstrand, J. Previous injury as a risk factor for injury in elite football: A prospective study over two consecutive seasons. *Br. J. Sports Med.* **2006**, *40*, 767–772. [CrossRef] [PubMed]
6. Van Beijsterveldt, A.; van de Port, I.G.; Vereijken, A.; Backx, F. Risk factors for hamstring injuries in male soccer players: A systematic review of prospective studies. *Scand. J. Med. Sci. Sports* **2013**, *23*, 253–262. [CrossRef] [PubMed]
7. Bowen, L.; Gross, A.S.; Gimpel, M.; Bruce-Low, S.; Li, F.-X. Spikes in acute: Chronic workload ratio (ACWR) associated with a 5–7 times greater injury rate in English Premier League football players: A comprehensive 3-year study. *Br. J. Sports Med.* **2020**, *54*, 731–738. [CrossRef]
8. Garrett, W.E., Jr. Muscle strain injuries. *Am. J. Sports Med.* **1996**, *24*, S2–S8. [CrossRef]
9. Ekstrand, J.; Hägglund, M.; Waldén, M. Epidemiology of Muscle Injuries in Professional Football. *Am. J. Sports Med.* **2011**, *39*, 1226–1232. [CrossRef]
10. Hallen, A.; Ekstrand, J. Return to play following muscle injuries in professional footballers. *J. Sports Sci.* **2014**, *32*, 1229–1236. [CrossRef]
11. Hägglund, M.; Waldén, M.; Ekstrand, J. Risk Factors for Lower Extremity Muscle Injury in Professional Soccer: The UEFA Injury Study. *Am. J. Sports Med.* **2013**, *41*, 327–335. [CrossRef] [PubMed]
12. Ekstrand, J.; Hagglund, M.; Walden, M. Injury incidence and injury patterns in professional football: The UEFA injury study. *Br. J. Sports Med.* **2011**, *45*, 553–558. [CrossRef] [PubMed]
13. Young, A. The relative isometric strength of type I and type II muscle fibres in the human quadriceps. *Clin. Physiol.* **1984**, *4*, 23–32. [CrossRef]
14. Neumann, D.A. Kinesiology of the hip: A focus on muscular actions. *J. Orthop. Sports Phys. Ther.* **2010**, *40*, 82–94. [CrossRef] [PubMed]
15. Mendiguchia, J.; Alentorn-Geli, E.; Brughelli, M. Hamstring strain injuries: Are we heading in the right direction? *Br. J. Sports Med.* **2012**, *46*, 81–85. [CrossRef]
16. Lewis, C.L.; Sahrmann, S.A.; Moran, D.W. Anterior hip joint force increases with hip extension, decreased gluteal force, or decreased iliopsoas force. *J. Biomech.* **2007**, *40*, 3725–3731. [CrossRef]
17. Lewindon, D.; Lee, J. Muscle injuries. In *Sports Injury Prevention and Rehabilitation. Integrating Medicine and Science for Performance Solutions*; Joyce, D., Lewindon, D., Eds.; Routledge: Abingdon, UK, 2016; pp. 106–120.
18. Svensson, K.; Eckerman, M.; Alricsson, M.; Magounakis, T.; Werner, S. Muscle injuries of the dominant or non-dominant leg in male football players at elite level. *Br. J. Sports Med.* **2016**, *50*, e4. [CrossRef]
19. Ueblacker, P.; Mueller-Wohlfahrt, H.-W.; Ekstrand, J. Epidemiological and clinical outcome comparison of indirect ('strain') versus direct ('contusion') anterior and posterior thigh muscle injuries in male elite football players: UEFA Elite League study of 2287 thigh injuries (2001–2013). *Br. J. Sports Med.* **2015**, *49*, 1461–1465. [CrossRef]

20. Eirale, C.; Farooq, A.; Smiley, F.A.; Tol, J.L.; Chalabi, H. Epidemiology of football injuries in Asia: A prospective study in Qatar. *J. Sci. Med. Sport* **2013**, *16*, 113–117. [CrossRef]
21. Orchard, J.W.; Jomaa, M.C.; Orchard, J.J.; Rae, K.; Hoffman, D.T.; Reddin, T.; Driscoll, T. Fifteen-week window for recurrent muscle strains in football: A prospective cohort of 3600 muscle strains over 23 years in professional Australian rules football. *Br. J. Sports Med.* **2020**, *54*, 1103–1107. [CrossRef]
22. Hägglund, M.; Waldén, M.; Bengtsson, H.; Ekstrand, J. Re-injuries in professional football: The UEFA Elite Club Injury Study. In *Return to Play in Football*; Springer: Berlin/Heidelberg, Germany, 2018; pp. 953–962.
23. Bubnov, R.; Yevseenko, V.; Semeniv, I. Ultrasound guided injections of Platelets Rich Plasma for muscle injury in professional athletes. Comparative study. *Med. Ultrason.* **2013**, *15*, 101–105. [CrossRef]
24. Chellini, F.; Tani, A.; Zecchi-Orlandini, S.; Sassoli, C. Influence of Platelet-Rich and Platelet-Poor Plasma on Endogenous Mechanisms of Skeletal Muscle Repair/Regeneration. *Int. J. Mol. Sci.* **2019**, *20*, 683. [CrossRef] [PubMed]
25. Mariani, E.; Pulsatelli, L. Platelet concentrates in musculoskeletal medicine. *Int. J. Mol. Sci.* **2020**, *21*, 1328. [CrossRef] [PubMed]
26. Valera-Garrido, F.; Minaya-Muñoz, F. Fundamentos y principios de la electrolisis percutánea musculoesquelética. In *Fisioterapia Invasiva*, 2nd ed.; Elsevier: Barcelona, Spain, 2016; Chapter 16; pp. 390–391.
27. Valera-Garrido, F.; Minaya-Muñoz, F.; Sánchez-Ibáñez, J.M.; García-Palencia, P.; Valderrama-Canales, F.; Medina-Mirapeix, F.; Polidori, F. Comparison of the acute inflammatory response and proliferation of dry needling and electrolysis percutaneous intratissue in healthy rat Achilles tendons. *Br. J. Sports Med.* **2013**, *47*, e2. [CrossRef]
28. Abat, F.; Sánchez-Sánchez, J.L.; Martín-Nogueras, A.M.; Calvo-Arenillas, J.I.; Yajeya, J.; Méndez-Sánchez, R.; Monllau, J.C.; Gelber, P.-E. Randomized controlled trial comparing the effectiveness of the ultrasound-guided galvanic electrolysis technique (USGET) versus conventional electro-physiotherapeutic treatment on patellar tendinopathy. *J. Exp. Orthop.* **2016**, *3*, 34. [CrossRef]
29. Valera-Garrido, F.; Minaya-Muñoz, F.; Medina-Mirapeix, F. Ultrasound-guided percutaneous needle electrolysis in chronic lateral epicondylitis: Short-term and long-term results. *Acupunct. Med.* **2014**, *32*, 446–454. [CrossRef]
30. Rodríguez-Huguet, M.; Góngora-Rodríguez, J.; Rodríguez-Huguet, P.; Ibañez-Vera, A.J.; Rodríguez-Almagro, D.; Martín-Valero, R.; Díaz-Fernández, Á.; Lomas-Vega, R. Effectiveness of Percutaneous Electrolysis in Supraspinatus Tendinopathy: A Single-Blinded Randomized Controlled Trial. *J. Clin. Med.* **2020**, *9*, 1837. [CrossRef]
31. Fernández-Rodríguez, T.; Fernández-Rolle, Á.; Truyols-Domínguez, S.; Benítez-Martínez, J.C.; Casaña-Granell, J. Prospective randomized trial of electrolysis for chronic plantar heel pain. *Foot Ankle Int.* **2018**, *39*, 1039–1046. [CrossRef]
32. Abat, F.; Valles, S.-L.; Gelber, P.-E.; Polidori, F.; Jorda, A.; García-Herreros, S.; Monllau, J.-C.; Sanchez-Ibáñez, J.-M. An experimental study of muscular injury repair in a mouse model of notexin-induced lesion with EPI® technique. *BMC Sports Sci. Med. Rehabil.* **2015**, *7*, 7. [CrossRef]
33. Santafé, M.; Margalef, R.; Minaya-Muñoz, F.; Valera-Garrido, F. Action of galvanic current on an experimentally generated muscle lesion: Preliminary findings. *Rev. Fisioter. Invasiva* **2019**, *2*, 108–109.
34. Valera-Garrido, F.; Minaya-Muñoz, F.; Sánchez-Ibáñez, J.M. Efecto de la electrolisis percutánea en las roturas musculares agudas. Caso clínico de la lesión de "tennis leg". In Proceedings of the II Congreso Regional de Fisioterapia de la Región de Murcia, Murcia, Spain, 3–4 May 2012.
35. Jiménez-Rubio, S.; Valera-Garrido, F.; Minaya-Muñoz, F.; Navandar, A. Ultrasound-guided percutaneous needle electrolysis and rehab & reconditioning program following a hamstring injury reduces return to play time in professional soccer players: A case series. *Rev. Fisioter. Invasiva* **2020**, *3*, 2–6.
36. Brughelli, M.; Nosaka, K.; Cronin, J. Application of eccentric exercise on an Australian Rules football player with recurrent hamstring injuries. *Phys. Ther. Sport* **2009**, *10*, 75–80. [CrossRef] [PubMed]
37. Mendiguchia, J.; Alentorn-Geli, E.; Idoate, F.; Myer, G.D. Rectus femoris muscle injuries in football: A clinically relevant review of mechanisms of injury, risk factors and preventive strategies. *Br. J. Sports Med.* **2013**, *47*, 359–366. [CrossRef]
38. Jiménez-Rubio, S.; Navandar, A.; Rivilla-García, J.; Paredes-Hernández, V. Validity of an on-Field Readaptation Program Following a Hamstring Injury in Professional Soccer. *J. Sport Rehabil.* **2019**, *28*, 1–7. [CrossRef]

39. Mendiguchia, J.; Martinez-Ruiz, E.; Edouard, P.; Morin, J.B.; Martinez-Martinez, F.; Idoate, F.; Mendez-Villanueva, A. A Multifactorial, Criteria-Based Progressive Algorithm for Hamstring Injury Treatment. *Med. Sci. Sports Exerc.* **2017**. [CrossRef]
40. van Dyk, N.; Bahr, R.; Whiteley, R.; Tol, J.L.; Kumar, B.D.; Hamilton, B.; Farooq, A.; Witvrouw, E. Hamstring and Quadriceps Isokinetic Strength Deficits Are Weak Risk Factors for Hamstring Strain Injuries: A 4-Year Cohort Study. *Am. J. Sports Med.* **2016**, *44*, 1789–1795. [CrossRef]
41. van Dyk, N.; Farooq, A.; Bahr, R.; Witvrouw, E. Hamstring and ankle flexibility deficits are weak risk factors for hamstring injury in professional soccer players: A prospective cohort study of 438 players including 78 injuries. *Am. J. Sports Med.* **2018**, *46*, 2203–2210. [CrossRef]
42. Guillodo, Y.; Bouttier, R.; Saraux, A. Value of sonography combined with clinical assessment to evaluate muscle injury severity in athletes. *J. Athl. Train.* **2011**, *46*, 500–504. [CrossRef]
43. Mohamad, H.A.S.; Ashril, Y.; Mohamed, M.A.R. Pattern of muscle injuries and predictors of return-to-play duration among Malaysian athletes. *Singap. Med. J.* **2013**, *54*, 587–591.
44. Renoux, J.; Brasseur, J.-L.; Wagner, M.; Frey, A.; Folinais, D.; Dibie, C.; Maiza, D.; Crema, M.D. Ultrasound-detected connective tissue involvement in acute muscle injuries in elite athletes and return to play: The French National Institute of Sports (INSEP) study. *J. Sci. Med. Sport* **2019**, *22*, 641–646. [CrossRef]
45. Hall, M.M. Return to play after thigh muscle injury: Utility of serial ultrasound in guiding clinical progression. *Curr. Sports Med. Rep.* **2018**, *17*, 296–301. [CrossRef]
46. Peetrons, P. Ultrasound of muscles. *Eur. Radiol.* **2002**, *12*, 35–43. [CrossRef]
47. Valera-Garrido, F.; Minaya-Muñoz, F. Aplicaciones clínicas de la electrolisis percutánea. In *Fisioterapia Invasiva*, 2nd ed.; Elsevier: Barcelona, Spain, 2016; Chapter 17; p. 425.
48. Hegyi, A.; Gonçalves, B.A.; Finni, T.; Cronin, N.J. Individual Region-and Muscle-specific Hamstring Activity at Different Running Speeds. *Med. Sci. Sports Exerc.* **2019**, *51*, 2274–2285. [CrossRef]
49. Oranchuk, D.J.; Storey, A.G.; Nelson, A.R.; Cronin, J.B. Scientific Basis for Eccentric Quasi-Isometric Resistance Training: A Narrative Review. *J. Strength Cond. Res.* **2019**, *33*, 2846–2859. [CrossRef]
50. King, E.; Franklyn-Miller, A.; Richter, C.; O'Reilly, E.; Doolan, M.; Moran, K.; Strike, S.; Falvey, É. Clinical and biomechanical outcomes of rehabilitation targeting intersegmental control in athletic groin pain: Prospective cohort of 205 patients. *Br. J. Sports Med.* **2018**, *52*, 1054–1062. [CrossRef]
51. Serner, A.; Weir, A.; Tol, J.L.; Thorborg, K.; Lanzinger, S.; Otten, R.; Hölmich, P. Return to Sport After Criteria-Based Rehabilitation of Acute Adductor Injuries in Male Athletes: A Prospective Cohort Study. *Orthop. J. Sports Med.* **2020**, *8*, 1–11. [CrossRef] [PubMed]
52. Taberner, M.; Allen, T.; Constantine, E.; Cohen, D. From control to chaos to competition. Building a pathway for return to performance following ACL reconstruction. *Aspetar Sports Med. J.* **2020**, *9*, 84–94.
53. Schache, A.G.; Dorn, T.W.; Williams, G.P.; Brown, N.A.; Pandy, M.G. Lower-limb muscular strategies for increasing running speed. *J. Orthop. Sports Phys. Ther.* **2014**, *44*, 813–824. [CrossRef]
54. Carlesso, L.C.; Macdermid, J.C.; Santaguida, L.P. Standardization of adverse event terminology and reporting in orthopaedic physical therapy: Application to the cervical spine. *J. Orthop. Sports Phys. Ther.* **2010**, *40*, 455–463. [CrossRef] [PubMed]
55. Balius, R.; Maestro, A.; Pedret, C.; Estruch, A.; Mota, J.; Rodriguez, L.; García, P.; Mauri, E. Central aponeurosis tears of the rectus femoris: Practical sonographic prognosis. *Br. J. Sports Med.* **2009**, *43*, 818–824. [CrossRef]
56. Jiménez-Rubio, S.; Navandar, A.; Rivilla-García, J.; Paredes-Hernández, V.; Gómez-Ruano, M.Á. Improvements in Match-Related Physical Performance of Professional Soccer Players After the Application of an on-Field Training Program for Hamstring Injury Rehabilitation. *J. Sport Rehabil.* **2019**, *1*, 1. [CrossRef]
57. Järvinen, T.A.; Järvinen, M.; Kalimo, H. Regeneration of injured skeletal muscle after the injury. *Muscles Ligaments Tendons J.* **2013**, *3*, 337. [CrossRef]
58. Knowles, B. Reconditioning. A performance-based response to an injury. In *Sports Injury Prevention and Rehabilitation Integrating Medicine and Science for Performance Solutions*; Joyce, D., Lewindon, D., Eds.; Routledge: London, UK; New York, NY, USA, 2016; pp. 3–10.
59. Buchheit, M.; Laursen, P.B. High-intensity interval training, solutions to the programming puzzle. *Sports Med.* **2013**, *43*, 927–954. [CrossRef]

60. Valera-Garrido, F.; Minaya-Muñoz, F.; Ramírez-Martínez, P.; Medina-i-Mirapeix, F. Adverse effects associated to the application of ultrasound-guided percutaneous needle electrolysis. *Rev. Fisioter. Invasiva* **2019**, *2*, 115–116.
61. Mathes, T.; Pieper, D. Clarifying the distinction between case series and cohort studies in systematic reviews of comparative studies: Potential impact on body of evidence and workload. *BMC Med. Res. Methodol.* **2017**, *17*, 107. [CrossRef]

Publisher's Note: MDPI stays neutral with regard to jurisdictional claims in published maps and institutional affiliations.

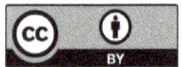

© 2020 by the authors. Licensee MDPI, Basel, Switzerland. This article is an open access article distributed under the terms and conditions of the Creative Commons Attribution (CC BY) license (http://creativecommons.org/licenses/by/4.0/).

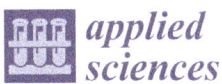

Review

Effectiveness of Training Prescription Guided by Heart Rate Variability Versus Predefined Training for Physiological and Aerobic Performance Improvements: A Systematic Review and Meta-Analysis

Juan Pablo Medellín Ruiz [1,*], Jacobo Ángel Rubio-Arias [2], Vicente Javier Clemente-Suarez [3,4] and Domingo Jesús Ramos-Campo [1]

1. Sport Science Faculty, Catholic University of Murcia, 30107 Murcia, Spain; djramos@ucam.edu
2. LFE Research Group, Department of Health and Human Performance, Faculty of Physical Activity and Sport Science-INEF, Universidad Politécnica de Madrid, 28040 Madrid, Spain; ja.rubio@upm.es
3. Faculty of Sports Sciences, Universidad Europea de Madrid, 28670 Madrid, Spain; vctxente@yahoo.es
4. Grupo de Investigación en Cultura, Educación y Sociedad, Universidad de la Costa, 080002 Barranquilla, Colombia
* Correspondence: m_juanpablo9@hotmail.com

Received: 27 October 2020; Accepted: 26 November 2020; Published: 29 November 2020

Abstract: A systematic review and meta-analysis were performed to determine if heart rate variability-guided training (HRV-g), compared to predefined training (PT), maximizes the further improvement of endurance physiological and performance markers in healthy individuals. This analysis included randomized controlled trials assessing the effects of HRV-g vs. PT on endurance physiological and performance markers in untrained, physically active, and well-trained subjects. Eight articles qualified for inclusion. HRV-g training significantly improved maximum oxygen uptake (VO_2max) (MD = 2.84, CI: 1.41, 4.27; $p < 0.0001$), maximum aerobic power or speed (WMax) (SMD = 0.66, 95% CI 0.33, 0.98; $p < 0.0001$), aerobic performance (SMD = 0.71, CI 0.16, 1.25; $p = 0.01$) and power or speed at ventilatory thresholds (VT) VT1 (SMD = 0.62, CI 0.04, 1.20; $p = 0.04$) and VT2 (SMD = 0.81, CI 0.41, 1.22; $p < 0.0001$). However, HRV-g did not show significant differences in VO_2max (MD = 0.96, CI −1.11, 3.03; $p = 0.36$), WMax (SMD = 0.06, CI −0.26, 0.38; $p = 0.72$), or aerobic performance (SMD = 0.14, CI −0.22, 0.51; $p = 0.45$) in power or speed at VT1 (SMD = 0.27, 95% CI 0.16, 0.70, $p = 0.22$) or VT2 (SMD = 0.18, 95% CI −0.20, 0.57; $p = 0.35$), when compared to PT. Although HRV-based training periodization improved both physiological variables and aerobic performance, this method did not provide significant benefit over PT.

Keywords: autonomic nervous system; cardiac autonomic regulation; cardiorespiratory fitness; daily training; endurance

1. Introduction

To maximize the physical fitness of athletes, correct management of training program variables (i.e., volume, intensity, frequency, density, etc.) is needed [1]. The optimal training dosage promotes physiological adaptations and reduces the risk of injury and overtraining syndrome, finally improving athletic performance [2]. The rational distribution of training sessions would be the pillar to obtain the correct physiological modifications in athletes [3]. Therefore, several training periodization strategies have been applied to manage the training load and obtain performance enhancement [4]. However, the relationship between training stimulus and physiological responses depends on the individual and varies widely [5]. Thus, to provide correct feedback to the training process and its optimization, the physiological monitoring of the athlete's individual response to the training program plays an essential role [6]. This way, the physiological monitorization allows the correct management of the training load, according to the athlete's individual response [6].

Recently, the autonomic nervous system analysis has been commonly used to manage the training load [7,8] and the endurance training prescription [9–14]. Heart rate variability (HRV) has been widely used, since it reflects the balance between sympathetic and parasympathetic modulation, showing autonomic nervous system (ANS) regulation [15–19]. After physical exercise, the ANS decreases the sympathetic activity and produces a rapid restoration of vagal tone (parasympathetic component) that allows performance improvements [20]. However, due to the misbalance between intensity, volume, and density of training, nonfunctional training loads produce a nonfunctional overreach, promoting a reduction in vagal indices of HRV and impairing the recovery process [21]. Consequently, changes in ANS regulation, assessed by HRV, can identify the relationship between training (stress) and recovery status. Thus, HRV can support the training process as an internal load marker or a long-term monitoring indicator [2].

Lately, a systematic literature review (five randomized controlled trials) critically discussed the potential of heart rate variability-guided training (HRV-g) as an intervention to improve aerobic performance in athletes [2]. Limitations of this previous work include the analysis of the effect of HRV-g only on runners. Only in 2018 and 2019, three additional randomized controlled trials [10,11,22] using cyclists or skiers were published, representing almost half of the total number of studies that were available until then. A potential limitation of a systematic review is that it does not include a data synthesis and statistical analysis to determine the summary effect of the intervention on the outcome's measures; it implies that results obtained in the literature review [2] could be oversized without a specific statistical analysis that offers a more accurate and general picture of the HRV-guided effects on aerobic performance. This highlighted the growing interest in the HRV-guided potential and the need to conduct a large meta-analysis; hence, it is necessary to systematically analyze the effect of this type of training as an intervention to improve aerobic performance in trained and untrained participants.

The aim of this study was to perform a systematic review and meta-analysis to determine if endurance HRV-g maximizes aerobic performance and/or aerobic physiological adaptation, compared to a predefined training (PT) program.

2. Materials and Methods

2.1. Study Design

The methodological process was based on the recommendations indicated by the PRISMA (preferred reporting items for systematic review and meta-analysis) statement [23]. All phases of the meta-analysis were conducted in duplicate. For the meta-analysis, only randomized controlled trials that investigated the effects of training prescription guided by HRV on any physiological (i.e., maximum oxygen uptake—VO_2max) or aerobic performance variables (performance at VO_2max, performance at VT1 and VT2, or performance test) were considered. The study was registered in PROSPERO (International Prospective Register of Systematic Reviews) (www.crd.york.ac.uk/prospero/index.asp, identifier CRD42020204461).

2.2. Data Sources and Search Profile

A comprehensive literature search was performed using PubMed–Medline, Web of Science, and the Cochrane Library databases. The search was performed without date restriction and was completed on 15 August 2020. The following combination of terms was used: "HRV or heart rate variability", "autonomic nervous system", "parasympathetic nervous system", "cardiac autonomic regulation", and "vagal activity". The Boolean operator "AND" was used to combine these descriptors with "training guided", "training periodization", or "exercise prescription".

2.3. Data Extraction and Selection Criteria

The following inclusion criteria were considered: randomized clinical trials, studies examining the effects of endurance training prescription guided by HRV on physiological or performance variables, studies that include a control group with a PT program, studies published in English, and studies that should report information on variables in one baseline and one post-treatment measure. Conversely, studies were excluded if they were not an original fully published work, if they did not specify the tests utilized or detailed the training program, and if they did not provide numerical data.

The articles analyzed were reviewed separately by two authors (J.P.M.R. and D.J.R.C.). Studies that fulfilled the inclusion criteria were coded and recorded on an Excel spreadsheet. In addition, the substantive aspects were extracted for Table 1: authors, country, methodology, number of participants per group, age, gender, level of physical activity, and methodological aspects; similarly, for Table 2: HRV variable, decision-making algorithm, volume, intensity distribution, frequency, load, and duration of the experiment. Finally, pre- and post-intervention means and the standard deviation of the studies included in the quantitative analysis were recorded.

2.4. Outcomes

The primary outcome was VO_2max. The secondary outcomes analyzed were (1) maximum aerobic power or speed (WMax) as a performance indicator in the VO_2max, (2) aerobic performance as an extrapolated value from a field test (i.e., 40 km time trial, 3 and 5 km running test), and (3) power or velocity at VT1 (WVT1) and VT2 (WVT2) as the performance variables at those points.

2.5. Evaluation of the Methodology of the Studies Selected

The methodological quality of the selected studies was assessed with the Cochrane risk-of-bias tool [24] that includes the following parameters: (1) random sequence generation (selection bias), (2) allocation concealment (selection bias), (3) blinding of participants and personnel (performance bias), (4) blinding of outcome assessment (detection bias), (5) incomplete outcome data (attrition bias), (6) selective reporting (reporting bias), and (7) other bias. For each study, each item was described as having either a low, an unclear, or a high risk of bias. In addition, the Egger's test was used to assess publication bias.

2.6. Data Synthesis and Statistical Analysis

The meta-analysis and the statistical analysis were conducted using the Review Manager software (RevMan 5.2; Cochrane Collaboration, Oxford, UK). A random-effects model was applied to determine the effect of endurance training prescription guided by HRV on physiological or performance variables. The effects of training on these outcomes between HRV-g and PT groups were expressed as mean differences (MD) or standard mean differences (SMD) and their 95% confidence intervals (CI). The inverse of variance model was used for the analysis. The heterogeneity between the studies was evaluated through the I^2 statistic and between-study variance, using the tau-square (τ^2) [25]. The I^2 values between 30 and 60% were considered as moderate levels of heterogeneity. Additionally, a value of τ^2 more than one suggests the presence of substantial statistical heterogeneity. The publication bias was evaluated through an asymmetry test as estimated from a funnel plot. A p value of less than 0.05 was considered to be statistically significant.

3. Results

3.1. General Characteristics of the Studies

A total of 849 studies were identified from the databases and no items were included from other sources. After removing duplicated articles from the different databases, 605 titles and abstracts were screened, 593 were excluded, and 12 were screened as full texts. Finally, statistical analysis was performed on 8 studies [9–12,22,26–28] (Figure 1).

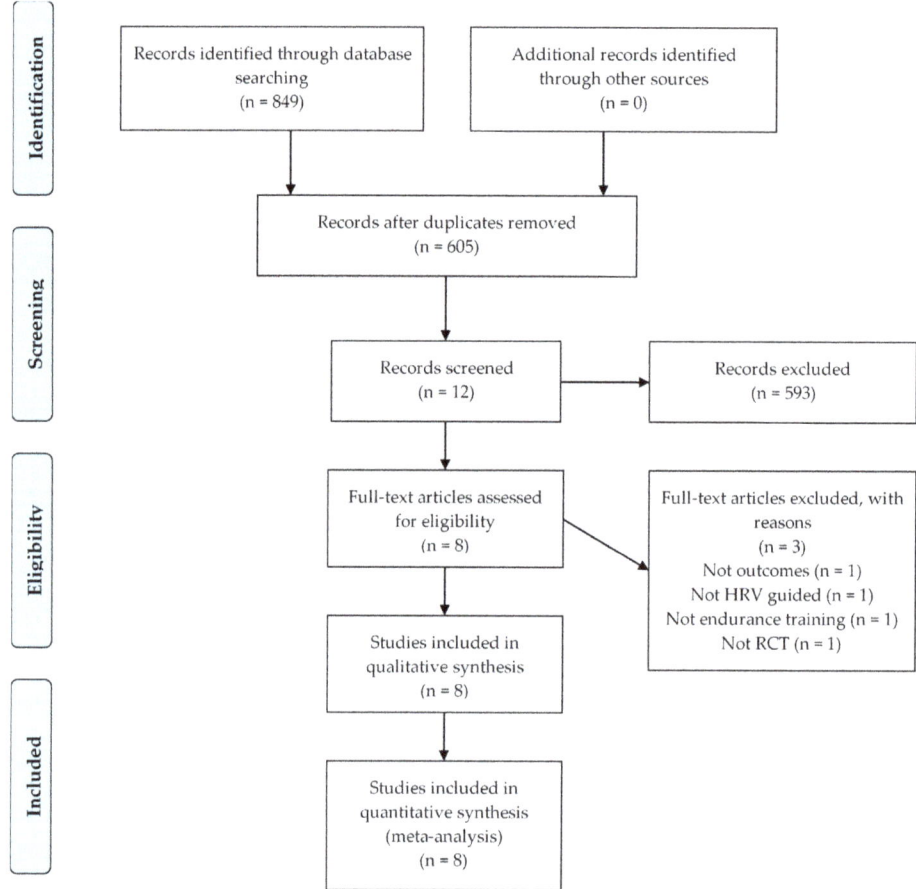

Figure 1. PRISMA flow diagram for studies included.

Table 1 provides an overview of the participants' characteristics of the studies included in the quantitative analysis. The total participants was 190 (males and females), mostly trained or active subjects. The mean age ranged from 20.5 ± 1.3 to 39.2 ± 5.3 years (men: 21.8 ± 0.3 to 39.2 ± 5.3; women: from 20.5 ± 1.3 to 35.0 ± 7.0). Training experience was reported in some articles and it ranged from 11.3 ± 3 to 15.0 ± 8 years. In addition, VO_2max values were between 35.0 ± 5.0 and 66.7 ± 5.9 mL/kg/min.

Table 1. Characteristics of the studies included in the meta-analysis.

Study, Year of Publication	Country of the Study	Groups	n	Type of Athletes	Sex	Age (Years)
Da Silva et al. [28]	Canada	HRV-g	15	Untrained	Females	25.8 ± 3.1
		PT	15			27.7 ± 3.6
Javaloyes et al. [11]	Spain	HRV-g	9	Trained cyclist	Males	39.2 ± 5.3
		PT (TP)	8			37.6 ± 7.1
Javaloyes et al. [10]	Spain	HRV-g	8	Trained cyclist	Not specified	28.1 ± 13.2
		PT (BP)	7			30.8 ± 10.5
Kiviniemi et al. [27]	Finland	HRV-g-I	14	Actives	50% Males	♂35 ± 4 ♀33 ± 4
		HRV-g-II	10		Females	35 ± 4.0
		PT	14		50% Males	♂37 ± 3 ♀34 ± 4
Kiviniemi et al. [9]	Finland	HRV-g	8	Recreational endurance runners	Males	31 ± 6.0
		PT (TP)	9			32 ± 5.0
Nuuttila et al. [12]	Finland	HRV-g	13	Endurance trained	Males	29.0 ± 4.0
		PT (BP)	11			31.0 ± 5.0
Schmitt et al. [22]	France	HRV-g +SH	9	Elite Nordic skiers	M = 7; W = 2	M = 22.9 ± 4.3; W = 20.5 ± 0.7
		PT+SH	9		M = 6; W = 3	M = 21.8 ± 1.3; W = 24.3 ± 4.9
Vesterinen et al. [26]	Finland	HRV-g	13	Recreational endurance runners *	M = 10; W = 10	M = 34 ± 8.0
		PT (TP)	18		M = 10; W = 10	W = 35 ± 7.0

M = men; W = women; SH = sleeping in hypoxia; BP: block periodization; TP: training periodization. * There were 9 dropouts, gender is not specified.

The intervention programs were eight weeks long [10–12,26–28], except for Kiviniemi et al. [9] (four weeks) and Schmitt et al. [22] (15 days); the frequency of training was between 3 to 6.3 sessions per week. Regarding the distribution of time by intensity zones, the studies that reported these variables ranged from 49 to 84% in zone 1, from 12 to 39% in zone 2, and from 3 to 13% in zone 3 [10–12,26]. The predominant method of analysis for HRV monitoring was time domain, followed by frequency domain. Remarkably, only one study used nonlinear measures (Table 2).

Table 2. Characteristics of the training intervention of studies included in the meta-analysis.

	Group	Type of HRV-g	Duration	Training Distribution (% Time)			Training Volume (Hours)	Training Volume (km)	Training Frequency	Training Load
				Z1	Z2	Z3				
Da Silva et al. [28]	HRV-g	Ref: 10-day average rMSSD. If rMSSD < mean rMSSD-1SD: MT; If not: HIT	8 weeks	-	-	-	-	-	3	-
	PT								3	
Javaloyes et al. [11]	HRV-g	SWC of rMSSD7D: If rMSSD7D outside the SWC: low intensity or rest	8 weeks	66	24	10	9.3 ± 2.8	-	-	-
	PT (TP)			64	27	9	8.8 ± 2.8			
Javaloyes et al. [10]	HRV-g	SWC of rMSSD7D: If rMSSD7D outside the SWC: low intensity or rest	8 weeks	49	39	12	11.1 ± 3.1	-	-	1033.3 ± 312.5 a.u.
	PT (BP)			54	33	13	11.4 ± 3.1			1028.8 ± 214.5 a.u.
Kiviniemi et al. [27]	HRV-g-I	Ref: 10-day average SD1. HRV-I: If SD1 ≥ SD1 ref:VG; SD1 ↓ SD SD1 ref:MD; If SD1 ↓ 2 consecutive days: rest; HRV-II = HRV-I but only VT if SD1 > SD1 ref.	8 weeks							♂515 ± 49 ♀390 ± 42 TRIMPS × week
	HRV-g-II								5.0 ± 0.3	314 ± 46 TRIMPS × week
	PT								♂5.3 ± 0.6 ♀5.0 ± 0.8	♂492 ± 91 ♀343 ± 107 TRIMPS × week
Kiviniemi et al. [9]	HRV-g	Ref: 10-day average HF power. If HF > HF ref ↓ load; If HF ↓ 2 consecutive days: rest	4 weeks	-	-	-	-	36 ± 4	-	463 ± 74 TRIMPS × week
	PT (TP)							38 ± 6		529 ± 49 TRIMPS × week
Nuuttila et al. [12]	HRV-g	LIT if QRT was higher than ref	8 weeks	82 ± 8	15 ± 6	3 ± 3	5.7 ± 2.1	-	6.3 ± 1.4	-
	PT (BP)			84 ± 7	12 ± 5	4 ± 3	6.0 ± 1.9		6.1 ± 0.4	
Schmitt et al. [22]	HRV-g+SH	If HF ↑ or →: ↑ load; If HF ↓ ≥30%: ↓ load; If HF ↓ 2 consecutive days: rest	15 days	-	-	-	-	-	-	3365 ± 425 a.u.
	PT+SH									3481 ± 179 a.u.
Vesterinen et al. [26]	HRV-g	SWC of rMSSD7D: If rMSSD7D outside the SWC: low intensity or rest	8 weeks	83 ± 27	14 ± 25	3 ± 5	6.5 ± 2.8	42 ± 22	6.1 ± 1.8	-
	PT (TP)			84 ± 12	13 ± 10	3 ± 4	6.3 ± 2.5	41 ± 20	5.6 ± 1.6	

a.u.: arbitrary units; HF: high frequencies; HIT: high-intensity training; MT: moderate training; Ref: reference; rMSSD: root of the mean squared differences of successive R-R-intervals; rMSSD7D: 7-day rolling average of vagal-mediated square; QRT: quick recovery test using rMSSD; SWC: smallest worthwhile change; TRIMPS: training impact; VT: vigorous training.

3.2. Heterogeneity and Risk of Bias Assessment

Risk of bias assessment is shown in Figure 2. The high risk of bias specified that none of the studies blinded the participants (performance bias) or the evaluators (detection bias). Visual inspection of the funnel plots showed an absence of asymmetry. Moreover, the Egger test demonstrated an absence of significant asymmetry in PT and HRV-g in VO$_2$max (PT: −0.369, $p = 0.712$; HRV-g: −0.752, $p = 0.452$), WMax (PT: −0.539, $p = 0.590$; HRV-g: 0.103, $p = 0.918$), Performance (PT: −0.273, $p = 0.785$; HRV-g: −0.07, $p = 0.944$), WVT1 (PT: 0.095, $p = 0.924$; HRV-g: 1.898, $p = 0.058$), and WVT2 (PT: 1.542, $p = 0.123$; HRV-g: 1.598, $p = 0.110$) (Figure 3).

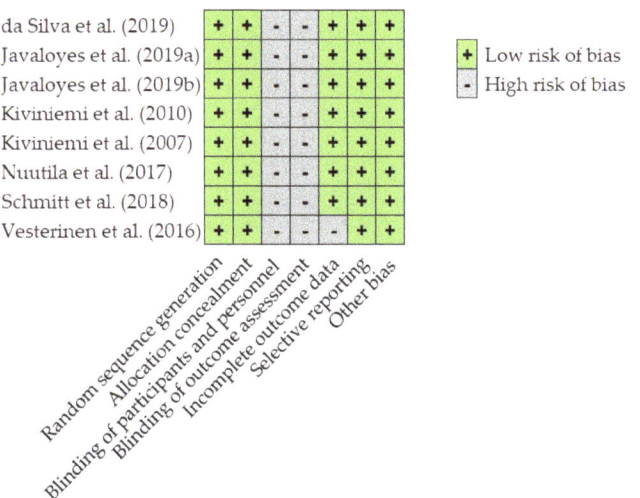

Figure 2. Risk of bias in the included randomized controlled trials.

3.3. Meta-Analyses

Regarding cardiorespiratory fitness, a significant improvement in VO$_2$max in participants who trained using HRV-g (MD = 2.84, 95% CI 1.41, 4.27; $p < 0.0001$) and PT (MD = 1.80, 95% CI 0.24, 3.36; $p = 0.02$) was found after training (Figure 4a). Thus, HRV-g and PT led to a significant increase in maximum aerobic power or speed (HRV-g: SMD = 0.66, 95% CI 0.33, 0.98; $p < 0.0001$, PT: SMD = 0.48, 95% CI 0.12, 0.83; $p = 0.009$) (Figure 5a) after training. Moreover, aerobic performance increased after HRV-g (SMD = 0.71, 95% CI 0.16, 1.25; $p = 0.01$) and PT programs (SMD = 0.47, 95% CI 0.07, 0.86; $p = 0.02$) (Figure 6a); however, no significant differences in training were observed for VO$_2$max (MD = 0.96, 95% CI −1.11, 3.03; $p = 0.36$), maximum aerobic power or speed (SMD=0.06, 95% CI −0.26, 0.38; $p = 0.72$), or aerobic performance (SMD = 0.14, 95% CI −0.22, 0.51; $p = 0.45$) (Figure 4b, Figure 5b, and Figure 6b, respectively).

Concerning power or speed at VT1 and VT2, performance at VT1 increased significantly after HRV-g programs (SMD = 0.62, 95% CI 0.04, 1.20; $p = 0.04$) but not after PT (SMD = 0.17, 95% CI −0.25, 0.59; $p = 0.42$) (Figure 7a). In addition, performance at VT2 improved significantly after HRV-g (SMD = 0.81, 95% CI 0.41, 1.22; $p < 0.0001$) and PT (SMD = 0.53, 95% CI 0.13, 0.93; $p = 0.009$) training programs (Figure 8a). Nevertheless, no significant differences were observed between both training methods in performance at VT1 (SMD = 0.27, 95% CI −0.16, 0.70; $p = 0.22$) and VT2 (SMD = 0.18, 95% CI −0.20, 0.57; $p = 0.35$) (Figures 7b and 8b, respectively).

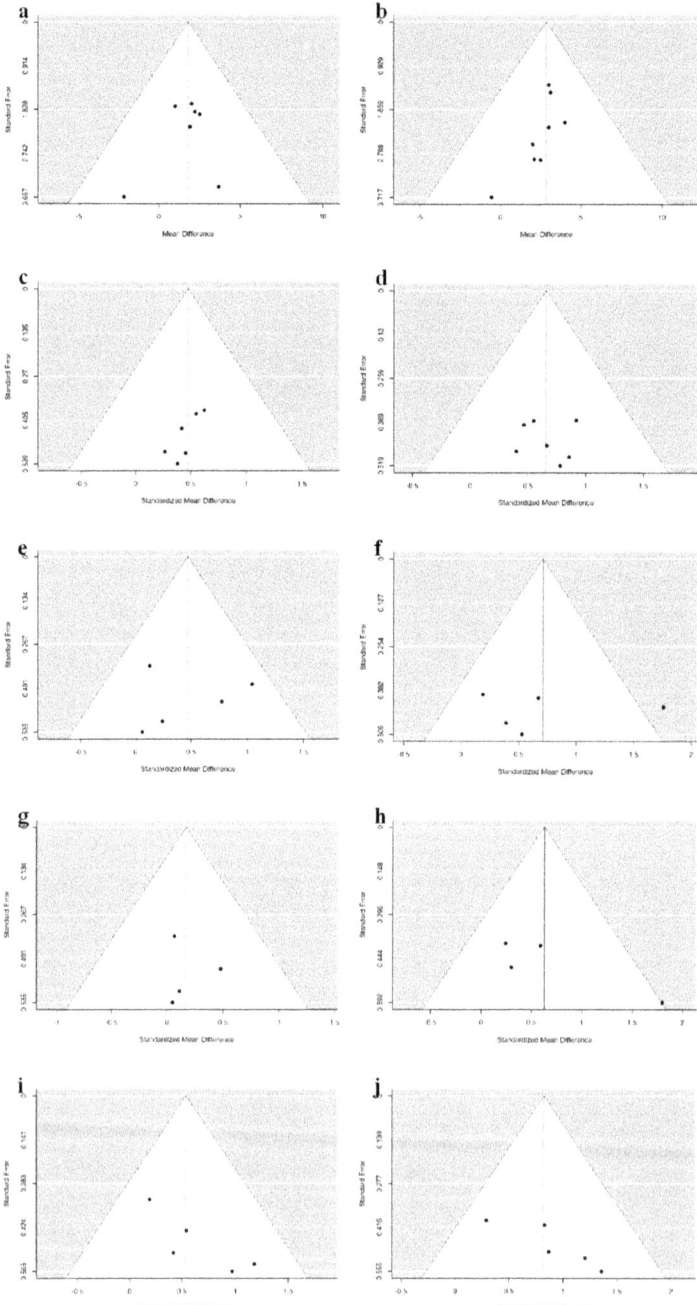

Figure 3. Test for funnel plot asymmetry. (**a**) VO$_2$max PT; (**b**) VO$_2$max HRV-g; (**c**) WMax PT; (**d**) WMax HRV-g; (**e**) Performance PT; (**f**) Performance HRV-g; (**g**) WVT1 PT; (**h**) WVT1 HRV-g; (**i**) WVT2 PT; (**j**) WVT2 HRV-g.

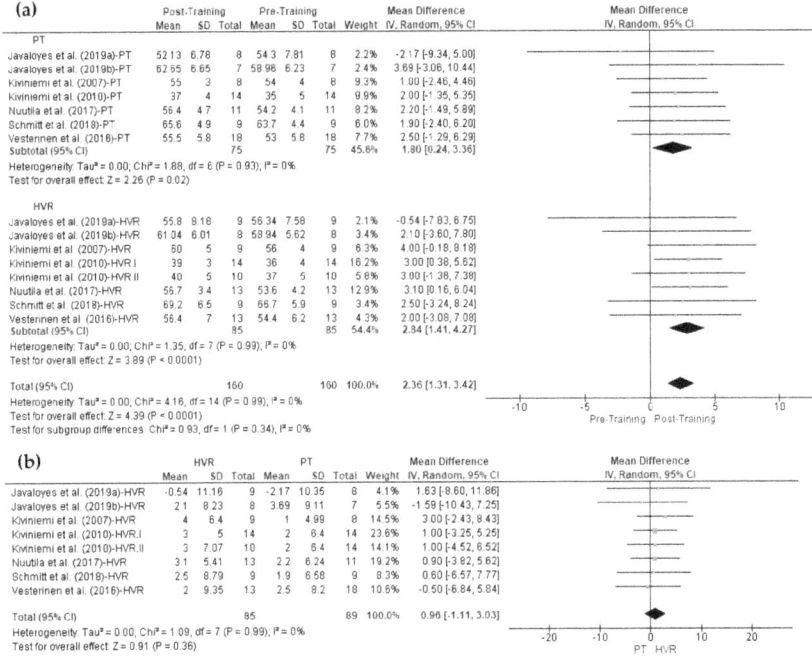

Figure 4. (a) Effects of endurance training on VO$_2$max pre-training vs. post-training; (b) effects of endurance training on VO$_2$max HRV-g vs. PT.

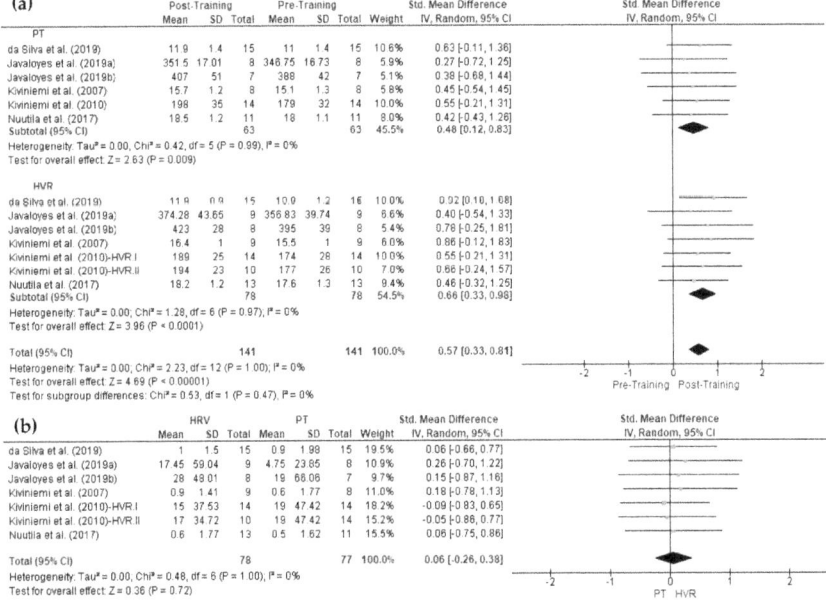

Figure 5. (a) Effects of endurance training on WMax pre-training vs. post-training; (b) effects of endurance training on WMax HRV-g vs. PT.

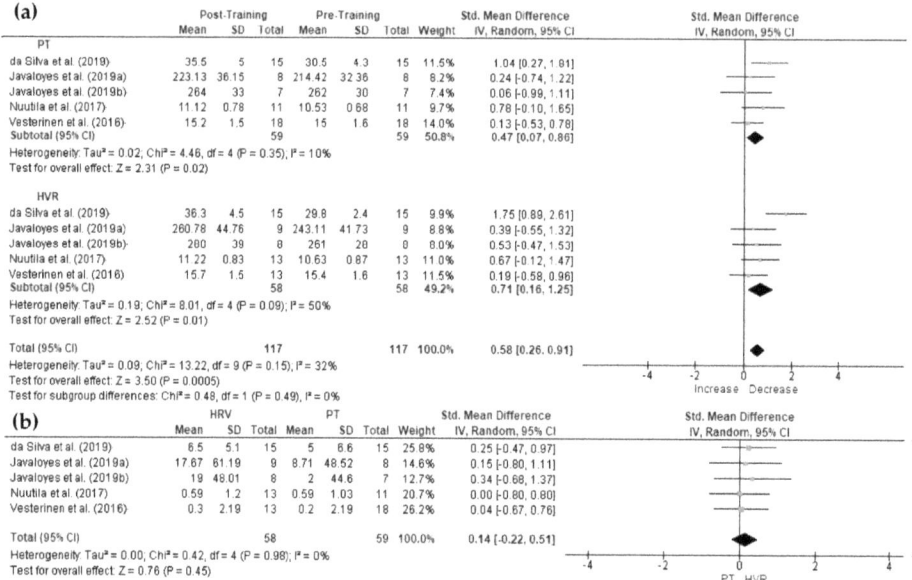

Figure 6. (a) Effects of endurance training on aerobic performance pre-training vs. post-training; (b) effects of endurance training on aerobic performance HRV-g vs. PT.

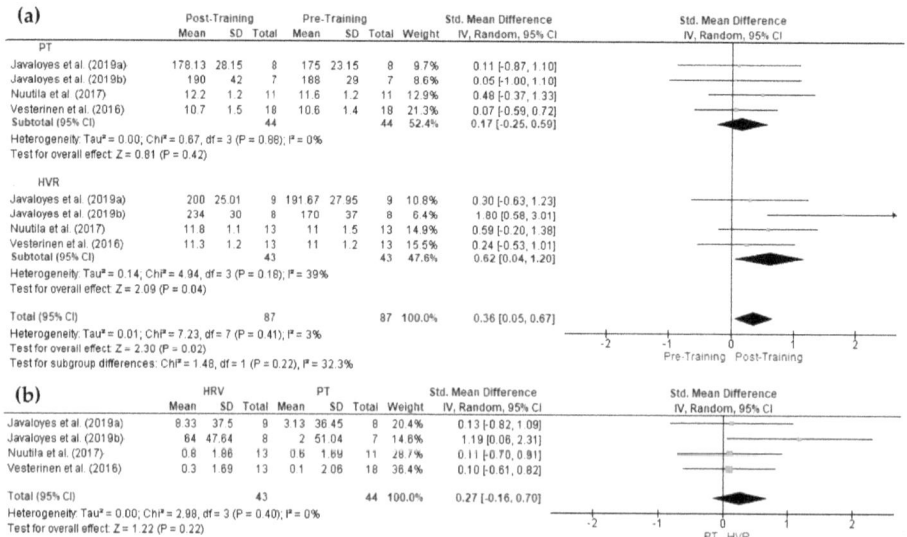

Figure 7. (a) Effects of endurance training on WVT1 pre-training vs. post-training; (b) effects of endurance training on WVT1 HRV-g vs. PT.

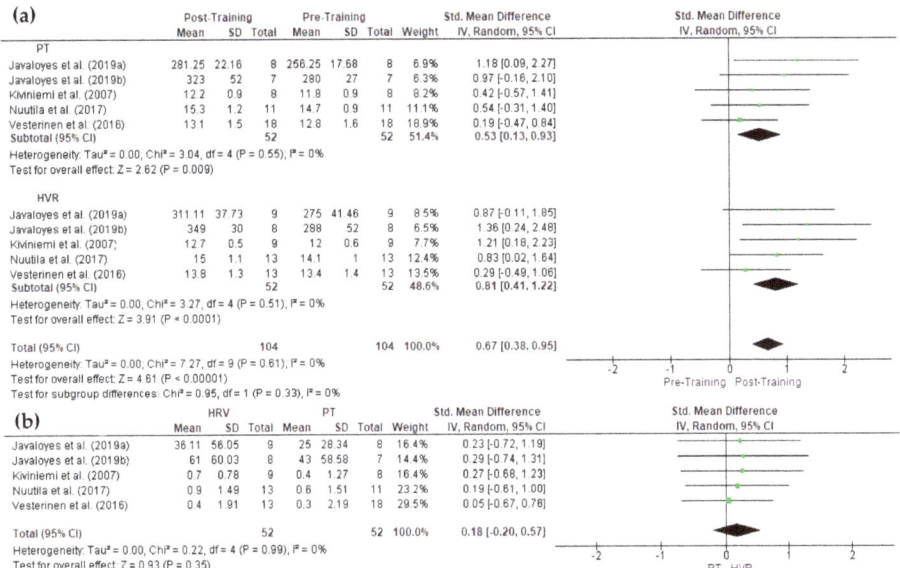

Figure 8. (a) Effects of endurance training on WVT2 pre-training vs. post-training; (b) effects of endurance training on WVT2 HRV-g vs. PT.

4. Discussion

This systematic review with meta-analysis aimed to determine if endurance HRV-g maximizes aerobic performance and/or aerobic physiological adaptation, compared to a PT program. The major findings indicate that HRV-g significantly improves VO_2max, maximum aerobic power or speed, performance at VT1 and VT2, and aerobic performance in running or cycling field test; however, these adaptations were not significantly greater than PT programs. Although these findings do not appear to support the use of HRV-g over PT programs, this study also highlights notable differences in the methodologies used between studies, which may impact the potential efficacy of HRV-g. Despite that both forms of training promote physiological adaptations and improve performance, most parameters related to aerobic performance and aerobic physiological indexes were improved further following HRV-based training.

One of the key physiological variables that determines endurance performance is VO_2max [29], showing that high-level endurance athletes can achieve a large VO_2max [10]. Therefore, a common aim of endurance training programs is to improve VO_2max. This way, it was found how both training programs significantly increase cardiorespiratory fitness (VO_2max) (HRV-g: MD = 2.84, $p < 0.0001$; ~5%) and PT (MD = 1.80, $p = 0.02$; ~3%). It could be assumed that both types of training models led to improvements in VO_2max, because there were no significant differences between PT and HRV-g ($p = 0.36$); but some factors could modulate the results obtained. Hence, the intensity training distribution and the fitness level of participants could play a key role in the VO_2max improvements. Although VO_2max has been improved in untrained [30], recreational [9,26], and trained athletes [10,22], the trainability and the increase of this parameter are limited in trained athletes [11]; specifically, only one study did not find an increase in VO_2max [11] and, remarkably, it used a trained cyclist sample. In addition, the intensity training distribution used by Javaloyes et al. [11] was a pyramidal distribution (~60% VT1, 30% VT2, 10% VO_2max).

In another study [26] with low fitness level (recreational athletes), participants spent much more time in zone 1 (below VT1) (~80% of total training program) and less time in zone 3 (VO_2max or higher) (~3% of total training program). While only one study found an improvement in VO_2max with trained athletes [10], that study applied an intensity distribution with a pyramidal distribution (~52% VT1, 35% VT2, 13% VO$_2$max). Thus, it seems that high intensity training (Z3) has to be higher in trained athletes than in untrained or recreational athletes; it is a fact that new periodization models are highlighted and defined as a crucial factor to increase athletes' performance [3,4]. For this reason, the use of HRV-g training could optimize the improvement in VO$_2$max (as the trend to higher increases in this training condition have shown; $p = 0.36$), because if the high-intensity training is individualized and it is performed when the athlete is in optimal autonomic homeostasis, it could lead to an improved adaptive response to training [11].

Regarding aerobic performance measured by field test and maximum aerobic power or speed, both training programs led to a similar increase. Nevertheless, one of the characteristics of the HRV-g is the individualization of the training, making this strategy less variable, with fewer nonresponders than PT programs. For example, Vesterinen et al. [26] found that the HRV-g had lower dispersion of results in a 3000 m test (−1 to +6%) than the PT group (−4 to +8%). Similarly, Javaloyes et al. [10,11] reported less variation in their two studies of 40 km time trial following HRV-based training, compared to PT program. Therefore, participants have a greater probability to increase their aerobic performance and reduce the risk of injury and overtraining by following a day-to-day training based on HRV-g. Additionally, in some of the studies included in the present review, the number of high-intensity training sessions of the participants in HRV-g programs varied according to the individual's recovery response of HRV. For example, the number of high-intensity training (HIT) sessions ranged from 11 to 21 in PT and from 5 to 24 sessions in the HRV-g program of Vesterinen et al. [26]. Although previous research reported a nonsignificant correlation between the training adaptation and the number of HIT sessions [26], this finding suggests that the use of HRV-g to manage the inclusion of a HIT session in the program could increase the effectiveness of the training and could diminish the variation in the adaptation.

Regarding performance (power or speed) at VT, results showed that WVT1 increased in the HRV-g but not in the PT; hence, performance at VT2 improved significantly after HRV-g and PT programs. Furthermore, the meta-analysis showed a trend towards higher WVT1 ($p = 0.22$; Δ 13%) and WVT2 ($p = 0.35$; Δ 10%) improvements after HRV-g than PT (Δ 2.2%; Δ 7%, respectively). These statistical trends that showed greater effects for HRV-g than PT were in line with the results reported by the studies included in the present review [11,12,31,32]. Some possible reasons to explain these findings could be related to the aforementioned training intensity distribution developed by each training group, which could affect the results.

In some of the studies included, HRV-g led to a lower proportion of moderate and greater intensity training (as did HIT), in comparison to PT [11]; while in another study, higher moderate intensity training was performed by HRV-g, compared to the PT [10]. Besides, as it was explained above, the individualization and adjustment of the training load by HRV-g reduced the number of nonresponders to training, increasing the number of athletes that improved their VT1 and VT2. Therefore, HRV, as a monitoring tool, would allow taking the principle of individualization of the load a step further.

Notably, the main findings of the present meta-analysis reported that the aerobic performance and aerobic physiological adaptations after HRV-g are not significantly greater than those observed after the PT, and only some trends were found. It could be considered that the HRV-g program, in comparison to the PT, may have a small impact, or some confounding variables may adjust its magnitude. This way, the duration of the training program is one variable to emphasize. It seems that the length needed to achieve meaningful increases in performance using the HRV-g training program could be shorter than the PT, due to the individualized training and the greater training quality, but the duration of the published studies (all of them with less than eight weeks) seems to be very short to obtain a significant difference. Therefore, longitudinal randomized controlled trials, using programs with more duration, are needed to obtain more conclusive results.

The HRV measurement protocol applied in each study included in the present review is another factor to highlight. Different variables to assess HRV were found: (a) time domain variables (root mean square of successive differences of RR intervals—rMSSD) [10,11,26,28]; (b) frequency domain variables (high frequency—HF, low frequency—LF) [9,22]; and (c) nonlinear variables (standard deviation of the intervals to the transverse diameter (short axis) of the ellipse—SD1) [27]. Therefore, frequency domain variables identify some types of fatigue [33], whereas rMSSD has been suggested as a global fatigue measurement [34]. In addition, the HRV assessment ranged from ultrashort records of 90 s [10,11] to 15 min [22], depending on the HRV variables analyzed. Thus, recording time shorter than five minutes was applied if the study used rMMSD as an indicator, while longer records were reported if the study used a frequency-based or a nonlinear variable [35,36]. Moreover, frequency domain variables were more influenced by breathing patterns than time-domain analysis [37]; there were divergencies in the participants measurement postures that included sitting [28], supine lying [10–12,26], standing, or a combination of some of them (lying + standing [22]; sitting + standing [9,27]). It seems that the supine position measures showed lower daily coefficient of variation than standing measures [38], but a standing position was recommended previously [2]. Therefore, the posture differences could also affect the HRV results obtained in the studies and, consequently, to the present meta-analysis.

There are several limitations in this meta-analysis related to the available randomized controlled trials (RCTs) and the divergent methodologies employed, including (i) the small number of studies; (ii) the different intensity training distribution, training programs, and modalities applied in the studies; (iii) the lack of systematic information about the training load performed in most of the study; (iv) the different methodologies applied to assess HRV; (v) the small number of studies using trained athletes to obtain a more specific picture about the effect of this type of training in this population; and (vi) the lack of longer studies to analyze the chronic effect of HRV-g (the duration of the studies was <8 weeks). Additionally, readers should take into consideration that the sport modality (running, cycling, or skiing) can influence the aerobic enhancement and this fact could modify the results obtained in the present review. In addition, it was found that the available evidence has high risk of bias primarily due to the low quality of available RCTs. Therefore, to develop further studies with a better-quality design, and before a more comprehensive training trend, trained athletes' samples are needed in order to analyze the effect of longer interventions (>8 weeks).

According to the results obtained in the present study, while no significant benefits were observed for HRV-g compared with PT, small effects were evident in the larger increases in aerobic performance and physiological adaptations following HRV-g. This suggests that some individuals may benefit more from HRV-g compared with PT, which would be important in well-trained athletic cohorts, where small changes in physical attributes are difficult to achieve and the individualization of the training plays a key role. Further research is required to investigate these responses in more detail, but it appears that the efficacy of HRV-g strategies have been affected by large variations in the structure of the training program (intensity distribution, duration, volume, etc.) performed and the methodology used to assess HRV. Hence, practitioners and coaches must use HRV with caution, due to the factors that affect its measurement. In terms of practical applications, HRV assessment should be carried out daily in the morning, standing or lying in a supine position, in a standardized condition (e.g., with an empty urinary bladder and spontaneous breathing) and using a validated sensor to assess HRV. In addition, it seems that the rMSSD should be the indicator of HRV, since it produces fewer disturbances in the athlete's daily routine and has several advantages, such as its quick and easy accessibility, and the lower sensitivity for the breathing pattern in comparison with spectral variables.

5. Conclusions

The current systematic review with meta-analysis concludes that HRV-g produces significant improvements in endurance performance and aerobic physiological adaptations. However, these adaptations are not significantly higher than in PT. Nevertheless, the findings from this meta-analysis are likely affected by the divergent methodologies employed in studies, specifically, in the HRV assessment, the training program, and the participant's characteristics. Therefore, the results of this meta-analysis reinforce the importance of additional detailed studies to analyze the effects of this novel training method.

Author Contributions: Conceptualization, D.J.R.-C. and J.Á.R.-A.; methodology, J.P.M.R.; formal analysis, D.J.R.-C. and J.Á.R.-A.; investigation, J.P.M.R.; resources, J.Á.R.-A.; data curation, J.Á.R.-A.; writing—original draft preparation, J.P.M.R., D.J.R.-C. and V.J.C.-S.; writing—review and editing, D.J.R.-C., J.Á.R.-A. and V.J.C.-S; supervision, D.J.R.-C. All authors have read and agreed to the published version of the manuscript.

Funding: This research received no external funding.

Conflicts of Interest: The authors declare no conflict of interest.

References

1. Clemente-Suárez, V.J.; Delgado-Moreno, R.; González, B.; Ortega, J.; Ramos-Campo, D.J. Amateur endurance triathletes' performance is improved independently of volume or intensity based training. *Physiol. Behav.* **2019**, *205*, 2–8. [CrossRef]
2. Düking, P.; Zinner, C.; Reed, J.L.; Holmberg, H.; Sperlich, B. Predefined vs. data guided training prescription based on autonomic nervous system variation: A systematic review. *Scand. J. Med. Sci. Sport.* **2020**, *30*, 2291–2304. [CrossRef]
3. Martín, J.P.G.; Clemente-Suárez, V.J.; Ramos-Campo, D.J. Hematological and running performance modification of trained athletes after reverse vs. block training periodization. *Int. J. Environ. Res. Public Health* **2020**, *17*, 4825. [CrossRef]
4. Clemente-Suarez, V.J.; Ramos-Campo, D.J. Effectiveness of reverse vs. traditional linear training periodization in triathlon. *Int. J. Environ. Res. Public Health* **2019**, *16*, 2807. [CrossRef] [PubMed]
5. Roos, L.; Taube, W.; Brandt, M.; Heyer, L.; Wyss, T. Monitoring of daily training load and training load responses in endurance sports: What do coaches want? *Schweiz. Z. Sportmed. Sporttraumatol.* **2013**, *61*, 30–36.
6. Halson, S.L. Monitoring training load to understand fatigue in athletes. *Sport. Med.* **2014**, *44*, 139–147. [CrossRef]
7. Achten, J.; Jeukendrup, A.E. Heart rate monitoring: Applications and limitations. *Sport. Med.* **2003**, *33*, 517–538. [CrossRef]
8. Bourdon, P.C.; Cardinale, M.; Murray, A.; Gastin, P.; Kellmann, M.; Varley, M.C.; Gabbett, T.J.; Coutts, A.J.; Burgess, D.J.; Gregson, W.; et al. Monitoring athlete training loads: Consensus statement. *Int. J. Sport. Physiol. Perform.* **2017**, *12*, 161–170. [CrossRef]
9. Kiviniemi, A.M.; Hautala, A.J.; Kinnunen, H.; Tulppo, M.P. Endurance training guided individually by daily heart rate variability measurements. *Eur. J. Appl. Physiol.* **2007**, *101*, 743–751. [CrossRef]
10. Javaloyes, A.; Sarabia, J.M.; Lamberts, R.P.; Plews, D.; Moya-Ramon, M. Training prescription guided by heart rate variability vs. block periodization in welltrained cyclists. *J. Strength Cond. Res.* **2019**, *34*, 1511–1518. [CrossRef]
11. Javaloyes, A.; Sarabia, J.M.; Lamberts, R.P.; Moya-Ramon, M. Training prescription guided by heart-rate variability in cycling. *Int. J. Sport. Physiol. Perform.* **2019**, *14*, 23–32. [CrossRef]
12. Nuuttila, O.P.; Nikander, A.; Polomoshnov, D.; Laukkanen, J.A.; Häkkinen, K. Effects of HRV-guided vs. predetermined block training on performance, HRV and serum hormones. *Int. J. Sport. Med.* **2017**, *38*, 909–920. [CrossRef]
13. Botek, M.; McKune, A.J.; Krejci, J.; Stejskal, P.; Gaba, A. Change in performance in response to training load adjustment based on autonomic activity. *Int. J. Sport. Med.* **2014**, *35*, 482–488. [CrossRef] [PubMed]
14. Carrasco-Poyatos, M.; González-Quílez, A.; Martínez-González-moro, I.; Granero-Gallegos, A. HRV-guided training for professional endurance athletes: A protocol for a cluster-randomized controlled trial. *Int. J. Environ. Res. Public Health* **2020**, *17*, 5465. [CrossRef]
15. Clemente-Suarez, V.J. Periodized training achieves better autonomic modulation and aerobic performance than non-periodized training. *J. Sport. Med. Phys. Fitness* **2018**, *58*, 1559–1564. [CrossRef]
16. Aubert, A.E.; Seps, B.; Beckers, F. Heart rate variability in athletes. *Sport. Med.* **2003**, *33*, 889–919. [CrossRef]

17. Yanlin, C.; Fei, H.; Shengjia, X. Training variables and autonomic nervous system adaption. *Chin. J. Tissue Eng. Res. Zhongguo Zu Zhi Gong Cheng Yan Jiu* **2020**, *24*, 312–319. [CrossRef]
18. Buchheit, M.; Chivot, A.; Parouty, J.; Mercier, D.; Al Haddad, H.; Laursen, P.B.; Ahmaidi, S. Monitoring endurance running performance using cardiac parasympathetic function. *Eur. J. Appl. Physiol.* **2010**, *108*, 1153–1167. [CrossRef]
19. Camm, A.J.; Malik, M.; Bigger, J.T.; Breithardt, G.; Cerutti, S.; Cohen, R.J.; Coumel, P.; Fallen, E.L.; Kennedy, H.L.; Kleiger, R.E.; et al. Heart rate variability: Standards of measurement, physiological interpretation, and clinical use. Task Force of the European society of cardiology and the North American society of pacing and electrophysiology. *Eur. Heart J.* **1996**, *17*, 1043–1065. [CrossRef]
20. Palak, K.; Furgała, A.; Biel, P.; Szyguła, Z.; Thor, P.J. Influence of physical training on the function of Autonomic nervous system in professional swimmers. *Med. Sport.* **2013**, *17*, 119–124. [CrossRef]
21. Buchheit, M. Monitoring training status with HR measures: Do all roads lead to Rome? *Front. Physiol.* **2014**, *5*, 73. [CrossRef]
22. Schmitt, L.; Willis, S.J.; Fardel, A.; Coulmy, N.; Millet, G.P. Live high–train low guided by daily heart rate variability in elite Nordic-skiers. *Eur. J. Appl. Physiol.* **2018**, *118*, 419–428. [CrossRef]
23. Liberati, A.; Altman, D.G.; Tetzlaff, J.; Mulrow, C.; Gøtzsche, P.C.; Ioannidis, J.P.; Clarke, M.; Devereaux, P.J.; Kleijnen, J.; Moher, D.; et al. The PRISMA statement for reporting systematic reviews and meta-analyses of studies that evaluate health care interventions: Explanation and elaboration. *J. Clin. Epidemiol.* **2009**, *62*, e1–e34. [CrossRef]
24. Higgins, J.P.; Altman, D.G.; Gøtzsche, P.C.; Jüni, P.; Moher, D.; Oxman, A.D.; Savović, J.; Schulz, K.F.; Weeks, L.; Sterne, J.A.; et al. The Cochrane collaboration's tool for assessing risk of bias in randomised trials. *BMJ* **2011**, *343*, 5928. [CrossRef]
25. Higgins, J.P.; Thompson, S.G.; Deeks, J.J.; Altman, D.G. Measuring inconsistency in meta-analyses. *BMJ* **2003**, *327*, 557. [CrossRef]
26. Vesterinen, V.; Nummela, A.; Heikura, I.; Laine, T.; Hynynen, E.; Botella, J.; Häkkinen, K. Individual endurance training prescription with heart rate variability. *Med. Sci. Sport. Exerc.* **2016**, *48*, 1347–1354. [CrossRef]
27. Kiviniemi, A.M.; Hautala, A.J.; Kinnunen, H.; Nissilä, J.; Virtanen, P.; Karjalainen, J.; Tulppo, M.P. Daily exercise prescription on the basis of hr variability among men and women. *Med. Sci. Sport. Exerc.* **2010**, *42*, 1355–1363. [CrossRef]
28. Da Silva, D.F.; Ferraro, Z.M.; Adamo, K.B.; Machado, F.A. Endurance running training individually guided by HRV in ultrained women. *J. Strength Cond. Res.* **2019**, *33*, 736–746. [CrossRef]
29. Frandsen, J.; Vest, S.D.; Larsen, S.; Dela, F.; Helge, J.W. Maximal fat oxidation is related to performance in an ironman triathlon. *Int. J. Sport. Med.* **2017**, *38*, 975–982. [CrossRef]
30. Tamburs, N.Y.; Rebelo, A.C.S.; Cesar, M.D.C.; Catai, A.M.; Takahashi, A.C.D.M.; Andrade, C.P.; Porta, A.; Silva, E.D. Relationship between heart rate variability and VO_2 peak in active women. *Rev. Bras. Med. Esporte* **2014**, *20*, 354–358. [CrossRef]
31. Vesterinen, V.; Hakkinen, K.; Hynynen, E.; Mikkola, J.; Hokka, L.; Nummela, A. Heart rate variability in prediction of individual adaptation to endurance training in recreational endurance runners. *Scand. J. Med. Sci. Sport.* **2013**, *23*, 171–180. [CrossRef]
32. Kiviniemi, A.M.; Tulppo, M.P.; Eskelinen, J.J.; Savolainen, A.M.; Kapanen, J.; Heinonen, I.H.A.; Hautala, A.J.; Hannukainen, J.C.; Kalliokoski, K.K. Autonomic function predicts fitness response to short-term high-intensity interval training. *Int. J. Sport. Med.* **2015**, *36*, 915–921. [CrossRef]
33. Schmitt, L.; Regnard, J.; Parmentier, A.L.; Mauny, F.; Mourot, L.; Coulmy, N.; Millet, G.P. Typology of fatigue by heart rate variability analysis in elite Nordic-skiers. *Int. J. Sport. Med.* **2015**, *36*, 999–1007. [CrossRef]
34. Schmitt, L.; Regnard, J.; Millet, G.P. Monitoring fatigue status with HRV measures in elite athletes: An avenue beyond RMSSD? *Front. Physiol.* **2015**, *6*, 343. [CrossRef]
35. Bourdillon, N.; Schmitt, L.; Yazdani, S.; Vesin, J.M.; Millet, G.P. Minimal window duration for accurate HRV recording in athletes. *Front. Neurosci.* **2017**, *11*. [CrossRef]
36. Melo, H.M.; Martins, T.C.; Nascimento, L.M.; Hoeller, A.A.; Walz, R.; Takase, E. Ultra-short heart rate variability recording reliability: The effect of controlled paced breathing. *Ann. Noninvasive Electrocardiol.* **2018**, *23*, e12565. [CrossRef]

37. Saboul, D.; Pialoux, V.; Hautier, C. The impact of breathing on HRV measurements: Implications for the longitudinal follow-up of athletes. *Eur. J. Sport Sci.* **2013**, *13*, 534–542. [CrossRef]
38. Sandercock, G.R.H.; Bromley, P.D.; Brodie, D.A. The reliability of short-term measurements of heart rate variability. *Int. J. Cardiol.* **2005**, *103*, 238–247. [CrossRef]

Publisher's Note: MDPI stays neutral with regard to jurisdictional claims in published maps and institutional affiliations.

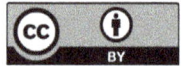

© 2020 by the authors. Licensee MDPI, Basel, Switzerland. This article is an open access article distributed under the terms and conditions of the Creative Commons Attribution (CC BY) license (http://creativecommons.org/licenses/by/4.0/).

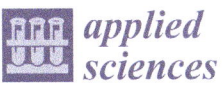

Article

Exercise Training of Secreted Protein Acidic and Rich in Cysteine *(Sparc)* KO Mice Suggests That Exercise-Induced Muscle Phenotype Changes Are SPARC-Dependent

Abdelaziz Ghanemi [1,2], Aicha Melouane [1,2], Mayumi Yoshioka [2] and Jonny St-Amand [1,2,*]

[1] Department of Molecular Medicine, Faculty of Medicine, Laval University, Québec, QC G1V 0A6, Canada; abdelaziz.Ghanemi@crchudequebec.ulaval.ca (A.G.); rimca@live.fr (A.M.)
[2] Functional Genomics Laboratory, Endocrinology and Nephrology Axis, CHU de Québec-Université Laval Research Center, Québec, QC G1V 4G2, Canada; mayumi.yoshioka@crchudequebec.ulaval.ca
* Correspondence: jonny.st-amand@crchudequebec.ulaval.ca; Tel.: +1-418-654-2296; Fax: +1-418-654-2761

Received: 1 December 2020; Accepted: 15 December 2020; Published: 20 December 2020

Featured Application: This work highlights secreted protein acidic and rich in cysteine (SPARC) and its pathways as pharmacological targets/tools for conditions and diseases in which muscle properties enhancement would provide therapeutic benefits.

Abstract: We previously identified secreted protein acidic and rich in cysteine *(Sparc)* as an exercise-induced gene in young and elderly individuals. Via this animal experiment, we aim to identify selected implications of SPARC mainly within the muscle in the contexts of exercise. Mice were divided into eight groups based on three variables (age, genotype and exercise): Old (O) or young (Y) × *Sparc* knock-out (KO) or wild-type (WT) × sedentary (Sed) or exercise (Ex). The exercised groups were trained for 12 weeks at the lactate threshold (LT) speed (including 4 weeks of adaptation period) and all mice were sacrificed afterwards. Body and selected tissues were weighed, and lactate levels in different conditions measured. Expression of skeletal muscle (SM) collagen type I alpha 1 chain (COL1A1) and mitochondrially encoded cytochrome c oxidase I (MT-CO1) in addition to SM strength (grip power) were also measured. Ageing increased the body and white adipose tissue (WAT) weights but decreased SM weight percentage (to body weight) and MT-CO1 expression (in WT). Exercise increased SM COL1A1 in WT mice and MT-CO1 expression, as well as weight percentage of the tibialis anterior muscle, and decreased WAT weight (trend). Compared to WT mice, *Sparc* KO mice had lower body, muscle and WAT weights, with a decrease in SM MT-CO1 and COL1A1 expression with no genotype effect on lactate levels in all our blood lactate measures. *Sparc* KO effects on body composition, adiposity and metabolic patterns are toward a reduced WAT and body weight, but with a negative metabolic and functional phenotype of SM. Whereas such negative effects on SM are worsened with ageing, they are relatively improved by exercise. Importantly, our data suggest that the exercise-induced changes in the SM phenotype, in terms of increased performance (metabolic, strength and development), including lactate-induced changes, are SPARC-dependent.

Keywords: secreted protein acidic and rich in cysteine *(Sparc)*; exercise; muscle performance; metabolic phenotype; lactate; ageing

---

1. Secreted Protein Acidic and Rich in Cysteine as an Exercise-Induced Gene

The modern lifestyle, characterized by the lack of physical activity combined with an unhealthy diet, leads to an increase in health problems typical of our era such as obesity and diabetes. In addition, the improvement of health care systems increased the life expectancy and, therefore, geriatric health problems, such as sarcopenia, are also increasing. Interestingly, exercise is considered as a "panacea" for many of these problems [1]. Whereas exercise benefits have been widely documented, many exercise-related molecular mechanisms are yet to be fully elucidated. In addition to its direct metabolic implications, skeletal muscles (SM) represent secretary organs producing myokine, such as secreted protein acidic and rich in cysteine (SPARC) [2]. Within the exercise context, functional genomics studies (mainly but not only in the energy metabolism context [3]) have identified genes related to physical activity among which we have *SPARC/Sparc*. Indeed, beyond the known implications of SPARC in wound healing and tissue repair [4,5], this gene was characterized (for the first time) as an exercise-induced gene [6] and also as an electrical pulse stimulation (considered as an in vitro model of exercise)-induced gene in muscular cells [7]. Moreover, SPARC secretion is induced by exercise [8–10] after which the concentrations of myokines (including SPARC, interleukin 6 and fibroblast growth factor) increase in the circulation [11]. Therefore, we hypothesize that at least some of the exercise benefits and biological consequences, mainly the muscular phenotype adaptation to exercise, would be mediated by SPARC or the pathways it controls. Therefore, in this study we aim to explore the implication of *Sparc* (via it knock-out (KO)) in mice with a focus on exercise effects on muscles. In addition, age was also introduced as a variable in this study. Therefore, we would find out the combinatory impacts of *Sparc* KO, exercise and age on selected patterns related to SM physiological properties and metabolic performance. We explore the lactate levels and their implications with the SM phenotype changes (both structural and metabolic) in a SPARC-dependent way.

2. Animal Experimental Design, Material and Methods

Our study was carried out on male mice and involved both wild-type (WT) mice (C57BL/6J, the most commonly used strain for genetic and/or transgenic study that also consistently showed the highest level of voluntary wheel-running [12]) and *Sparc* KO mice (129/Sv-C57BL/6J) fed with chow diet (Teklad global 18% protein rodent diets [13]). Mice had access to food and water ad libitum during the whole experimental period (except for fasting periods during which they had access to water only). WT mice were from the Jackson Laboratory (https://www.jax.org/) and *Sparc* KO mice were generated via in vitro fertilization using *Sparc* KO mice sperm generously provided by Dr. Amy D. Bradshaw. *Sparc* KO mice of Dr. Amy D. Bradshaw were generated as previously described [14,15]. Each age-group of mice (young (Y) and old (O)) was divided based on the genotype (KO or WT) to obtain 4 groups: Y-KO, Y-WT, O-KO, O-WT. Finally, each of these 4 groups was further subdivided into two groups according to whether they were exercising (Ex) or sedentary (Sed) mice. Therefore, our experimental design included 8 groups: Y-WT-Sed, Y-WT-Ex, Y-KO-Sed, Y-KO-Ex, O-WT-Sed, O-WT-Ex, O-KO-Sed and O-KO-Ex. Each group had 11 to 12 mice (n). Mice were housed at the animal facility of the CHU de Québec-Université Laval Research Center (12-h light/dark cycle) and periodically checked by animal care technicians for health and wellness. The exercise groups were trained during the dark phase.

The exercising mice were trained during 12 weeks (starting at the age of 9 weeks for Y mice and 66 weeks for O mice) on running wheels (Lafayette instrument Co, Lafayette, IN, USA) placed horizontally (no angle adjustment). Whereas Y mice were sacrificed at the age of 21 weeks, old mice were sacrificed at the age of 78 weeks. Mice were sacrificed following a 12-h fasting (postprandial period) by cardiac puncture following isoflurane inhalation anesthesia. The coming sub-sections detail the measures performed before, during and after the training, as well as on and after the sacrifice day.

All animal experimentation was conducted in accord with the guidelines of the Canadian Council on Animal Care and approved by the Animal Protection Committee of Laval University (Identifications: 2014165 and 2014168). Mice with any type of illness were immediately euthanized by cervical dislocation and excluded from the study. Mice found with anatomical abnormalities (during the sacrifice) were also excluded from the study.

2.1. Mice Exercise Protocol and Running Speed Determination

At the beginning of the training, mice had an adaptation period of 4 weeks. During those 4 weeks, mice performed the incremental exercise. They were trained through a progressive (gradual) increase in both running speed and duration (up to their maximum endurance) throughout this adaptation step, at the end of which we determined the speed at the lactate threshold (LT). The LT level [16] is a parameter indicating the level of physical activity corresponding to the metabolic point at which the muscle production of lactate starts to increase and overcome the blood clearance of lactate. This indicates that the energy produced via oxidative phosphorylation is insufficient to meet energetic needs and, therefore, the muscles trigger anaerobic energy production that generates lactate at a level superior to its blood clearance. At the end of the adaptation period, LT levels were determined following a measure of running speed-dependent blood lactate level curves, based on previously reported protocols [12,17]. Briefly, the mouse run at a determined speed for 4 min, after which we immediately measure the blood lactate level (within 1 min), after that it ran at the next speed (higher) and again the blood lactate speed was measured. We repeated this procedure until the mouse was not able to run (cannot maintain the speed). At the end, we obtained the curve representing blood lactate levels corresponding to the different running speeds, based on which we obtained the speed at the LT. The blood lactate levels were measured, as described in the next section (**1.2**). The LT speed was chosen as a parameter for our study, based on evidence showing that exercise at LT generates metabolic and functional benefits, including improved insulin sensitivity, peripheral glucose effectiveness, lipid profile, blood pressure, physiological fitness [18–21] and body fat weight percentage decrease [6]. The LT was determined for each mouse of the exercise groups. After that, for each set of mice trained at the same period, the running speed of the 8 remaining weeks of training was a value chosen among the average values (range) of all the mice of that set.

The training was at those values close to the LT levels (LT speed) because it was the LT level that was the speed used during the study in which *SPARC* has been characterised as an exercise-induced gene [6]. In addition, the exercise frequency of our study (60 min/day, five times/week) was also similar to the same study [6]. However, we extended the duration from 6 weeks to 12 weeks to be able to easily see the impacts with significant differences between groups. The literature reported studies exploring the effect of exercise in which mice were both trained for longer periods (over 12 weeks) with the same frequency (60 min/day, five times/week) [22] and also at least as young and as old (3 and 19 months of age) [23] as the mice in this study. In addition, the life span for C57BL/6 mice is around 104 weeks (26 months) [24,25]. Therefore, our choices of mice ages, exercise speed and frequency were within a range of the mice's abilities and did not damage their muscles, nor were they limited by physiological parameters. Importantly, since LT speed was chosen, based on evidence showing that exercise at LT generates metabolic and functional benefits, our study will provide additional data for molecular and biochemical explanations of such training benefits.

During mouse training, and unlike other protocols, no electrical [17] or any potentially harmful stimulations were used to force the mice to run. Only a light air stimulation (using a small hand air pump) was applied for mice in some cases to ensure, as much as possible, that all mice ran during the same period and at the same speed throughout the same training period (optimize the protocol for similar exercise amounts). Moreover, mice were always handled gently when taken from the cage to the training device and vice versa. In addition, sedentary mice were also transported to the exercise training room and kept in their cages, while exercising mice were trained so that all mice received a similar environmental (light, noise, etc.) stimuli. Thus, any possible impacts of stress or environmental stimuli on the performed measures were reduced to minimum.

The last training session was 48 h prior to the sacrifice so that the measures we obtained during the sacrifice and those performed on tissues afterwards did not reflect any possible acute effect of exercise, such as dehydration or neuroendocrine changes that could impact gene expression, post-exercise energy intake or expenditure, etc. Our study aimed to investigate the effects of the 12 weeks of exercise (chronic).

2.2. Fasting Lactate and Oral Glucose Gavage-Dependant Lactate Levels

As a resting metabolic indicator in the muscle, blood lactate levels were measured before and after glucose (prepared from 45% solution, Sigma-Aldrich Canada Co., Oakville, ON, Canada) oral gavage (2 mg of glucose per 1 g of body weight). Mice were fasted for 6 h prior to the glucose gavage. Each measure had 5 time points (0, 15, 30, 60 and 120 min after glucose gavage) allowing us to obtain a curve and calculate the area under the curve (AUC). This test was performed three times (a total of three AUCs)—before the training, at week 5 and the end of week 12 of the training. In addition, we also measured blood lactate (single measure) at the sacrifice day (following 12 h fasting) and at the end of the last training session. Blood lactate levels were measured via tail pricking with a needle to collect blood samples on lactate test strips that were then inserted into the lactate meter (Lactate scout, Sports Resource Group, Inc., Minneapolis, MN, USA).

2.3. Grip Power Test

At the end of the training period, the muscle strengths of all the mice were evaluated through performing a grip power test with a grip strength meter (Columbus Instruments International, Columbus, OH, USA). The grip strength was measured by allowing a mouse to grab (with four limbs) pull bar assemblies attached to the force transducer while the mouse was pulled horizontally by the tail away from the bars, similar to what has been previously described [26,27]. The peak force applied by the mouse (g) was then shown on a digital display.

This test was conducted five times (5 min apart) for each mouse, after which the forces (both mean and maximum) were calculated both as absolute values as well as being normalized to the body weights of the corresponding mice.

2.4. Body and Tissue Weights

Body and selected tissues were weighted at the sacrifice day. The selected tissues were the brain, pituitary gland, hypothalamus, liver, heart, aorta, white adipose tissue (WAT), SMs (gastrocnemius, soleus, tibialis anterior and extensor digitorum longus muscles). The values are reported both as tissue weights as well as a weight percentages (normalized) to the body weights of the corresponding mice.

2.5. Western Blotting

We measured the SM (tibialis anterior muscle) expression of two proteins—collagen alpha 1 type I (COL1A1) and mitochondrially encoded cytochrome c oxidase I (MT-CO1). Whereas COL1A1 is important in the structure of the muscle [28], MT-CO1 is an indicator of mitochondrial oxidative phosphorylation [29]. At the day of sacrifice, the tibialis anterior muscle was removed and quickly put in liquid nitrogen (snap frozen) then moved to −80 °C and kept until the protein extraction procedure. To measure the expression of both COL1A1 and MT-CO1, total proteins were extracted from the tibialis anterior muscle, using a radio-immunoprecipitation assay (RIPA) buffer and protease inhibitors cocktail (Sigma-Aldrich Canada Co., Oakville, ON, Canada) and followed by a protein quantification of each protein extract using Bio-Rad protein assay (Bio-Rad Laboratories Ltd., Mississauga, ON, Canada). Fifteen (MT-CO1) or ten (COL1A1) micrograms of proteins were separated by sodium dodecyl sulfate polyacrylamide gel electrophoresis (SDS-PAGE) using the TGX Stain-Free FastCast acrylamide solutions (Bio-Rad Laboratories Ltd., Mississauga, ON, Canada), and the trihalo compound in the gels was activated under UV light. Then, total proteins were transferred to polyvinylidene fluoride (PVDF) membranes (Bio-Rad Laboratories Ltd., Mississauga, ON, Canada), and gels (before and after the transfer) and membranes were visualized under UV light by using the AlphaImager TM 1220 (Alpha Innotech Co., San Leandro, CA, USA).

Membranes were blocked using the Pierce™ Protein-Free (TBS) blocking buffer (Life Technologies Inc., Burlington, ON, Canada), incubated with 1/400 (sc-8784R for COL1A1 and sc-48143 for MT-CO1) dilution of primary antibodies (Santa Cruz Biotechnology Inc., Dallas, TX, USA) and secondary antibodies (sc-2004 for COL1A1 and sc-2350 for MT-CO1, 1/10000 dilution: Santa Cruz Biotechnology Inc., Dallas, TX, USA), and finally visualized with the Clarity™ Western ECL Blotting Substrate on a film (Bio-Rad Laboratories Ltd., Mississauga, ON, Canada). The visualized total proteins on the membranes and target proteins on the films were quantified using ImageJ software (ImageJ bundled with 64-bit Java 1.8.0_172, U. S. National Institutes of Health, Bethesda, MD, USA) [30]. The methodology of lane and band quantifications, followed by expression evaluations, was performed according to Taylor et al. [31,32] as we have detailed in one of our previous works [33].

2.6. Statistical Analyses and Sample Size Determination

The data were analyzed by three-way (age, genotype and exercise) and the four-way (for the lactate AUC) ANOVA. When the ANOVA revealed a significant interaction between two or three variables, the Tukey Kramer post hoc test was performed to identify the significant difference between the groups ($p < 0.05$). A trend corresponds to $0.05 \leq p < 0.1$. In the results section, all the effects are significant ($p < 0.05$), unless mentioned as a trend.

The number of mice (11–12 mice per experimental condition) was based on the results of power analysis by setting the statistical power at 80% ($\alpha = 0.05$ and $\beta = 0.2$) with our previous study, which used the same strain of WT mice [34].

3. Results

3.1. Exercise Patterns, Running Speed and Lactate Concentrations

Tables 1 and 2 report the data collected during the 4 weeks of incremental exercise, the weeks of the LT speed training and the day of sacrifice. During the 4 weeks of incremental exercise, we have the effect of age on both LT speed (Y > O) and blood lactate level at rest (O > Y). However, for lactate at rest, this genotype effect is attributed to the *Sparc* KO mice since, for the WT, there is no difference between Y and O mice, but for the *Sparc* KO mice, O mice have a higher lactate concentration at rest than Y mice (significant effects of genotype×age interaction). We also have the effect of age (Y > O) for both the mean exercise speed as well as the total exercise distance during the 12 weeks of training. The same effect of age (Y > O) is observed during the last training session for both speed and lactate concentration, measured at the end of that last running hour (Table 1).

In Table 2, we notice effect of age (Y > O) for blood lactate level (trend) on the sacrifice day (measured after 12 h of fasting). For the curve of post glucose–gavage lactate concentrations at different time points (0, 15, 30, 60 and 120 min), we only have an effect of the age (Y > O). The value of the AUC was measured three times—before the training and at week 5 and the end of the week 12 of the training. Each time, mice had a 6 h fasting period prior to glucose gavage.

Table 1. Summary of wheel exercise training.

		Young		Old		2-Way ANOVA			
		Wild-type	Knockout	Wild-type	Knockout	A	G	A × G	
During an incremental exercise test (wk 4)									
LT speed	m/min	8.7 ± 0.4	7.8 ± 0.5	5.5 ± 0.6	5.4 ± 0.4	Y > O	-	-	
Lactate at rest	mM	2.8 ± 0.2	2.6 ± 0.2	3.1 ± 0.4	3.8 ± 0.2	O > Y	-	KO: O > Y	
Lactate at LT	mM	3.2 ± 0.2	3.1 ± 0.3	3.4 ± 0.4	3.3 ± 0.5	-	-	-	
During LT training (wk 1–12)									
Mean exercise speed	m/min	7.5 ± 0.2	7.6 ± 0.2	5.5 ± 0.0	5.3 ± 0.0	Y > O	-	-	
Total exercise time	min	3332 ± 52	3353 ± 45	3334 ± 1	3335 ± 3	-	-	-	
Total exercise distance	m	24,903 ± 763	25,445 ± 670	18,219 ± 41	17,811 ± 156	Y > O	-	-	
During the last LT training (wk 12)									
Speed	m/min	7.8 ± 0.2	7.9 ± 0.2	5.5 ± 0.0	5.3 ± 0.1	Y > O	-	-	
Lactate	mM	2.7 ± 0.3	2.9 ± 0.3	2.1 ± 0.2	2.5 ± 0.2	Y > O	-	-	

Data are mean ± SEM. Number of mice: 11–12 mice per experimental condition. Abbreviations: A, age; G, genotype; KO, knockout; LT, lactate threshold; m, meter; min, minute; mM, millimolar; O, old; wk, week; Y, young. -: No effect.

Table 2. Fasting and post glucose-gavage blood lactate levels.

	Young				Old				ANOVA							
	Wild-type		Knockout		Wild-type		Knockout									
	Sedentary	Exercise	Sedentary	Exercise	Sedentary	Exercise	Sedentary	Exercise	A	G	Ex	A × G	A × Ex	G × Ex	A × G × Ex	
At sacrifice (12 h fast)																
Blood lactate mM	1.09 ± 0.12	0.88 ± 0.08	1.28 ± 0.38	1.24 ± 0.15	0.89 ± 0.07	0.99 ± 0.13	0.98 ± 0.08	0.75 ± 0.04	Y > O*	-	-	-	-	-	-	
Post glucose gavage (6 h fast)																
AUC									Y > O	-	-	-	3-way	-	-	
Blood lactate													4-way			
Pre	615 ± 35	498 ± 63	479 ± 29	533 ± 44	429 ± 29	424 ± 24	473 ± 39	461 ± 54								
At wk 5	529 ± 32	509 ± 34	503 ± 41	519 ± 38	422 ± 27	450 ± 42	479 ± 44	392 ± 32								
After 12 wks	465 ± 34	391 ± 27	452 ± 22	486 ± 45	440 ± 56	381 ± 20	414 ± 35	371 ± 28								

Data are mean ± SEM. Number of mice: 11—12 mice per experimental condition. Abbreviations: A, age; AUC, area under the curve; Ex, Exercise; G, genotype; h, hour; KO, knockout; mM, millimolar; O, old; wk, week; Y, young. *: Trend ($0.05 \leq p < 0.1$). -: No effect.

3.2. Body and Tissue Weights

Mice were weighed the morning of the sacrifice. During the sacrifice, tissues were removed and weighed as well (Table 3). Analyzed data are both as absolute values (weight) and percentages of the tissues weights to the body weight.

We found the effect of age (O > Y) on body weight as well as on the weights of pituitary gland, hypothalamus, liver, heart, and WAT, in addition to the weight percentage of WAT; the opposite effect of age (Y > O) on the weight percentages (to the body weight) of the brain, heart, aorta, SM and tibialis anterior muscle. We also found an effect (trend) of age (Y > O) on the weights of both SM and the tibialis anterior muscle.

We found an effect of genotype (WT > KO) on the body, aorta, WAT, SM and tibialis anterior muscle weights, and another effect (KO > WT) on the brain weight and weight percentage, liver and heart (both weight percentage). Coming to the last variable, exercise, we also report these exercise effects—Sed > Ex (trend) for body weight and liver weight percentage and WAT weight. Ex > Sed (trend) for weight percentages of both the brain and the hypothalamus. Ex > Sed for tibialis anterior muscle weight and Sed > Ex for liver weight.

3.3. Muscle Strength (Grip Power Tests)

As a measure of muscle strength for the four limbs (simultaneously), the grip power tests results (Table 4) show effect of the age (Y > O) for the both the mean and the maximum grip power as well as for the percentage of each of these two values (mean and the maximum grip power) on body weight. We also have an effect of the genotype (WT > KO) for both mean and the maximum grip powers. For the effect of exercise, we have a trend (Ex > Sed) for the percentage of the maximum grip power to the body weight.

3.4. COL1A1 and MT-CO1 Expressions in Tibialis Anterior Muscle

Protein expression of both COL1A1 and MT-CO1 was measured in the SM tibialis anterior muscle. The results (Figure 1) indicate an effect of genotype (WT > KO) on both proteins and an effect of exercise (Ex > Sed) on COL1A1 (trend) and MT-CO1. For the interactions, we found one between genotype and exercise for COL1A1 (Ex > Sed in WT) and one between age and genotype for MT-CO1 (high in Y-WT).

Table 3. Body and tissue weights.

		Young				Old				3-Way ANOVA							
		Wild-type		Knockout		Wild-type		Knockout									
		Sedentary	Exercise	Sedentary	Exercise	Sedentary	Exercise	Sedentary	Exercise	A	G	Ex	A × G	A × Ex	G × Ex	A × G × Ex
Body weight	g	29.5 ± 0.7	28.9 ± 1.0	27.8 ± 0.6	25.0 ± 0.8	37.4 ± 2.1	35.2 ± 1.0	31.3 ± 1.5	30.4 ± 0.7	O > Y	WT > KO	Sed > Ex *	-	-	-	-
Tissues weights																
Brain	mg	430 ± 2	430 ± 6	448 ± 4	445 ± 3	432 ± 7	436 ± 2	451 ± 4	446 ± 4	-	KO > WT	-	-	-	-	WT-Sed: Y > O, WT-Ex: Y > O, KO-Ex: Y >> O
	%	1.47 ± 0.03	1.50 ± 0.05	1.62 ± 0.04	1.80 ± 0.05	1.18 ± 0.05	1.25 ± 0.03	1.48 ± 0.07	1.47 ± 0.02	Y > O	KO > WT	Ex > Sed *	-	-	-	-
Pituitary gland	mg	1.52 ± 0.20	1.49 ± 0.10	1.47 ± 0.10	1.33 ± 0.10	1.77 ± 0.16	1.76 ± 0.13	1.78 ± 0.04	1.65 ± 0.12	O > Y	-	-	-	-	-	-
	%	0.0052 ± 0.0007	0.0052 ± 0.0003	0.0053 ± 0.0004	0.0054 ± 0.0004	0.0049 ± 0.0006	0.0050 ± 0.0004	0.0059 ± 0.0003	0.0055 ± 0.0005	-	-	-	-	-	-	-
Hypothalamus	mg	8.7 ± 0.7	9.1 ± 0.6	8.0 ± 0.5	8.9 ± 0.8	10.7 ± 0.9	10.8 ± 0.8	9.4 ± 0.8	11.0 ± 0.5	O > Y	-	Ex > Sed *	-	-	-	-
	%	0.030 ± 0.003	0.032 ± 0.003	0.029 ± 0.002	0.036 ± 0.003	0.030 ± 0.003	0.031 ± 0.003	0.030 ± 0.003	0.036 ± 0.002	-	-	Sed > Ex	-	-	-	-
Liver	mg	984 ± 27	954 ± 33	964 ± 35	899 ± 30	1370 ± 136	1114 ± 28	1174 ± 82	1101 ± 24	O > Y	KO > WT	Sed > Ex *	-	Sed: O > Y *	Ex: KO > WT	WT-Sed: O > Y, WT-Ex: Y > O *, KO-Ex: O > Y
	%	3.34 ± 0.04	3.31 ± 0.09	3.54 ± 0.09	3.60 ± 0.04	3.59 ± 0.14	3.17 ± 0.04	3.71 ± 0.12	3.62 ± 0.05	-						
Heart	mg	138 ± 3	149 ± 7	146 ± 6	131 ± 4	159 ± 6	135 ± 4	152 ± 5	159 ± 7	O > Y	-	-	KO: O > Y	-	-	-
	%	0.47 ± 0.01	0.51 ± 0.01	0.53 ± 0.02	0.53 ± 0.01	0.43 ± 0.01	0.38 ± 0.01	0.50 ± 0.02	0.52 ± 0.02	Y > O	KO > WT	-	WT: Y >> O	-	-	WT-Sed: Y > O, WT-Ex: Y >> O
Aorta	mg	12.8 ± 1.5	12.0 ± 1.5	12.9 ± 1.3	9.0 ± 0.6	13.0 ± 1.5	12.3 ± 1.0	9.7 ± 1.0	9.9 ± 0.7	-	WT > KO	-	-	-	-	-
	%	0.044 ± 0.006	0.042 ± 0.006	0.047 ± 0.005	0.037 ± 0.003	0.034 ± 0.003	0.035 ± 0.003	0.031 ± 0.003	0.032 ± 0.002	Y > O	-	-	-	-	-	-
White adipose tissue **	mg	1021 ± 206	812 ± 126	955 ± 138	684 ± 125	2913 ± 362	2649 ± 175	1804 ± 226	1505 ± 164	O > Y	WT > KO	Sed > Ex *	WT: O >> Y, KO: O > Y	-	-	-
	%	3.36 ± 0.58	2.72 ± 0.36	3.36 ± 0.44	2.63 ± 0.38	7.52 ± 0.65	7.44 ± 0.32	5.51 ± 0.50	4.85 ± 0.43	O > Y	WT > KO	-	WT: O >> Y, KO: O > Y	-	-	-
Skeletal muscle ***	mg	532 ± 11	524 ± 15	432 ± 8	413 ± 7	508 ± 11	510 ± 6	416 ± 8	417 ± 7	Y > O *	WT > KO	-	-	-	-	-

Table 3. Cont.

		Young				Old				3-Way ANOVA						
		Wild-type		Knockout		Wild-type		Knockout								
		Sedentary	Exercise	Sedentary	Exercise	Sedentary	Exercise	Sedentary	Exercise	A	G	Ex	A × G	A × Ex	G × Ex	A × G × Ex
Tibialis anterior muscle	mg	1.81 ± 0.04	1.82 ± 0.05	1.56 ± 0.04	1.67 ± 0.05	1.39 ± 0.05	1.46 ± 0.05	1.36 ± 0.06	1.38 ± 0.03	Y > O	WT > KO	-	WT: Y >> O, KO: Y > O	-	-	-
	%	0.45 ± 0.01	0.48 ± 0.01	0.42 ± 0.01	0.46 ± 0.01	0.36 ± 0.02	0.36 ± 0.01	0.36 ± 0.01	0.39 ± 0.02	Y > O*	WT > KO	-	-	-	-	WT-Ex: Y > O
										Y > O	-	Ex > Sed	WT: Y >> O, KO: Y > O	-	-	-

Data are mean ± SEM. Number of mice: 11–12 mice per experimental condition. Abbreviations: A, age; Ex, exercise; G, genotype; g, gram; KO, knockout; mg, milligram; O, old; Sed, sedentary; WT, wild-type; Y, young. *: Trend ($0.05 \leq p < 0.1$); **: Inguinal and abdominal adipose tissues; ***: Gastrocnemius, soleus, tibialis anterior and extensor digitorum longus muscles. %: percentage to the body weight. -: No effect.

Table 4. Grip Power at the End of Week 12.

		Young				Old				3-Way ANOVA						
		Wild-Type		Knockout		Wild-Type		Knockout								
		Sedentary	Exercise	Sedentary	Exercise	Sedentary	Exercise	Sedentary	Exercise	A	G	Ex	A × G	A × Ex	G × Ex	A × G × Ex
Grip power																
Mean	g	240 ± 12	248 ± 11	226 ± 10	208 ± 11	216 ± 8	220 ± 8	182 ± 8	203 ± 9	Y > O	WT > KO	-	-	-	-	-
	g/BW	8.2 ± 0.5	8.6 ± 0.4	8.1 ± 0.4	8.4 ± 0.4	5.8 ± 0.4	6.1 ± 0.2	5.9 ± 0.5	6.6 ± 0.3	Y > O	-	-	-	-	-	-
Max	g	308 ± 12	301 ± 11	277 ± 11	250 ± 9	250 ± 8	257 ± 9	210 ± 8	235 ± 10	Y > O	WT > KO	-	-	-	-	-
	g/BW	10.5 ± 0.4	10.5 ± 0.4	10.0 ± 0.4	10.1 ± 0.4	6.7 ± 0.5	7.2 ± 0.3	6.8 ± 0.5	7.6 ± 0.3	Y > O	-	Ex > Sed *	-	-	-	-

Data are mean ± SEM. Number of mice: 11–12 mice per experimental condition. Abbreviations: A, age; BW, body weight; Ex, exercise; G, genotype; g, gram; KO, knockout; O, old; Sed, sedentary; WT, wild-type; Y, young. *: Trend ($0.05 \leq p < 0.1$). -: No effect.

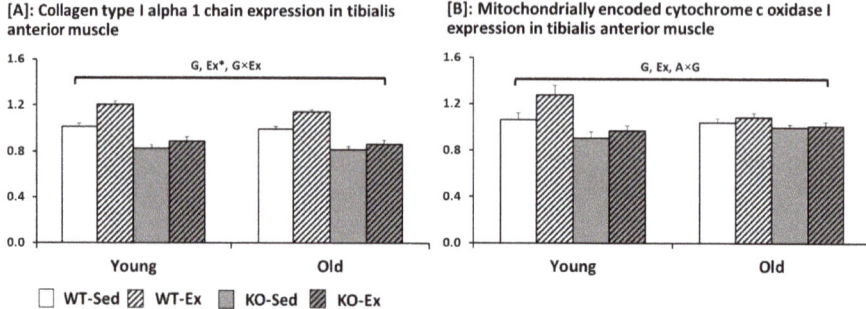

Figure 1. Expression of both collagen type I alpha 1 chain (COL1A1) (**A**) and mitochondrially encoded cytochrome c oxidase I (MT-CO1) (**B**) in the tibialis anterior muscle. The results indicate an effect of genotype^G (WT > KO) for both proteins and an effect of exercise^{Ex} (Ex > Sed) for COL1A1 (trend) and MT-CO1. For the interactions, we have one between genotype and exercise$^{G \times Ex}$ for COL1A1 (Ex > Sed in WT) and one between age and genotype$^{A \times G}$ for MT-CO1 (high in Y-WT). All data are mean ± SEM. The number of mice: 11–12 mice per experimental condition. Abbreviations: A, age; Ex, exercise; G, genotype; KO, knockout; O, old; Sed, sedentary; WT, wild-type; Y, young. *: Trend (0.05 ≤ p < 0.1).

4. Discussion and Interpretation

As per Table 1, there is no effect in the genotype for the LT speed (in all the performed measures both during the 4 weeks of adaptation and during the 8 weeks of LT training), exercise speed, exercise time, exercise distance and even lactate concentrations during exercise. This has a key importance, since it means that mice of the two different genotypes (KO and WT) had equal amounts of exercise training (speed, distance, time and frequency) and blood lactate levels. Therefore, genotypes effects seen for the other measures will be, indeed, due to the genotype itself (consequence of *Sparc* KO) rather than difference in the exercise amount.

SPARC (osteonectin or BM-40) is a three-modular-domain [35,36] calcium binding extracellular matrix-associated glycoprotein [37,38]. The *Sparc* gene localized to the central region of chromosome 11 in mice [39] and in the chromosomal site at 5q31–q33 in humans [40]. It is well known for its roles in extracellular matrix (ECM) organization, growth, cellular differentiation, cell–matrix communication, wound healing, cell cycle and tissue response to injury [35,36,41–43]. SPARC is also implicated in metabolism [44,45], cancer [46] and inflammatory [47] homeostasis. Importantly, for the SM, a key metabolic tissue and the key organ for the exercise performance, SPARC represents an important element for its development [28] and function [7].

Indeed, SPARC is known for its importance is SM development and regeneration (satellite cells/myoblasts. myotubes and muscle fibers) [48]. Moreover, whereas during embryogenesis SPARC is highly expressed, its expression is mainly restricted to tissues undergoing changes and remodeling during adulthood [35,49–51] which indicates its importance for exercising muscle; which does undergo remodeling as an adaptation to exercise [52,53]. Importantly, SPARC modulates actin cytoskeleton within the SM structure which results in defective force recovery following in vitro fatigue stimulation in muscle from *Sparc* KO mice [54]; but in normal and uninjured muscles, SPARC is not detectable [48]. This further indicates the importance of SPARC in the context of healing, repair, remodeling and development, especially that the ECM (important for the cellular remodeling, for instance) repair, disassembly and degradation is mediated by SPARC [55]. These impacts on regeneration and during embryogenesis suggest that SPARC deficiency could impact some tissue development and growth, as illustrated by the loss of bone mass (osteopenia) in *Sparc* KO mice [56].

Another structural importance for SPARC in SM derives from its ability to interact with collagens. It interacts with collagen I and procollagen I [57], binds to fibrillar collagens [58], maintains SM stiffness (collagen accumulation regulation) [59] and specifically binds several molecules, including collagen types I, III and IV [60]. SPARC deficiency has also been shown to reduce the expression of different types of collagen such as collagen type I in mesangial cells [61], collagen in skin [62] and fibrillar collagen accumulation in tibialis anterior muscle [59].

Moving from SPARC-related structural muscle properties to metabolic implications, SPARC has been shown to be required for the expression of the exercise-induced (in vitro model of) mitochondrial enzymes (oxidative phosphorylation) [28] and is suggested to enhance the muscle mitochondrial biogenesis [63] as supported by the fact that small interfering RNA (siRNA) of *SPARC* reduces 5-aminoimidazole-4-carboxamide-1-β-Dribofuranoside (AICAR)-stimulated adenosine monophosphate-activated protein kinase (AMPK) phosphorylation [64], which is known to induce mitochondrial biogenesis via the activation/induction of peroxisome proliferator-activated receptor gamma coactivator 1 alpha (PPARGC1A, also known as PGC1α) [65–67], a master regulator of mitochondrial biogenesis. Importantly, knowing the importance of the mitochondria during regeneration [68,69], SPARC would impact regeneration. In addition, SPARC regulates glucose transporter type 4 expression [64] and improves glucose tolerance [70]. These are selected illustrations of SPARC importance and implications for the metabolism, mainly for the SM that we focus on in our study.

For other tissues, the implication of SPARC in tissue regeneration and development (including tissue repair, cell turnover, cellular differentiation and remodeling) [35,38,44,71,72], especially with the known implications of SPARC in the functions of stem cells [73,74] and other types of cells such as erythroid progenitors [74], could indicate that SPARC-deficient mice could exhibit impairments in terms of development for certain tissues under selected conditions.

4.1. Lactate Concentrations among the Indicators of Muscles Metabolic Performance

Lactate is not just produced by SM and WAT [75] but it is also consumed by muscles [76] with special metabolic patterns [77] and serves as a gluconeogenic precursor [78]. Therefore, the blood lactate levels represent the outcome of the balance between the production and the consumption (clearance) of lactate [79] mainly (but not only) by SM [80]. The production of lactate by SM does not always mean insufficient energy production through oxidative phosphorylation, but could also be due to the lack of oxygen [81], as illustrated by the production of lactate in the adipose tissue of obese subjects as a consequence of hypoxia in this adipose tissue [75]. Importantly, exercise-produced lactate both upregulates the expression cytochrome oxidase gene and protein expression and is a mitochondrial biogenesis activation signal [79]. All these changes seem to result from negative feedback, aiming to increase the oxidative phosphorylation ability and, therefore, reduce lactate production and increase its clearance (usage). The liver and heart also contribute to lactate clearance and, whereas myocardia oxidases lactate as a fuel, the brain also takes it when its levels increase in the blood and the liver uptakes it to form glucose [80]. The fact that no genotype effect has been seen for lactate levels, at similar amount of exercise indicates that *Sparc* KO mice are able to maintain the lactate concentrations at a homeostatic level (similar to that of WT mice) in spite of the impaired muscular functions (compared to WT mice), suggesting a compensatory effect of other tissues to re-balance blood lactate (as we detail below). This compensatory pathway highlights the importance of lactate blood homeostasis.

4.2. Body and Tissue Weights (Table 3)

The importance of SPARC is tissue development, embryogenesis, regeneration, its interaction with collagen and ECM, in addition to its role in collagen accumulation [59] would explain why *Sparc* KO reduces body weight and SM weights, including the tibialis anterior muscle (correlated with what Omi et al. reported [59]) in addition to other tissues (aorta and WAT), as a result of regeneration and development deficiency, similar to the decrease in bone mass (osteopenia) as a result of SPARC deficiency [56]. However, the observed increased weights or weight percentages of other tissues, such as the brain, liver and heart in *Sparc* KO mice, could result from feedback signals. Indeed, the reduced development and metabolic deficiency in *Sparc* KO mice would lead to the production of signals aiming to correct this developmental and metabolic deficiency (resulting from muscle low oxidation capacity, myokines secretion reduction, etc). Such signal effects would target selected tissues (those increased with *Sparc* KO, such as the brain, which is the center of numerous neuroendocrine signals and in which Compolongo et al., have shown that the neuronal activity levels of *Sparc* KO mice are increased in the brain region dentate gyrus [82] which could support the hypothesis of such signals in *Sparc* KO mice) and either be nonspecific or with insufficient impacts on other tissues (those for which *Sparc* KO does not reduce the weights). For instance, the increased heart weight percentage in *Sparc* KO mice could be adaptive to the fact that these mice have reduced oxidative phosphorylation ability (as shown by the low MT-CO1 expression) and would have more muscle-produced lactate. The developed heart could be an adaptation to the increased lactate production in order to increase the circulation and, therefore, increase lactate clearance, which could be taken by the liver to form glucose [80], which could also explain the increased weight (percentage) of the liver in *Sparc* KO mice. Therefore, although *Sparc* KO mice SM produced more lactate (weak oxidation capacity), they have the same blood lactate levels as WT mice because they would compensate via increased lactate blood clearance through enhanced blood circulation (increased heart weight percentage) combined to an increased intake by the liver (increased weight percentage), the brain (increased weight and weight percentage) and probably other tissues leading to that weight/weight percentage increase in those tissues in *Sparc* KO mice. This correlates with the liver weight percentage for which we have Ex-KO>Ex-WT, meaning that, in the exercised groups, the liver (weight percentage) of *Sparc* KO mice is superior to the liver (weight percentage) of WT mice (even though both had similar amount of training). This could indicate more tissue glycogen storage [83] (in a hydrated form that adds more water weight to the liver [84]) built from glucose made of the taken lactate because the *Sparc* KO mice SM would produce more lactate (weak oxidative phosphorylation reflected by the decrease in MT-CO1 expression in the *Sparc* KO mice) but clear it better through an increased blood circulation (increased heart weight percentage in *Sparc* KO) combined with lactate uptake (clearance) by the liver [80] and also by the brain [80] (that also increased in weight in *Sparc* KO mice) to compensate the low oxidation ability of the SM (supposed to contribute to lactate clearance but remains insufficient in terms of lactate clearance in *Sparc* KO mice). Overall, there is no genotype-related difference in lactate level because there would be compensation. Indeed, whereas WT mice have good muscle lactate clearance (with low lactate production), *Sparc* KO mice (although they have higher lactate production) have increased lactate clearance via the liver, brain, heart (that have increased weight percentage, compared to those in WT mice), etc.

Furthermore, the known implications of SPARC in the functions of erythroid progenitors [74] could suggest that *Sparc* KO mice would have reduced hemoglobin (low blood cells cancer) and, therefore, reduced oxygen transport ability. This would require one to increase the blood supply to different tissues to compensate low blood oxygenation via increased blood circulation that would require a developed cardiac pump and, thus, explains the increased weight (percentage) of the heart in *Sparc* KO mice; such low oxygenation further worsens the weak oxidative phosphorylation capacity in SM that *Sparc* KO mice already have.

The other tissues patterns (age- and exercise-dependant) are in accordance with the known effects of both ageing and exercise on diverse tissues. For instance, the increased brain and hypothalamus weight percentages (trend) with exercise fits with the ability of exercise to enhance neurogenesis [23,85,86], the exercise also reduces (trend) both body weight and liver weight percentage and WAT weight, whereas it increases the tibialis anterior muscle weight percentage. All these elements correlate with the ability of exercise to increase energy usage (WAT lipids and liver glycogen) as well as muscle weight. Regarding the tibialis anterior muscle, in addition to its increase (weight percentage) with exercise, it decreases with both age (weight percentage) and *Sparc* KO (weight). It is for these patterns in changes according to genotype, age and exercise that we have chosen the tibialis anterior muscle to measure the expression of COL1A1 and MT-CO1; which allowed us to make a correlation between the genotype-dependent changes in muscle weight and power and the corresponding changes in the expression of these two proteins, depending on SPARC expression. Additionally, the decrease in brain weight percentage with ageing correlates with age-related neurodegeneration and related diseases [87,88], which are improved by exercise [89–91] and that, also, correlate with our data, showing an increase (trend) in the brain weight percentage with exercise.

Interleukin 6 (among other myokine) is produced by the muscles during exercise [92,93], which reduces appetite [94] and WAT [93]. This correlates with our results, indicating an effect (trend) of exercise on reducing the body weight and WAT weight percentage, but without any interaction effect on genotype and exercise. This indicates that SPARC absence would not impact the ability of exercise to reduce adiposity. The possibilities could be whether the effect of SPARC is partial since (in *Sparc* KO mice) the WAT weight is lower in Y mice compare to O mice, or there are other SPARC-independent pathways linking myokine to adiposity reduction, such as IL-6 or also because both WT and *Sparc* KO mice spent similar amounts of exercise, leading to similar exercise-induced energy expenditure (would have similar impacts of reducing the WAT).

For the WAT, both for the age and age × genotype (both in WT and *Sparc* KO mice), we always found an increase in adiposity (weight and weight percentage) with ageing. In addition, there is also a reduction in the muscle mass (percentage) with age and for both WT and *Sparc* KO mice, which corresponds to the classical ageing profile (decreased muscle mass and increased adiposity) along with increased body weight with ageing [95–98], as our data show. It is worth noting that, while looking into the effects of genotype × age, both for the decrease in SM mass percentage and the increase in WAT weight (as well as weight percentage), we notice that these ageing-induced changes (musculature decrease and adiposity decrease), are more important in O mice than in Y mice. This could be explained by the implication of SPARC in these changes. Indeed, since *SPARC* expression is downregulated by ageing [8], the consequences of its KO would be more important in Y mice compared to O mice, where its expression is already reduced by ageing.

This ageing effect on SM explains the results of Table 1, showing that ageing reduces the LT speed (adaptation phase), mean exercise speed, total exercise distance (12 weeks of training) and both running speed and the lactate concentration of the last running session at the end of the 12 weeks training. However, the lactate at rest level (week 4 of the adaptation phase), which increases with age, indicates a reduced aerobic metabolic performance of the muscle. Importantly, the effect of genotype × age interaction reveals that the age effect comes from the *Sparc* KO mice rather than WT mice, meaning that it is the *Sparc* KO in O mice that leads to an increase in the resting lactate compared to both WT mice and KO-Y mice. This also explains, in part, how ageing is both a risk factor for numerous diseases and health conditions [99–103].

Since Norose et al. reported that, when handled, *Sparc* KO mice reduced physical activity [104], we deduce that our *Sparc* KO mice had reduced energy expenditure (compared to WT mice), but with a lower body and WAT weights they most probably had less food intake compared to the WT mice. This could indicate an effect (direct or indirect) of *Sparc* KO on appetite. This appetite (in addition to the physical activity patter), both impacting the body weight, could be explained by the increased levels of anxiety and reduced depression-related behaviors in *Sparc* KO mice [82]. Such variations in mood states would impact food intake and energy balance [105,106] and, therefore, body and tissue weights.

4.3. Protein Expressions (Figure 1) and Muscle Strength (Table 4)

The reduced expression of COL1A1 in *Sparc* KO mice fits with what Omi et al. reported [59] and confirms the importance of SPARC for COL1A1 expression, as we have previously shown [28], and as reported by Norose et al. [104] and Bradshaw et al. [107].

In addition, MT-CO1 decreased expression with *Sparc* KO highlights the implication of SPARC in mitochondrial enzyme expression [28] and mitochondrial regeneration [63], whereas MT-CO1 increases expression with exercise, which fits with our previous gene expression studies, showing an increase in oxidative phosphorylation genes with training at LT intensity [6], which further validates the choice of the exercise speed in this study.

Sparc KO mice have been reported as passive and with reduced physical activity compared to WT mice [104], this would indicate weak muscles and correlates with reduced grip power (both mean and maximum) in *Sparc* KO mice compared to WT mice of our study. The importance of SPARC in myoblast fusion [28] and, more important, the interaction of SPARC with actin in SM (actin cytoskeleton modulator) [54] also support our data, indicating a decrease in muscle strength with SPARC deficiency. This SPARC deficiency also reduced COL1A1 expression; indicating an impact on muscle structure (for which collage is a key element) and correlated with the *Sparc* KO-induced muscle strength decrease.

The effect of age (Y > O) on the muscle strength and the effect of exercise (Ex > Sed, trend of the percentage of maximum grip power) is an additional illustration of how ageing worsened the effects of SPARC deficiency (reduce the muscle power) while exercise improved it (increase in both SM strength and expression of both COL1A1 and MT-CO1 with exercise represents muscle adaptation to exercise).

5. Conclusions and Hypothetical Mechanisms

Sparc KO effects are toward a reduced body and WAT weights with a negative SM phenotype (metabolism and strength). Such negative effects worsen with ageing but relatively improve through exercise (Figure 2). While exercise reduces risk factor for many diseases, ageing increases those risks [108].

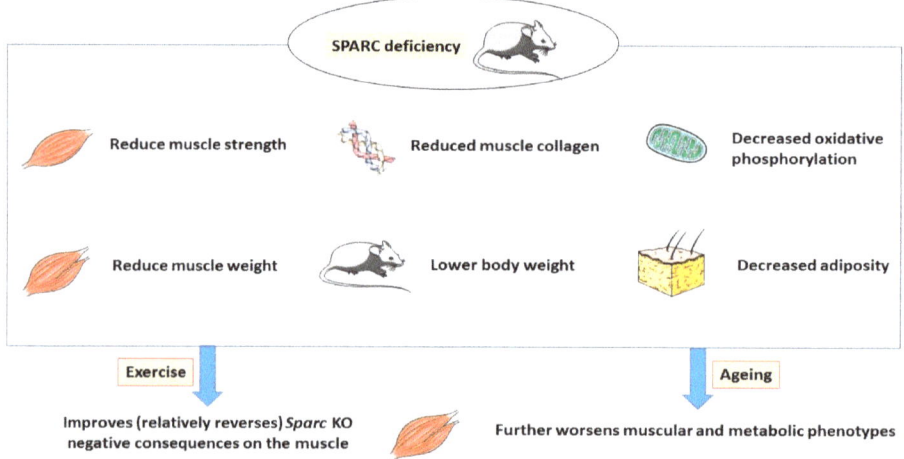

Figure 2. SPARC-deficiency impacts. Our data highlight that *Sparc* KO effects are toward a reduced body and white adipose tissue weights with a negative skeletal muscle phenotype (metabolic and strength). Such negative effects worsen with ageing but relatively improve through exercise. Abbreviations: KO, knockout; SPARC, secreted protein acidic and rich in cysteine.

Within this context, Aoi et al. reported 24 genes (including *SPARC*) that are both upregulated by exercise and downregulated by ageing [8] suggesting, once more, that some of the exercise-induced benefits such as mitochondrial biogenesis [109] could be SPARC-dependent or partially mediated by SPARC. It is within this perspective that we developed our hypothesis.

The exercise-produced lactate induces both an up-regulation of the expression of the cytochrome oxidase gene and protein, as well as a mitochondrial biogenesis activation signal [79], and since *Sparc* KO did not induce any genotype effect on the different lactate levels we measured (both WT and *Sparc* KO mice had statistically similar lactate levels) but reduced the expression of the MT-CO1 (WT and *Sparc* KO mice have similar lactate levels but WT mice express more MT-CO1 than *Sparc* KO mice), we hypothesize that the exercise-produced lactate-induced cytochrome oxidase upregulation and mitochondrial biogenesis activation do require SPARC (Figure 3A). This would, at least in part, explain why SPARC deficiency reduces tumor growth. Indeed, cancer cells require glycolytic energy and produce lactate, leading to lower pH, compared to normal tissue extracellular pH [110,111], and lactate would be an attempt to increase oxidative phosphorylation capacity via improving mitochondrial biogenesis. However, in the absence of SPARC this lactate-induced mitochondrial biogenesis remains limited, which worsens the tumor bioenvironment and results in tumor progress inhibition. This concept of lactate-related signaling correlates with the theory presenting lactate as a signaling molecule "lactormone" in the context of lactate shuttle [112,113] of lactate formation, utilization and exchange between tissues [114].

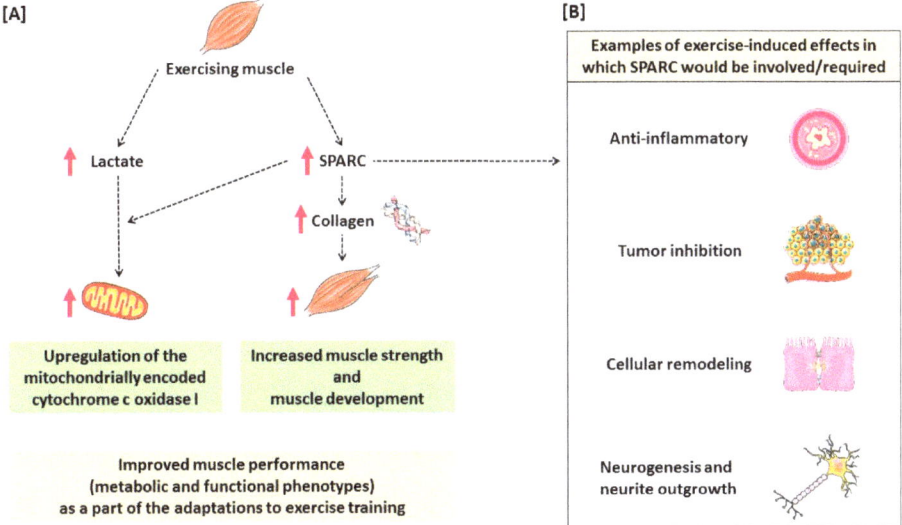

Figure 3. Hypothetical mechanisms linking SPARC to the exercise-induced SPARC-mediated changes in the skeletal muscle phenotype. [**A**] Exercise induces the secretion and expression of SPARC as well as the production of lactate. Our data suggest that, whereas SPARC enhances collagen expression and muscle strength, the lactate increases mitochondrial enzyme expression in a SPARC-dependant manner (probably via mitochondrial biogenesis induction) and, therefore, the oxidative phosphorylation capacity. [**B**] The similarities between exercise benefits and effects shown to be regulated or modulated by SPARC, such as inflammation, cancer growth, metabolic and structural remodeling of the skeletal muscle, and even neurite outgrowth and neurogenesis, all suggest that part of exercise benefits would be mediated by or dependent on SPARC expression. Abbreviation: SPARC, secreted protein acidic and rich in cysteine.

The results of Figure 1B further support our hypothesis that SPARC-dependent exercise impacts SM. Indeed, whereas there is a significant effect of exercise (increase in COL1A1 expression) in WT mice (WT-Ex > WT-Sed), there is no such effect in *Sparc* KO mice (both KO-Ex and KO-Sed mice have statistically similar expression of COL1A1). This also correlates with the genotype-induced decrease in COL1A1 expression (WT > KO) although both WT and *Sparc* KO mice had equal amounts of exercise (as detailed in the introduction of Section 4), therefore, indicating that exercise-induced COL1A1 is SPARC-dependent (Figure 3A). Moreover, since exercise-induced COL1A1 seems SPARC-dependent, and based on the importance of collagens in the SM structure (and fibrillar collagen I is reported to bind SPARC [115]) and development [116], this could also explain, in part, the low tibialis anterior muscle weight in *Sparc* KO mice compared to WT mice, even though all mice had similar amounts of exercise. Thus, this also suggests that SM development (tibialis anterior weight percentage increase; Table 3), as a part to the adaptation to exercise, would also be SPARC-dependent (Figure 3A).

These conclusions are based on the fact that, as per Table 1, there is no effect of the genotype for LT speed, exercise speed, exercise time, exercise distance and lactate concentrations during exercise. This means that mice of two different genotypes (*Sparc* KO and WT) had equal amounts of training (similar speed, distance, time and frequency). Therefore, genotype effects seen for MT-CO1, COL1A1 (Figure 1) and grip power (Table 4) are, indeed, due to the genotype itself (*Sparc* KO) rather than the difference in the exercise amount; suggesting that these exercise-induced changes are SPARC-dependent/mediated. Such exercise-induced effects in the muscle represent a part of the adaptation via increasing the respiratory capacity, mitochondrial content [52] and contractile properties of the SM [53].

In addition to these SPARC-mediated effects, the similarity of exercise benefits and the effects shown to be regulated or modulated by SPARC, such as inflammation [22,47], cancer growth [8,46], metabolic and structural remodeling of the SM [53], and even neurite outgrowth [117,118] and neurogenesis [85,119], all suggest that some of the exercise benefits would indeed be mediated by or dependent on SPARC expression (Figure 3B).

6. Implications and Perspectives

Our data suggest that the benefits of exercise would also be reduced in *Sparc* KO mice, not only because some of exercise benefits are directly mediated via SPARC, but also because physical performance and muscle performance is reduced as a result of *Sparc* KO (indirect effects). As an illustration, *Sparc* KO increases tumor growth [120,121], loss of SPARC increases cancer progression [122] and the tumorigenesis is prevented and suppressed by exercise-induced SPARC [8,123,124]. More generally, since SPARC is also a myokine secreted during exercise [2,8], exercise benefits including metabolic benefits and inflammation regulation would also be reduced with the *Sparc* KO since SPARC has been shown to play roles in metabolism [44], inflammation regulation [47] and cancer homeostasis [46]. Thus, its absence from circulation would impact tissues other than the SM. For instance, even some of the mechanisms underlying the beneficial effects of exercise that have been shown to involve factors other than SPARC, such as tumor growth suppression through interleukin 6 and epinephrine [92], would also be deficient in *Sparc* KO mice, since the absence of SPARC would reduce the ability of SM to correctly secrete the other myokines involved in the related pathways.

Overall, SM, both as a secretory organ [2] and a metabolic engine, represents the key tissue upon which exercise benefits depend. SPARC represents a "booster" of the SM, with beneficial effects on some other tissues as well. Therefore, SPARC and the pathways it governs would represent good targets to pharmacologically mimic the effects of SPARC, including improved muscle strength and metabolic performances. This is of a particular importance for individuals suffering from health problems, such as heart failure or physical handicap and, therefore, are unable to perform the required physical activity although they need it (reduce obesity, treat lipid disorders, etc.). In such a scenario we could imagine an "exercise pill", targeting SPARC-related pathways and inducing exercise-like effects that would also be of a high therapeutic importance for diseases, such as sarcopenia. Such a therapeutic goal still requires further investigations into the implications of SPARC, not only within the SM but also on other tissues and in the diverse aspects of homeostasis. This will both extend the expected benefits of such an "exercise pill" and anticipate the side effects to decide whether it would be better given as a systemic drug or rather target a specific tissue (that would be the SM based on this study) to optimize clinical efficiency. Importantly, the results obtained from studying SPARC/*Sparc* in mice would be expected to be valid in humans, due the high homology between mouse and human SPARC [104], which would reduce the bridge between results in animals and future clinical studies. Perspectives of the future studies on SPARC implications in SM metabolism and contractile properties, both for sedentary and exercise individuals, would be of great clinical importance not only for SM diseases but also for ageing-related health deterioration and, due to the importance of the SM in the energy homeostasis, energy balance-related pathologies such as obesity and diabetes.

Our study was conducted only on male mice. Therefore, we acknowledge the limitation of sex-determined factors. Similar studies in female subjects, as well as studies comparing male and female subjects, will add significant data of clinical importance, especially with the sex-related difference effects on SM and exercise patterns, such as exercise capacity [125], pinch force reproduction [126], maximal oxygen uptake [127], cardiac adaptation to exercise [125], as well as metabolism, including lactate levels [128,129], aerobic oxidation and anaerobic glycolysis [130]. The parameters illustrated by patterns, including differences between men/male animals and women/female animals in red pepper-induced metabolic phenotype (carbohydrate oxidation Vs lipid oxidation) [131,132], beta-oxidation [130], type I fiber percentage [133] and enzyme activities [134], explain beyond such sex-related differences in exercise and SM properties. Based on such sex-related differences, our results could also indicate that SPARC involvement in exercise-induced muscle phenotype changes could also be sex-dependent and points to a possible interaction between SPARC activities and sexual hormones based on the known impacts of sexual hormones on exercise patterns and the adaptation to exercise [135–137].

Our data indicate that the impacts of *Sparc* KO on body composition, adiposity and metabolic patterns point toward a reduced WAT and body weight, but with negative metabolic and functional phenotypes of SM. Whereas such negative effects on SM worsen with ageing, they are relatively improved by exercise. Importantly, we report, for the first time, evidence suggesting that the exercise-induced changes in the SM phenotype in terms of increased performance (metabolic, strength and development), including lactate-induced changes, are SPARC-dependent. Such important implications of SPARC highlight SPARC and its pathways as pharmacological targets/tools for conditions and diseases in which muscle properties enhancement would provide therapeutic benefits.

Author Contributions: Data curation, A.G., A.M., M.Y. and J.S.-A.; Formal analysis, A.G., A.M. and M.Y.; Funding acquisition, J.S.-A.; Investigation, A.G., A.M., M.Y. and J.S.-A.; Methodology, A.G., A.M., M.Y. and J.S.-A.; Project administration, M.Y. and J.S.-A.; Supervision, M.Y. and J.S.-A.; Validation, M.Y. and J.S.-A.; Visualization, A.G., A.M., M.Y. and J.S.-A.; Writing—original draft, A.G.; Writing—review & editing, A.G., A.M., M.Y. and J.S.-A. All authors have read and agreed to the published version of the manuscript.

Funding: This work was supported by the Canadian Institutes of Health Research (CIHR), Number: 201309MOP-311306-BCA-CFBA-40425.

Acknowledgments: We thank Amy D. Bradshaw for providing our research group with sperm of *Sparc* KO mice. Abdelaziz Ghanemi received a Merit scholarship for foreign students from the Ministry of Education and Higher Education of Quebec, Canada, The Fonds de recherche du Québec—Nature et technologies (FRQNT) is responsible for managing the program (Bourses d'excellence pour étudiants étrangers du Ministère de l'Éducation et de l'Enseignement supérieur du Québec, Le Fonds de recherche du Québec—Nature et technologies (FRQNT) est responsable de la gestion du programme). Figures 2 and 3 were created using images from http://smart.servier.com. Servier Medical Art by Servier is licensed under a Creative Commons Attribution 3.0 Unported License.

Conflicts of Interest: The authors declare no conflict of interest.

References

1. Pedersen, B.K. The physiology of optimizing health with a focus on exercise as medicine. *Annu. Rev. Physiol.* **2019**, *81*, 607–627. [CrossRef] [PubMed]
2. Aoi, W.; Sakuma, K. Skeletal muscle: Novel and intriguing characteristics as a secretory organ. *BioDiscovery* **2013**, *7*, e8942. [CrossRef]
3. Ghanemi, A.; Melouane, A.; Yoshioka, M.; St-Amand, J. Exercise and high-fat diet in obesity: Functional genomics perspectives of two energy homeostasis pillars. *Genes* **2020**, *11*, 875. [CrossRef] [PubMed]
4. Berryhill, B.L.; Kane, B.; Stramer, B.M.; Fini, M.E.; Hassell, J.R. Increased SPARC accumulation during corneal repair. *Exp. Eye Res.* **2003**, *77*, 85–92. [CrossRef]
5. Phan, E.; Ahluwalia, A.; Tarnawski, A.S. Role of SPARC—Matricellular protein in pathophysiology and tissue injury healing. Implications for gastritis and gastric ulcers. *Med. Sci. Monit.* **2007**, *13*, RA25–RA30.
6. Riedl, I.; Yoshioka, M.; Nishida, Y.; Tobina, T.; Paradis, R.; Shono, N.; Tanaka, H.; St-Amand, J. Regulation of skeletal muscle transcriptome in elderly men after 6 weeks of endurance training at lactate threshold intensity. *Exp. Gerontol.* **2010**, *45*, 896–903. [CrossRef]

7. Melouane, A.; Yoshioka, M.; Kanzaki, M.; St-Amand, J. Sparc, an EPS-induced gene, modulates the extracellular matrix and mitochondrial function via ILK/AMPK pathways in C2C12 cells. *Life Sci.* **2019**, *229*, 277–287. [CrossRef]
8. Aoi, W.; Naito, Y.; Takagi, T.; Tanimura, Y.; Takanami, Y.; Kawai, Y.; Sakuma, K.; Hang, L.P.; Mizushima, K.; Hirai, Y.; et al. A novel myokine, secreted protein acidic and rich in cysteine (SPARC), suppresses colon tumorigenesis via regular exercise. *Gut* **2013**, *62*, 882–889. [CrossRef]
9. Matsuo, K.; Sato, K.; Suemoto, K.; Miyamoto-Mikami, E.; Fuku, N.; Higashida, K.; Tsuji, K.; Xu, Y.; Liu, X.; Iemitsu, M.; et al. A mechanism underlying preventive effect of high-intensity training on colon cancer. *Med. Sci. Sports Exerc.* **2017**, *49*, 1805–1816. [CrossRef]
10. Norheim, F.; Raastad, T.; Thiede, B.; Rustan, A.C.; Drevon, C.A.; Haugen, F. Proteomic identification of secreted proteins from human skeletal muscle cells and expression in response to strength training. *Am. J. Physiol. Endocrinol. Metab.* **2011**, *301*, E1013–E1021. [CrossRef]
11. Garneau, L.; Parsons, S.A.; Smith, S.R.; Mulvihill, E.E.; Sparks, L.M.; Aguer, C. Plasma myokine concentrations after acute exercise in non-obese and obese sedentary women. *Front. Physiol.* **2020**, *11*, 18. [CrossRef] [PubMed]
12. Billat, V.L.; Mouisel, E.; Roblot, N.; Melki, J. Inter- and intrastrain variation in mouse critical running speed. *J. Appl. Physiol. (1985)* **2005**, *98*, 1258–1263. [CrossRef] [PubMed]
13. Available online: https://insights.envigo.com/hubfs/resources/data-sheets/2018s-datasheet-0915.pdf (accessed on 9 August 2020).
14. Norose, K.; Lo, W.K.; Clark, J.I.; Sage, E.H.; Howe, C.C. Lenses of SPARC-null mice exhibit an abnormal cell surface-basement membrane interface. *Exp. Eye Res.* **2000**, *71*, 295–307. [CrossRef] [PubMed]
15. Nie, J.; Bradshaw, A.D.; Delany, A.M.; Sage, E.H. Inactivation of SPARC enhances high-fat diet-induced obesity in mice. *Connect. Tissue Res.* **2011**, *52*, 99–108. [CrossRef]
16. Faude, O.; Kindermann, W.; Meyer, T. Lactate threshold concepts: How valid are they? *Sports Med.* **2009**, *39*, 469–490. [CrossRef]
17. Schefer, V.; Talan, M.I. Oxygen consumption in adult and AGED C57BL/6J mice during acute treadmill exercise of different intensity. *Exp. Gerontol.* **1996**, *31*, 387–392. [CrossRef]
18. Nishida, Y.; Tokuyama, K.; Nagasaka, S.; Higaki, Y.; Shirai, Y.; Kiyonaga, A.; Shindo, M.; Kusaka, I.; Nakamura, T.; Ishibashi, S.; et al. Effect of moderate exercise training on peripheral glucose effectiveness, insulin sensitivity, and endogenous glucose production in healthy humans estimated by a two-compartment-labeled minimal model. *Diabetes* **2004**, *53*, 315–320. [CrossRef]
19. Tanaka, H.; Shindo, M. The benefits of the low intensity training. *Ann. Physiol. Anthr.* **1992**, *11*, 365–368. [CrossRef]
20. Motoyama, M.; Sunami, Y.; Kinoshita, F.; Kiyonaga, A.; Tanaka, H.; Shindo, M.; Irie, T.; Urata, H.; Sasaki, J.; Arakawa, K. Blood pressure lowering effect of low intensity aerobic training in elderly hypertensive patients. *Med. Sci. Sports Exerc.* **1998**, *30*, 818–823.
21. Sunami, Y.; Motoyama, M.; Kinoshita, F.; Mizooka, Y.; Sueta, K.; Matsunaga, A.; Sasaki, J.; Tanaka, H.; Shindo, M. Effects of low-intensity aerobic training on the high-density lipoprotein cholesterol concentration in healthy elderly subjects. *Metabolism* **1999**, *48*, 984–988. [CrossRef]
22. Kawanishi, N.; Yano, H.; Mizokami, T.; Takahashi, M.; Oyanagi, E.; Suzuki, K. Exercise training attenuates hepatic inflammation, fibrosis and macrophage infiltration during diet induced-obesity in mice. *Brain Behav. Immun.* **2012**, *26*, 931–941. [CrossRef] [PubMed]
23. Van Praag, H.; Shubert, T.; Zhao, C.; Gage, F.H. Exercise enhances learning and hippocampal neurogenesis in aged mice. *J. Neurosci.* **2005**, *25*, 8680–8685. [CrossRef] [PubMed]
24. Rowlatt, C.; Chesterman, F.C.; Sheriff, M.U. Lifespan, age changes and tumour incidence in an ageing C57BL mouse colony. *Lab. Anim.* **1976**, *10*, 419–442. [CrossRef] [PubMed]
25. Kunstyr, I.; Leuenberger, H.G. Gerontological data of C57BL/6J mice. I. Sex differences in survival curves. *J. Gerontol.* **1975**, *30*, 157–162. [CrossRef] [PubMed]
26. Smith, J.P.; Hicks, P.S.; Ortiz, L.R.; Martinez, M.J.; Mandler, R.N. Quantitative measurement of muscle strength in the mouse. *J. Neurosci. Methods* **1995**, *62*, 15–19. [CrossRef]

27. Takeshita, H.; Yamamoto, K.; Nozato, S.; Inagaki, T.; Tsuchimochi, H.; Shirai, M.; Yamamoto, R.; Imaizumi, Y.; Hongyo, K.; Yokoyama, S.; et al. Modified forelimb grip strength test detects aging-associated physiological decline in skeletal muscle function in male mice. *Sci. Rep.* **2017**, *7*, 42323. [CrossRef]
28. Melouane, A.; Carbonell, A.; Yoshioka, M.; Puymirat, J.; St-Amand, J. Implication of SPARC in the modulation of the extracellular matrix and mitochondrial function in muscle cells. *PLoS ONE* **2018**, *13*, e0192714. [CrossRef]
29. Zong, S.; Wu, M.; Gu, J.; Liu, T.; Guo, R.; Yang, M. Structure of the intact 14-subunit human cytochrome c oxidase. *Cell Res.* **2018**, *28*, 1026–1034. [CrossRef]
30. Schneider, C.A.; Rasband, W.S.; Eliceiri, K.W. NIH Image to ImageJ: 25 years of image analysis. *Nat. Methods* **2012**, *9*, 671–675. [CrossRef]
31. Taylor, S.C.; Berkelman, T.; Yadav, G.; Hammond, M. A defined methodology for reliable quantification of Western blot data. *Mol. Biotechnol.* **2013**, *55*, 217–226. [CrossRef]
32. Taylor, S.C.; Posch, A. The design of a quantitative western blot experiment. *Biomed. Res. Int.* **2014**, *2014*, 361590. [CrossRef] [PubMed]
33. Ghanemi, A.; Melouane, A.; Mucunguzi, O.; Yoshioka, M.; St-Amand, J. Energy and metabolic pathways in trefoil factor family member 2 (Tff2) KO mice beyond the protection from high-fat diet-induced obesity. *Life Sci.* **2018**, *215*, 190–197. [CrossRef]
34. De Giorgio, M.R.; Yoshioka, M.; Riedl, I.; Moreault, O.; Cherizol, R.G.; Shah, A.A.; Blin, N.; Richard, D.; StAmand, J. Trefoil factor family member 2 (Tff2) KO mice are protected from high-fat diet-induced obesity. *Obesity (Silver Spring)* **2013**, *21*, 1389–1395. [CrossRef] [PubMed]
35. Bradshaw, A.D.; Sage, E.H. SPARC, a matricellular protein that functions in cellular differentiation and tissue response to injury. *J. Clin. Investig.* **2001**, *107*, 1049–1054. [CrossRef] [PubMed]
36. Brekken, R.A.; Sage, E.H. SPARC, a matricellular protein: At the crossroads of cell-matrix communication. *Matrix Biol.* **2001**, *19*, 816–827. [CrossRef]
37. Lane, T.F.; Sage, E.H. The biology of SPARC, a protein that modulates cell-matrix interactions. *FASEB J.* **1994**, *8*, 163–173. [CrossRef] [PubMed]
38. Yan, Q.; Sage, E.H. SPARC, a matricellular glycoprotein with important biological functions. *J. Histochem. Cytochem.* **1999**, *47*, 1495–1506. [CrossRef]
39. Mason, I.J.; Murphy, D.; Münke, M.; Francke, U.; Elliott, R.W.; Hogan, B.L. Developmental and transformation-sensitive expression of the Sparc gene on mouse chromosome 11. *EMBO J.* **1986**, *5*, 1831–1837. [CrossRef]
40. Swaroop, A.; Hogan, B.L.; Francke, U. Molecular analysis of the cDNA for human SPARC/osteonectin/BM-40: Sequence, expression, and localization of the gene to chromosome 5q31-q33. *Genomics* **1988**, *2*, 37–47. [CrossRef]
41. Brekken, R.A.; Sage, E.H. SPARC, a matricellular protein. At the crossroads of cell-matrix. *Matrix Biol.* **2000**, *19*, 569–580. [CrossRef]
42. Francki, A.; Motamed, K.; McClure, T.D.; Kaya, M.; Murri, C.; Blake, D.J.; Carbon, J.G.; Sage, E.H. SPARC regulates cell cycle progression in mesangial cells via its inhibition of IGF-dependent signaling. *J. Cell. Biochem.* **2003**, *88*, 802–811. [CrossRef]
43. Basu, A.; Kligman, L.H.; Samulewicz, S.J.; Howe, C.C. Impaired wound healing in mice deficient in a matricellular protein SPARC (osteonectin, BM-40). *BMC Cell Biol.* **2001**, *2*, 15. [CrossRef] [PubMed]
44. Ghanemi, A.; Melouane, A.; Yoshioka, M.; St-Amand, J. Secreted protein acidic and rich in cysteine and bioenergetics: Extracellular matrix, adipocytes remodeling and skeletal muscle metabolism. *Int. J. Biochem. Cell Biol.* **2019**, *117*, 105627. [CrossRef] [PubMed]
45. Ghanemi, A.; Yoshioka, M.; St-Amand, J. Secreted protein acidic and rich in cysteine: Metabolic and homeostatic properties beyond the extracellular matrix structure. *Appl. Sci.* **2020**, *10*, 2388. [CrossRef]
46. Ghanemi, A.; Yoshioka, M.; St-Amand, J. Secreted protein acidic and rich in cysteine and cancer: A homeostatic hormone? *Cytokine* **2020**, *127*, 154996. [CrossRef] [PubMed]
47. Ghanemi, A.; Yoshioka, M.; St-Amand, J. Secreted protein acidic and rich in cysteine and inflammation: Another homeostatic property? *Cytokine* **2020**, *133*, 155179. [CrossRef]

48. Jørgensen, L.H.; Petersson, S.J.; Sellathurai, J.; Andersen, D.C.; Thayssen, S.; Sant, D.J.; Jensen, C.H.; Schrøder, H.D. Secreted protein acidic and rich in cysteine (SPARC) in human skeletal muscle. *J. Histochem. Cytochem.* **2009**, *57*, 29–39. [CrossRef]
49. Holland, P.W.; Harper, S.J.; McVey, J.H.; Hogan, B.L. In vivo expression of mRNA for the Ca+++-binding protein SPARC (osteonectin) revealed by in situ hybridization. *J. Cell Biol.* **1987**, *105*, 473–482. [CrossRef]
50. Sage, H.; Vernon, R.B.; Decker, J.; Funk, S.; Iruela-Arispe, M.L. Distribution of the calcium-binding protein SPARC in tissues of embryonic and adult mice. *J. Histochem. Cytochem.* **1989**, *37*, 819–829. [CrossRef]
51. Framson, P.E.; Sage, E.H. SPARC and tumor growth: Where the seed meets the soil? *J. Cell. Biochem.* **2004**, *92*, 679–690. [CrossRef]
52. Holloszy, J.O. Muscle metabolism during exercise. *Arch. Phys. Med. Rehabil.* **1982**, *63*, 231–234. [PubMed]
53. Ferraro, E.; Giammarioli, A.M.; Chiandotto, S.; Spoletini, I.; Rosano, G. Exercise-induced skeletal muscle remodeling and metabolic adaptation: Redox signaling and role of autophagy. *Antioxid. Redox Signal.* **2014**, *21*, 154–176. [CrossRef] [PubMed]
54. Jørgensen, L.H.; Jepsen, P.L.; Boysen, A.; Dalgaard, L.B.; Hvid, L.G.; Ørtenblad, N.; Ravn, D.; Sellathurai, J.; Møller-Jensen, J.; Lochmüller, H.; et al. SPARC interacts with actin in skeletal muscle in vitro and in vivo. *Am. J. Pathol.* **2017**, *187*, 457–474. [CrossRef] [PubMed]
55. Chlenski, A.; Guerrero, L.J.; Salwen, H.R.; Yang, Q.; Tian, Y.; La Madrid, A.M.; Mirzoeva, S.; Bouyer, P.G.; Xu, D.; Walker, M.; et al. Secreted protein acidic and rich in cysteine is a matrix scavenger chaperone. *PLoS ONE* **2011**, *6*, e23880. [CrossRef] [PubMed]
56. Delany, A.M.; Amling, M.; Priemel, M.; Howe, C.; Baron, R.; Canalis, E. Osteopenia and decreased bone formation in osteonectin-deficient mice. *J. Clin. Investig.* **2000**, *105*, 915–923. [CrossRef] [PubMed]
57. Wang, H.; Fertala, A.; Ratner, B.D.; Sage, E.H.; Jiang, S. Identifying the SPARC binding sites on collagen I and procollagen I by atomic force microscopy. *Anal. Chem.* **2005**, *77*, 6765–6771. [CrossRef]
58. Giudici, C.; Raynal, N.; Wiedemann, H.; Cabral, W.A.; Marini, J.C.; Timpl, R.; Bächinger, H.P.; Farndale, R.W.; Sasaki, T.; Tenni, R. Mapping of SPARC/BM-40/osteonectin-binding sites on fibrillar collagens. *J. Biol. Chem.* **2008**, *283*, 19551–19560. [CrossRef]
59. Omi, S.; Yamanouchi, K.; Nakamura, K.; Matsuwaki, T.; Nishihara, M. Reduced fibrillar collagen accumulation in skeletal muscle of secreted protein acidic and rich in cysteine (SPARC)-null mice. *J. Vet. Med. Sci.* **2019**, *81*, 1649–1654. [CrossRef]
60. Sage, H.; Vernon, R.B.; Funk, S.E.; Everitt, E.A.; Angello, J. SPARC, a secreted protein associated with cellular proliferation, inhibits cell spreading in vitro and exhibits Ca+2-dependent binding to the extracellular matrix. *J. Cell Biol.* **1989**, *109*, 341–356. [CrossRef]
61. Francki, A.; Bradshaw, A.D.; Bassuk, J.A.; Howe, C.C.; Couser, W.G.; Sage, E.H. SPARC regulates the expression of collagen type I and transforming growth factor-beta1 in mesangial cells. *J. Biol. Chem.* **1999**, *274*, 32145–32152. [CrossRef]
62. Bradshaw, A.D.; Reed, M.J.; Sage, E.H. SPARC-null mice exhibit accelerated cutaneous wound closure. *J. Histochem. Cytochem.* **2002**, *50*, 1–10. [CrossRef] [PubMed]
63. Melouane, A.; Yoshioka, M.; St-Amand, J. Extracellular matrix/mitochondria pathway: A novel potential target for sarcopenia. *Mitochondrion* **2020**, *50*, 63–70. [CrossRef] [PubMed]
64. Song, H.; Guan, Y.; Zhang, L.; Li, K.; Dong, C. SPARC interacts with AMPK and regulates GLUT4 expression. *Biochem. Biophys. Res. Commun.* **2010**, *396*, 961–966. [CrossRef] [PubMed]
65. Lira, V.A.; Benton, C.R.; Yan, Z.; Bonen, A. PGC-1alpha regulation by exercise training and its influences on muscle function and insulin sensitivity. *Am. J. Physiol. Endocrinol. Metab.* **2010**, *299*, E145–E161. [CrossRef]
66. Jäger, S.; Handschin, C.; St-Pierre, J.; Spiegelman, B.M. AMP-activated protein kinase (AMPK) action in skeletal muscle via direct phosphorylation of PGC-1alpha. *Proc. Natl. Acad. Sci. USA* **2007**, *104*, 12017–12022. [CrossRef]
67. Wu, Z.; Puigserver, P.; Andersson, U.; Zhang, C.; Adelmant, G.; Mootha, V.; Troy, A.; Cinti, S.; Lowell, B.; Scarpulla, R.C.; et al. Mechanisms controlling mitochondrial biogenesis and respiration through the thermogenic coactivator PGC-1. *Cell* **1999**, *98*, 115–124. [CrossRef]
68. Smith, G.M.; Gallo, G. The role of mitochondria in axon development and regeneration. *Dev. Neurobiol.* **2018**, *78*, 221–237. [CrossRef]

69. Han, S.M.; Baig, H.S.; Hammarlund, M. Mitochondria localize to injured axons to support regeneration. *Neuron* **2016**, *92*, 1308–1323. [CrossRef]
70. Aoi, W.; Hirano, N.; Lassiter, D.G.; Björnholm, M.; Chibalin, A.V.; Sakuma, K.; Tanimura, Y.; Mizushima, K.; Takagi, T.; Naito, Y.; et al. Secreted protein acidic and rich in cysteine (SPARC) improves glucose tolerance via AMP-activated protein kinase activation. *FASEB J.* **2019**, *33*, 10551–10562. [CrossRef]
71. Bradshaw, A.D. The role of secreted protein acidic and rich in cysteine (SPARC) in cardiac repair and fibrosis: Does expression of SPARC by macrophages influence outcomes? *J. Mol. Cell. Cardiol.* **2016**, *93*, 156–161. [CrossRef]
72. McCurdy, S.; Baicu, C.F.; Heymans, S.; Bradshaw, A.D. Cardiac extracellular matrix remodeling: Fibrillar collagens and secreted protein acidic and rich in cysteine (SPARC). *J. Mol. Cell. Cardiol.* **2010**, *48*, 544–549. [CrossRef] [PubMed]
73. Cheng, L.; Sun, X.; Guo, J.; Lu, G. SPARC support the expansion of cord blood stem cells in vitro. *Cell Res.* **2008**, *18*, S49. [CrossRef]
74. Zhu, J.; Wang, L.Y.; Li, C.Y.; Wu, J.Y.; Zhang, Y.T.; Pang, K.P.; Wei, Y.; Du, L.Q.; Liu, M.; Wu, X.Y. SPARC promotes self-renewal of limbal epithelial stem cells and ocular surface restoration through JNK and p38-MAPK signaling pathways. *Stem Cells* **2020**, *38*, 134–145. [CrossRef] [PubMed]
75. Rooney, K.; Trayhurn, P. Lactate and the GPR81 receptor in metabolic regulation: Implications for adipose tissue function and fatty acid utilisation by muscle during exercise. *Br. J. Nutr.* **2011**, *106*, 1310–1316. [CrossRef] [PubMed]
76. Gladden, L.B. Muscle as a consumer of lactate. *Med. Sci. Sports Exerc.* **2000**, *32*, 764–771. [CrossRef] [PubMed]
77. Gladden, L.B. Lactate metabolism: A new paradigm for the third millennium. *J. Physiol.* **2004**, *558*, 5–30. [CrossRef]
78. Hashimoto, T.; Hussien, R.; Oommen, S.; Gohil, K.; Brooks, G.A. Lactate sensitive transcription factor network in L6 cells: Activation of MCT1 and mitochondrial biogenesis. *FASEB J.* **2007**, *21*, 2602–2612. [CrossRef]
79. Hashimoto, T.; Brooks, G.A. Mitochondrial lactate oxidation complex and an adaptive role for lactate production. *Med. Sci. Sports Exerc.* **2008**, *40*, 486–494. [CrossRef]
80. Gladden, L.B. A lactic perspective on metabolism. *Med. Sci. Sports Exerc.* **2008**, *40*, 477–485. [CrossRef]
81. Jacobs, I. Blood lactate. *Sports Med.* **1986**, *3*, 10–25. [CrossRef]
82. Campolongo, M.; Benedetti, L.; Podhajcer, O.L.; Pitossi, F.; Depino, A.M. Hippocampal SPARC regulates depression-related behavior. *Genes Brain Behav.* **2012**, *11*, 966–976. [CrossRef] [PubMed]
83. Leveille, G.A.; Chakrabarty, K. Diurnal variations in tissue glycogen and liver weight of meal-fed rats. *J. Nutr.* **1967**, *93*, 546–554. [CrossRef] [PubMed]
84. Kreitzman, S.N.; Coxon, A.Y.; Szaz, K.F. Glycogen storage: Illusions of easy weight loss, excessive weight regain, and distortions in estimates of body composition. *Am. J. Clin. Nutr.* **1992**, *56* (Suppl. 1), 292s–293s. [CrossRef]
85. Ma, C.L.; Ma, X.T.; Wang, J.J.; Liu, H.; Chen, Y.F.; Yang, Y. Physical exercise induces hippocampal neurogenesis and prevents cognitive decline. *Behav. Brain Res.* **2017**, *317*, 332–339. [CrossRef] [PubMed]
86. Yuan, T.F.; Paes, F.; Arias-Carrión, O.; Ferreira Rocha, N.B.; de Sá Filho, A.S.; Machado, S. Neural mechanisms of exercise: Anti-depression, neurogenesis, and serotonin signaling. *CNS Neurol. Disord. Drug Targets* **2015**, *14*, 1307–1311. [CrossRef]
87. Uddin, M.S.; Hossain, M.F.; Mamun, A.A.; Shah, M.A.; Hasana, S.; Bulbul, I.J.; Sarwar, M.S.; Mansouri, R.A.; Ashraf, G.M.; Rauf, A.; et al. Exploring the multimodal role of phytochemicals in the modulation of cellular signaling pathways to combat age-related neurodegeneration. *Sci. Total Environ.* **2020**, *725*, 138313. [CrossRef]
88. Hung, C.W.; Chen, Y.C.; Hsieh, W.L.; Chiou, S.H.; Kao, C.L. Ageing and neurodegenerative diseases. *Ageing Res. Rev.* **2010**, *9* (Suppl. 1), S36–S46. [CrossRef]
89. Mahalakshmi, B.; Maurya, N.; Lee, S.-D.; Bharath Kumar, V. Possible neuroprotective mechanisms of physical exercise in neurodegeneration. *Int. J. Mol. Sci.* **2020**, *21*, 5895. [CrossRef]
90. Ang, E.-T.; Tai, Y.-K.; Lo, S.-Q.; Seet, R.; Soong, T.-W. Neurodegenerative diseases: Exercising toward neurogenesis and neuroregeneration. *Front. Aging Neurosci.* **2010**, *2*, 25. [CrossRef]

91. Liu, Y.; Yan, T.; Chu, J.M.; Chen, Y.; Dunnett, S.; Ho, Y.S.; Wong, G.T.; Chang, R.C. The beneficial effects of physical exercise in the brain and related pathophysiological mechanisms in neurodegenerative diseases. *Lab. Investig.* **2019**, *99*, 943–957. [CrossRef]
92. Pedersen, L.; Idorn, M.; Olofsson, G.H.; Lauenborg, B.; Nookaew, I.; Hansen, R.H.; Johannesen, H.H.; Becker, J.C.; Pedersen, K.S.; Dethlefsen, C.; et al. Voluntary running suppresses tumor growth through epinephrine- and IL-6-dependent NK cell mobilization and redistribution. *Cell Metab.* **2016**, *23*, 554–562. [CrossRef] [PubMed]
93. Wedell-Neergaard, A.S.; Lang Lehrskov, L.; Christensen, R.H.; Legaard, G.E.; Dorph, E.; Larsen, M.K.; Launbo, N.; Fagerlind, S.R.; Seide, S.K.; Nymand, S.; et al. Exercise-induced changes in visceral adipose tissue mass are regulated by IL-6 signaling: A randomized controlled trial. *Cell Metab.* **2019**, *29*, 844–855.e3. [CrossRef] [PubMed]
94. Ellingsgaard, H.; Hojman, P.; Pedersen, B.K. Exercise and health—Emerging roles of IL-6. *Curr. Opin. Physiol.* **2019**, *10*, 49–54. [CrossRef]
95. Sakuma, K.; Yamaguchi, A. Sarcopenic obesity and endocrinal adaptation with age. *Int. J. Endocrinol.* **2013**, *2013*, 204164. [CrossRef]
96. Candow, D.G.; Chilibeck, P.D. Differences in size, strength, and power of upper and lower body muscle groups in young and older men. *J. Gerontol. A Biol. Sci. Med. Sci.* **2005**, *60*, 148–156. [CrossRef]
97. Kalyani, R.R.; Corriere, M.; Ferrucci, L. Age-related and disease-related muscle loss: The effect of diabetes, obesity, and other diseases. *Lancet Diabetes Endocrinol.* **2014**, *2*, 819–829. [CrossRef]
98. Kim, T.N.; Choi, K.M. The implications of sarcopenia and sarcopenic obesity on cardiometabolic disease. *J. Cell. Biochem.* **2015**, *116*, 1171–1178. [CrossRef]
99. Dhingra, R.; Vasan, R.S. Age as a risk factor. *Med. Clin. N. Am.* **2012**, *96*, 87–91. [CrossRef]
100. Keenan, C.R.; White, R.H. Age as a risk factor for venous thromboembolism after major surgery. *Curr. Opin. Pulm. Med.* **2005**, *11*, 398–402. [CrossRef]
101. Koshiyama, M.; Tamaki, K.; Ohsawa, M. Age-specific incidence rates of atrial fibrillation and risk factors for the future development of atrial fibrillation in the Japanese general population. *J. Cardiol.* **2020**, *77*, 88–92. [CrossRef]
102. Zhang, H.; Rogers, K.; Sukkar, L.; Jun, M.; Kang, A.; Young, T.; Campain, A.; Cass, A.; Chow, C.K.; Comino, E.; et al. Prevalence, incidence and risk factors of diabetes in Australian adults aged ≥ 45 years: A cohort study using linked routinely-collected data. *J. Clin. Transl. Endocrinol.* **2020**, *22*, 100240. [CrossRef] [PubMed]
103. Mosher, C.L.; Weber, J.M.; Frankel, C.W.; Neely, M.L.; Palmer, S.M. Risk factors for mortality in lung transplant recipients aged ≥ 65 years: A retrospective cohort study of 5815 patients in the scientific registry of transplant recipients. *J. Heart Lung Transplant.* **2020**. [CrossRef]
104. Norose, K.; Clark, J.I.; Syed, N.A.; Basu, A.; Heber-Katz, E.; Sage, E.H.; Howe, C.C. SPARC deficiency leads to early-onset cataractogenesis. *Investig. Ophthalmol. Vis. Sci.* **1998**, *39*, 2674–2680. [PubMed]
105. Singh, M. Mood, food, and obesity. *Front. Psychol.* **2014**, *5*, 925. [CrossRef]
106. Ortolani, D.; Oyama, L.M.; Ferrari, E.M.; Melo, L.L.; Spadari-Bratfisch, R.C. Effects of comfort food on food intake, anxiety-like behavior and the stress response in rats. *Physiol. Behav.* **2011**, *103*, 487–492. [CrossRef] [PubMed]
107. Bradshaw, A.D.; Graves, D.C.; Motamed, K.; Sage, E.H. SPARC-null mice exhibit increased adiposity without significant differences in overall body weight. *Proc. Natl. Acad. Sci. USA* **2003**, *100*, 6045–6050. [CrossRef]
108. Sinclair, A.J.; Abdelhafiz, A.H. Cardiometabolic disease in the older person: Prediction and prevention for the generalist physician. *Cardiovasc. Endocrinol. Metab.* **2020**, *9*, 90–95. [CrossRef]
109. Islam, H.; Hood, D.A.; Gurd, B.J. Looking beyond PGC-1α: Emerging regulators of exercise-induced skeletal muscle mitochondrial biogenesis and their activation by dietary compounds. *Appl. Physiol. Nutr. Metab.* **2020**, *45*, 11–23. [CrossRef]
110. Su, J.; Chen, X.; Kanekura, T. A CD147-targeting siRNA inhibits the proliferation, invasiveness, and VEGF production of human malignant melanoma cells by down-regulating glycolysis. *Cancer Lett.* **2009**, *273*, 140–147. [CrossRef]

111. Gillies, R.J.; Raghunand, N.; Karczmar, G.S.; Bhujwalla, Z.M. MRI of the tumor microenvironment. *J. Magn. Reason. Imaging* **2002**, *16*, 430–450. [CrossRef]
112. Gladden, L.B. Current trends in lactate metabolism: Introduction. *Med. Sci. Sports Exerc.* **2008**, *40*, 475–476. [CrossRef] [PubMed]
113. Brooks, G.A. Lactate shuttles in nature. *Biochem. Soc. Trans.* **2002**, *30*, 258–264. [CrossRef] [PubMed]
114. Brooks, G.A. Current concepts in lactate exchange. *Med. Sci. Sports Exerc.* **1991**, *23*, 895–906. [CrossRef] [PubMed]
115. Sasaki, T.; Hohenester, E.; Göhring, W.; Timpl, R. Crystal structure and mapping by site-directed mutagenesis of the collagen-binding epitope of an activated form of BM-40/SPARC/osteonectin. *EMBO J.* **1998**, *17*, 1625–1634. [CrossRef]
116. Bailey, A.J. The role of collagen in the development of muscle and its relationship to eating quality. *J. Anim. Sci.* **1985**, *60*, 1580–1587. [CrossRef]
117. Au, E.; Richter, M.W.; Vincent, A.J.; Tetzlaff, W.; Aebersold, R.; Sage, E.H.; Roskams, A.J. SPARC from olfactory ensheathing cells stimulates Schwann cells to promote neurite outgrowth and enhances spinal cord repair. *J. Neurosci.* **2007**, *27*, 7208–7221. [CrossRef]
118. Lee, M.H.; Amin, N.D.; Venkatesan, A.; Wang, T.; Tyagi, R.; Pant, H.C.; Nath, A. Impaired neurogenesis and neurite outgrowth in an HIV-gp120 transgenic model is reversed by exercise via BDNF production and Cdk5 regulation. *J. Neurovirol.* **2013**, *19*, 418–431. [CrossRef]
119. Vincent, A.J.; Lau, P.W.; Roskams, A.J. SPARC is expressed by macroglia and microglia in the developing and mature nervous system. *Dev. Dyn.* **2008**, *237*, 1449–1462. [CrossRef]
120. Brekken, R.A.; Puolakkainen, P.; Graves, D.C.; Workman, G.; Lubkin, S.R.; Sage, E.H. Enhanced growth of tumors in SPARC null mice is associated with changes in the ECM. *J. Clin. Investig.* **2003**, *111*, 487–495. [CrossRef]
121. Puolakkainen, P.A.; Brekken, R.A.; Muneer, S.; Sage, E.H. Enhanced growth of pancreatic tumors in SPARC-null mice is associated with decreased deposition of extracellular matrix and reduced tumor cell apoptosis. *Mol. Cancer Res.* **2004**, *2*, 215–224.
122. Said, N.; Frierson, H.F.; Sanchez-Carbayo, M.; Brekken, R.A.; Theodorescu, D. Loss of SPARC in bladder cancer enhances carcinogenesis and progression. *J. Clin. Investig.* **2013**, *123*, 751–766. [CrossRef] [PubMed]
123. Liu, Y.P.; Hsiao, M. Exercise-induced SPARC prevents tumorigenesis of colon cancer. *Gut* **2013**, *62*, 810–811. [CrossRef] [PubMed]
124. Aoi, W. Possibility of the novel myokine SPARC: A mechanistic approach to colon cancer prevention by physical exercise. *Jpn. J. Phys. Fit. Sports Med.* **2013**, *62*, 263–271. [CrossRef]
125. Konhilas, J.P.; Maass, A.H.; Luckey, S.W.; Stauffer, B.L.; Olson, E.N.; Leinwand, L.A. Sex modifies exercise and cardiac adaptation in mice. *Am. J. Physiol. Heart Circ. Physiol.* **2004**, *287*, H2768–H2776. [CrossRef]
126. Li, L.; Li, Y.; Wang, H.; Chen, W.; Liu, X. Effect of force level and gender on pinch force perception in healthy adults. *Iperception* **2020**, *11*, 2041669520927043. [CrossRef]
127. Sundberg, S. Maximal oxygen uptake in relation to age in blind and normal boys and girls. *Acta Paediatr. Scand.* **1982**, *71*, 603–608. [CrossRef]
128. Hafen, P.S.; Vehrs, P.R. Sex-related differences in the maximal lactate steady state. *Sports* **2018**, *6*, 154. [CrossRef]
129. Zhang, J.; Ji, L. Gender differences in peak blood lactate concentration and lactate removal. *Ann. Sports Med. Res.* **2016**, *3*, 1088.
130. Green, H.J.; Fraser, I.G.; Ranney, D.A. Male and female differences in enzyme activities of energy metabolism in vastus lateralis muscle. *J. Neurol. Sci.* **1984**, *65*, 323–331. [CrossRef]
131. Yoshioka, M.; St-Pierre, S.; Suzuki, M.; Tremblay, A. Effects of red pepper added to high-fat and high-carbohydrate meals on energy metabolism and substrate utilization in Japanese women. *Br. J. Nutr.* **1998**, *80*, 503–510. [CrossRef]
132. Yoshioka, M.; Lim, K.; Kikuzato, S.; Kiyonaga, A.; Tanaka, H.; Shindo, M.; Suzuki, M. Effects of red-pepper diet on the energy metabolism in men. *J. Nutr. Sci. Vitam. (Tokyo)* **1995**, *41*, 647–656. [CrossRef] [PubMed]
133. Simoneau, J.A.; Bouchard, C. Human variation in skeletal muscle fiber-type proportion and enzyme activities. *Am. J. Physiol.* **1989**, *257*, E567–E572. [CrossRef] [PubMed]

134. Simoneau, J.A.; Lortie, G.; Boulay, M.R.; Thibault, M.C.; Thériault, G.; Bouchard, C. Skeletal muscle histochemical and biochemical characteristics in sedentary male and female subjects. *Can. J. Physiol. Pharm.* **1985**, *63*, 30–35. [CrossRef] [PubMed]
135. Di Luigi, L.; Romanelli, F.; Sgrò, P.; Lenzi, A. Andrological aspects of physical exercise and sport medicine. *Endocrine* **2012**, *42*, 278–284. [CrossRef] [PubMed]
136. Isacco, L.; Duché, P.; Boisseau, N. Influence of hormonal status on substrate utilization at rest and during exercise in the female population. *Sports Med.* **2012**, *42*, 327–342. [CrossRef] [PubMed]
137. Amelink, G.J.; Bär, P.R. Exercise-induced muscle protein leakage in the rat. Effects of hormonal manipulation. *J. Neurol. Sci.* **1986**, *76*, 61–68. [CrossRef]

Publisher's Note: MDPI stays neutral with regard to jurisdictional claims in published maps and institutional affiliations.

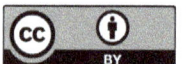

© 2020 by the authors. Licensee MDPI, Basel, Switzerland. This article is an open access article distributed under the terms and conditions of the Creative Commons Attribution (CC BY) license (http://creativecommons.org/licenses/by/4.0/).

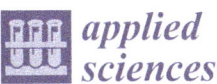

Article

Effects of High-Impact Weight-Bearing Exercise on Bone Mineral Density and Bone Metabolism in Middle-Aged Premenopausal Women: A Randomized Controlled Trial

Sung-Woo Kim [1], Myong-Won Seo [2], Hyun-Chul Jung [3] and Jong-Kook Song [2,*]

1. Department of Physical Education, Graduate School, Kyung Hee University (Global Campus), 1732 Deokyoungdaero, Giheung-gu, Yongin-si 17014, Gyeonggi-do, Korea; kswrha@khu.ac.kr
2. Department of Sports Science & Medicine, Graduate School of Physical Education, Kyung Hee University (Global Campus), 1732 Deokyoungdaero, Giheung-gu, Yongin-si 17014, Gyeonggi-do, Korea; myongwonseo@khu.ac.kr
3. Department of Coaching, College of Physical Education, Kyung Hee University (Global Campus), 1732 Deokyoungdaero, Giheung-gu, Yongin-si 17014, Gyeonggi-do, Korea; jhc@khu.ac.kr
* Correspondence: jksong@khu.ac.kr; Tel.: +82-31-201-2700

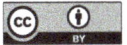

Abstract: This study examined the effects of high-impact weight-bearing exercise on bone mineral density (BMD) and bone metabolic markers in middle-aged premenopausal women. Forty middle-aged premenopausal women were initially enrolled, but thirty-one participants (40.34 ± 3.69 years) completed in the study. The subjects were randomly divided into two groups including the high-impact weight-bearing exercise group (HWE, n = 14) and control group (CON, n = 17). The HWE group participated in the exercise for 50 min a day, three days per week for four months, while the CON group maintained their regular lifestyle. The HWE program included 10 different high-impact weight-bearing exercises such as jumping and running. BMD was measured using DXA (Hologic, QDR 4500W, Marlborough, MA, USA). The bone metabolic markers including serum 25-(OH) D, intact parathyroid hormone (PTH), osteoprotegerin (OPG), osteopontin (OPN), receptor activator of nuclear factor κB ligand (RANKL), osteocalcin (OC), C-terminal telopeptide of type 1 collagen (CTX), and calcium were analyzed. The results showed that the BMDs of femur, lumbar, and forearm did not significantly change during the intervention period in both the HWE and CON groups. A significant decrease in bone formation markers such as OC ($F = 10.514$, $p = 0.003$, $\eta_p^2 = 0.266$) and an increase in bone resorption marker including CTX ($F = 8.768$, $p = 0.006$, $\eta_p^2 = 0.232$) were found only in the CON group, while these values did not change in the HWE group. There was a significant increase in serum 25-(OH) D ($F = 4.451$, $p = 0.044$, $\eta_p^2 = 0.133$) in the HWE group. Our findings suggest that four months of HWE is not sufficient to improve BMD and bone metabolic markers, but this impact exercise program may prevent the age-associated changes in bone turnover markers in middle-aged premenopausal women.

Keywords: high-impact weight-bearing exercise; bone mineral density; bone metabolic markers; serum 25-(OH) D; middle-aged premenopausal women

1. Introduction

Physical inactivity adversely affects some health conditions including osteoporosis, neurological diseases, type 2 diabetes, obesity, cardiovascular diseases (CVD), and sarcopenia [1]. In particular, osteoporosis has been reported worldwide as a serious public health problem in recent years. It is estimated that over 200 million women suffer from this disease, and there are approximately 75 million people experiencing osteoporosis in the USA, Europe, and Japan [2–6]. Bone loss is commonly accompanied by aging, which slowly increases bone loss after the age of 35 years, and the process of osteoporosis rises at an exponential rate after menopause [7]. Elderly women with hip fractures have a higher mortality rate of 10 to 20% than their counterparts, and osteoporosis has a much higher prevalence rate in women over 45 years of age than other diseases including breast cancer, diabetes mellitus, myocardial infarction [8,9]. Furthermore, the previous study suggested that the incidence of hip fracture would increase by 310% in men and 240% in women by 2050 due to the growth of the aging population and vulnerability to hip fracture with age [10]. Due to these clinical prescriptions, the diagnosis, consequences, monitoring of treatment, and therapy for osteoporosis are of crucial importance [11].

Analyzing bone turnover markers, an index of bone metabolism, are novel tools that detect bone remodeling dynamics including bone formation and resorption [12]. Bone remodeling is regulated by the activation of osteoclasts and osteoblasts and these biomarkers reflect the current status of bone turnover rate [11]. Bone turnover rate can be examined by analyzing bone formation markers such as bone-specific alkaline phosphatase, procollagen type 1 N propeptide, and osteocalcin (OC) and bone resorption markers including the N-terminal telopeptide of type 1 collagen and C-terminal telopeptide of type 1 collagen (CTX) [13]. It is also actively regulated by various factors such as osteopontin (OPN), osteoprotegerin (OPG), receptor activator of nuclear factor κB ligand (RANKL), parathyroid hormone (PTH), and vitamin D involved in the bone formation process [14–16]. RANKL is produced in osteoblasts and stromal cells and is the critical factor for the activation of mature osteoclasts and differentiation of monocyte-macrophage osteoclasts, which are precursors to multinucleated osteoclasts [10]. In contrast, OPG, one of the primary regulators of osteoclast-mediated bone resorption, is a factor observed in bone tissue [16]. OPN is a glycoprotein of the extracellular matrix of bone tissues that bind to hydroxyapatite and calcium, and it has been proposed as a mediator of atherosclerosis pathogenic pathways [16]. Vitamin D deficiency may be cause hyperthyroidism, resulting in increased bone turnover and bone loss [17,18]. According to the National Academy of Medicine, vitamin D deficient is defined as a level of serum 25(OH)D of 12 ng·mL^{-1}, whereas a level of 12 to <20 ng·mL^{-1} is considered to be inadequate, and a level of $\geq$20 ng·mL^{-1} defines vitamin D sufficiency [19]. Additionally, the elevated circulatory PTH levels may have negative effects [20]. However, several confounding factors determine the cause of the inverse relationship between serum 25(OH)D and PTH, and consistent results are not found in previous studies [20,21]. Calcium plays an important role as an essential nutrient for bone health [22]. However, previous studies have shown an excessively increased serum calcium relationship with an increased risk of cardiovascular disease [23–25]. These causes require an understanding of the potential impacts of serum calcium on bone health and care for health benefits. Thus, exploring the changes in bone turnover markers in response to exercise is essential for identifying mechanisms of the bone response [26].

The mechanical loading of high-impact physical activities (e.g., jumping and running) has been shown to increase bone mass in humans [27]. Additionally, impact activities such as high-intensity weight-bearing and jumping are more likely to be osteogenic than non-weight-bearing or low-impact activities such as swimming and walking [28]. Meta-analysis studies have shown that dynamic and resistance exercises are appropriate for increasing bone mineral density (BMD) in middle-aged women [29,30]. The majority of female participants that have been studied in impact exercise interventions were post-menopausal women because they represent the most popular group in which osteoporosis is manifested. Therefore, studies on pre-menopausal females are perceived to be in the greatest need [31–35]. However, a relatively small number of studies utilizing impact exercise training have targeted pre-menopausal women with combinations of supervised and home-based exercise sessions, which resulted in small positive effects [29,30,36]. Analyzing the bone turnover rate, an index of bone metabolism, plays an important role in understanding the biochemical activities in the bone and the changes in these markers can increase bone mineral density after weight-bearing exercise. It has been reported that acute, short-, and long-term exercise training increased the regulation bone remodeling markers such as OC, CTX, OPN, OPG, RANKL, PTH, and calcium [37–40]. Scott et al. [39] reported that acute weight-bearing exercise training increased serum levels of OPG, calcium, and PTH. Lester et al. [40] reported that combined aerobic and resistance exercise training for eight weeks significantly increased serum levels of OC in young women. Nevertheless, impact exercise training has not been explicitly directed at adult pre-menopausal women, despite the significant risk of developing osteoporosis after menopause.

Therefore, our study aimed to examine the effects of four months of high-impact weight-bearing exercise on BMD and bone metabolic markers in middle-aged premenopausal women.

2. Materials and Methods

2.1. Subjects

The power test was performed using G*Power 3.1.9.2 (Franz Faul, University of Kiel, Kiel, Germany) at the effect size of 0.3, the significant level of 0.05 (α = 0.05), and the power of 0.8 for all statistical tests. G*Power showed that 24 subjects had sufficient power for this study. Forty middle-aged premenopausal women aged 33–47 years were initially enrolled in the study. The exclusion criteria were specified as follows: (1) participated in regular exercise within the last three months; (2) users of pharmaceutical agents that directly affect bone, hypertension, and hyperlipidemia; and (3) blood pressure $\geq$ 140/90 mmHg. The subjects were randomly divided into two groups including HWE and CON. However, nine dropped out due to personal reasons and pregnancy; thus, thirty-one subjects completed the study (HWE: n = 14, CON: n = 17) (Table 1). All proceedings of the study were approved by the Institutional Review Board of Kyung Hee University (KHGIRB-19-226) and were conducted according to the Declaration of Helsinki.

Table 1. Physical characteristics and nutritional intake of subjects.

Variables	HWE		CON		F-Value		
	Pre	Post	Pre	Post	Time	Group	Interaction
Age (yrs)	40.3 ± 4.23	-	40.4 ± 3.31	-			
Body height (cm)	160.5 ± 4.74	-	161.2 ± 5.04	-			
Body weight (kg)	58.8 ± 10.98	57.9 ± 9.43	62.8 ± 11.73	63.3 ± 12.16	0.148	1.377	1.875
BMI (kg·m^{-2})	22.7 ± 3.62	22.3 ± 3.14	24.1 ± 4.14	24.3 ± 4.46	0.277	1.409	2.137
Total caloric intake (Kcal)	2151.20 ± 487.94	2027.71 ± 636.44	2328.61 ± 640.41	2274.09 ± 582.72	0.632	1.353	0.095
Carbohydrate (g)	293.29 ± 79.16	260.95 ± 89.44	297.46 ± 86.66	294.98 ± 85.55	1.409	0.497	1.036
Fat (g)	72.75 ± 19.01	73.82 ± 23.36	83.69 ± 25.82	80.00 ± 26.35	0.065	1.495	0.215
Protein (g)	98.08 ± 29.89	92.35 ± 29.98	113.30 ± 40.46	102.07 ± 31.60	1.665	1.498	0.175
Vitamin D (ug)	5.18 ± 4.47	4.57 ± 2.84	4.76 ± 2.26	6.02 + 5.30	0.109	0.260	0.900
Calcium (mg)	878.26 ± 242.49	854.96 ± 346.25	1051.38 ± 474.55	995.38 ± 575.03	0.224	1.352	0.038
Magnesium (mg)	163.6 ± 80.95	136.60 ± 53.77	124.24 ± 51.53	134.56 ± 63.81	0.270	1.650	1.350

Values are expressed as mean ± SD. HWE: high-impact weight-bearing exercise group, CON: control group, BMI: body mass index.

2.2. High-Impact Weight-Bearing Exercise Program

The training group performed the HWE program for 50 min a day (10:30 a.m.–11:20 a.m.), three days per week for four months. The training program was composed of 10 min of warm-up, 30 min of HWE, and 10 min of cool-down. The HWE comprised of the clap, walking, jumping burpee, jumping squat, running in place, wall press, bench stepping, jumping lunge, jumping jack, and push up [30]. The exercise intensity including exercise time increased progressively every four week period. The training intensity was set at 60–80% (mean: 136.9 ± 9.03 beat/min, range: 123–180 beat/min) of the heart rate reserve (HRR) and monitored every day by using a potable heart rate monitor (Polar RS400, Polar Electro Oy, Kempele, Finland). The detailed training program is shown in Table 2.

Table 2. High-impact weight-bearing exercise program for the four-months of the study.

Program	Contents	Phase (Weeks)	Set	Duration (min) Exercise Time	Duration (min) Rest Time	FITT
Warm-up	Dynamic stretching (Upper and lower body)			10		
Main exercise	Clap, Walking, Jumping burpee, Jumping squat, Running in place, Wall press, Bench stepping, Jumping lunge, Jumping jack, Push up	1–4 5–8 9–12 13–16	5 6 5 6	12.5 15 17 20	14 15 12 12.5	Frequency: 3 times/wk Intensity: 60–80% HRR Time: 50 min Type: HWE with music (1–8 wks: 15 s for each exercise) (9–16 wks: 20 s for each exercise)
Cool-down	Static stretching (Upper and lower body)			10		

HRR: heart rate reserve, FITT: frequency, intensity, time, type, HWE: high-impact weight-bearing exercise.

2.3. Anthropometric Measurements

The body height and body weight were measured, and body mass index (BMI) was calculated by dividing body weight (kg) by the square of body height (m^2). Body height was measured using a stadiometer to the nearest 0.1 cm (T.K.K. 11253, Takei Scientific Ins Co., Tokyo, Japan). Body weight was measured using a balance beam scale (Seca 700, Seca Co., Hamburg, Germany) to the nearest 0.1 kg.

2.4. Bone Mineral Density

BMD was measured using dual-energy x-ray absorptiometry (DXA), with a Hologic QDR 4500W bone densitometer (Hologic, Marlborough, MA, USA). All participants were scanned at three different sites of the BMD (e.g., femur, lumbar, and forearm). The same technician performed all tests. The intra-class correlation coefficient (ICC) was measured (femur BMD: 0.997; lumbar BMD: 0.990; forearm BMD: 0.987) [41].

2.5. Bone Metabolic Markers

Blood samples were collected before and after the four-month intervention period. Participants arrived at the laboratory in the morning between 08:30 a.m. and 09:30 a.m. after 12 h, overnight fasting, and avoiding severe physical activity or training the night before. Venous blood samples were taken 5 mL at the antecubital vein by a medical laboratory technologist and separated into each serum separate tube. The clotting of blood was separated using centrifugation with 3000 rpm for 15 min. The samples obtained were stored at −80 °C until analysis.

Serum 25-(OH) D was measured by a chemiluminescence microparticle immunoassay (CMIA) method (Architect i2000SR, Abbott, Singapore) with an ARCHITECT 25-(OH) vitamin D kit (Abbott Diagnostics, Lake Forest, IL, USA). The electrochemiluminescence immunoassay (ECLIA) method (E170, Roche, Germany) was used for intact PTH and CTX with an Elecsys PTH kit (Roche, Germany) and β-CrossLaps/serum kit (Roche, Germany). Bone metabolic markers including OPG, RANKL, and OPN were measured (VERSA Max, Molecular Device, Sunnyvale, CA, USA) by an enzyme-linked immunosorbent assay (ELISA) with OPG kit (ICL, Portland, OR, USA), RANKL kit (sRANKL ELISA, Immundiagnostik, Germany), and OPN kit (ICL, Portland, OR, USA). A radioimmunoassay (RIA) method (COBRA 5010 Quantum, USA) was used for analyzing OC, a marker of bone formation, with an OC kit (BRAHMS, Berlin, Germany). Calcium was measured by a homogeneous enzymatic colorimetric assay (HECA) method (c702, Germany) with a Calcium Gen.2 (Roche, Germany). The blood analysis was performed at the expertized research laboratory (Green Cross LabCell, Korea). The company is certified by the Korean Board for Accreditation and Conformity assessment.

2.6. Nutritional Intake

The dietary intake was assessed by three-day dietary records including twice on weekdays and once at the weekend in the first and the last weeks of the intervention. All data were analyzed by a computerized nutrient-intake assessment software program (CAN-PRO 4.0, Korean Nutrition Society, Seoul, Korea). The participants were instructed to maintain the same macronutrient distribution throughout the study.

2.7. Statistical Analysis

Statistical analyses were performed by using SAS software version 9.4 (SAS Institute, Cary, NC, USA). The mean, standard deviation, and 95% confidence interval (CI) were calculated. The normality of distribution of all dependent variables was verified using the Kolmogorov–Smirnov test. Two-way repeated-measures ANOVA was applied to determine the interaction effect for the group by the time during the intervention. If any significant interaction or main effects were observed, the independent t-test and paired t-test were applied to analyze the significant differences within groups and between groups. The effect size was computed as partial eta-squared values (η_p^2; small: ≥ 0.01, medium: ≥ 0.06, large: ≥ 0.14) [42]. The statistical significance level was set at 0.05.

3. Results

3.1. Bone Mineral Density

There were no significant interaction effects for group by time on femur BMD ($F = 0.458$, $p = 0.504$, $\eta_p^2 = 0.016$), lumbar BMD ($F = 0.009$, $p = 0.925$, $\eta_p^2 = 0.000$), and forearm BMD ($F = 0.048$, $p = 0.827$, $\eta_p^2 = 0.002$) during the intervention period (Table 3).

Table 3. Changes of bone mineral density (BMD) between pre- and post-tests in middle-aged premenopausal women.

Variables	HWE		CON		Time	Group	Interaction
	Pre (95% CI)	Post (95% CI)	Pre (95% CI)	Post (95% CI)		F-Value (ηp^2)	
Femur BMD (g/cm²)	0.891 ± 0.103 (0.838–0.946)	0.895 ± 0.103 (0.842–0.950)	0.898 ± 0.109 (0.846–0.952)	0.898 ± 0.113 (0.846–0.952)	0.515 (0.017)	0.015 (0.001)	0.458 (0.016)
Lumbar BMD (g/cm²)	1.036 ± 0.158 (0.956–1.122)	1.036 ± 0.167 (0.952–1.126)	1.009 ± 0.111 (0.957–1.062)	1.009 ± 0.112 (0.958–1.064)	0.003 (0.000)	0.290 (0.010)	0.009 (0.000)
Forearm BMD (g/cm²)	0.563 ± 0.036 (0.544–0.584)	0.560 ± 0.037 (0.541–0.581)	0.579 ± 0.041 (0.560–0.598)	0.576 ± 0.045 (0.555–0.596)	3.413 (0.105)	1.243 (0.041)	0.048 (0.002)

Values are expressed as mean ± SD. 95% CI: 95% confidence interval, BMD: bone mineral density, HWE: high-impact weight-bearing exercise, CON: control.

3.2. Bone Metabolic Markers

There were significant interaction effects for group by time on serum 25-(OH) D ($F = 4.451$, $p = 0.044$, $\eta_p^2 = 0.133$) and OC ($F = 10.514$, $p = 0.003$, $\eta_p^2 = 0.266$) (Figures 1 and 2). The post-test showed that serum 25-(OH) D concentration was increased significantly following the four-months of high impact weight-bearing exercise ($p < 0.01$), while no significant change was found in the CON group. OC level was not changed in the HWE group, but this value decreased significantly in the CON group ($p < 0.05$). There were significant time effects on intact PTH ($F = 4.447$, $p = 0.044$, $\eta_p^2 = 0.133$), OPN ($F = 5.480$, $p = 0.026$, $\eta_p^2 = 0.159$), CTX ($F = 8.768$, $p = 0.006$, $\eta_p^2 = 0.232$), and calcium ($F = 7.986$, $p = 0.008$, $\eta_p^2 = 0.216$) (Table 4).

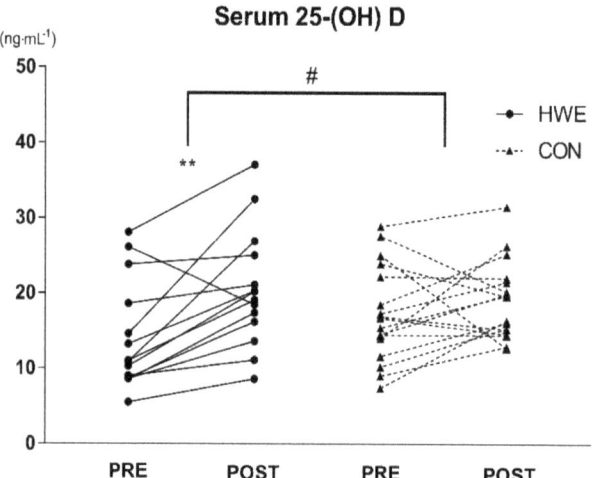

Figure 1. Serum 25-(OH) D before and after the four-month exercise program. For serum 25-(OH) D, statistical analyses revealed an increase between pre- and post-tests in the HWE group. HWE: high-impact weight-bearing exercise, CON: control. Significant difference between pre- and post-tests, ** $p < 0.01$. Significant interaction effect, # $p < 0.05$.

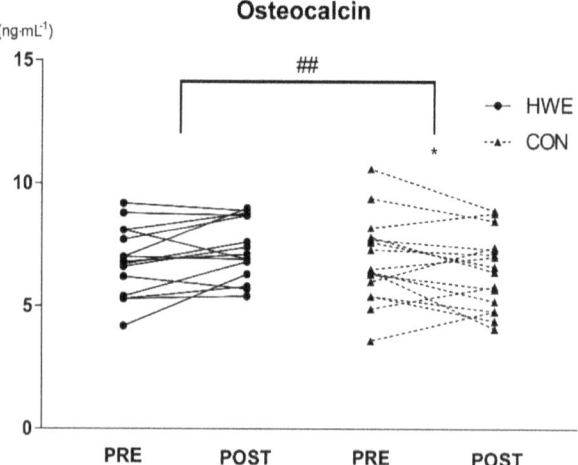

Figure 2. Osteocalcin before and after the four-month exercise program. For osteocalcin, statistical analyses revealed a decrease between pre- and post-tests in the CON group. HWE: high-impact weight-bearing exercise, CON: control. Significant difference between pre- and post-tests, * $p < 0.05$. Significant interaction effect, ## $p < 0.01$.

Table 4. Changes in bone metabolic markers between pre- and post-tests in middle-aged premenopausal women.

Variables	HWE		CON		F-value (ηp^2)		
	Pre (95% CI)	Post (95% CI)	Pre (95% CI)	Post (95% CI)	Time	Group	Interaction
25-(OH) D (ng·mL^{-1})	14.1 ± 7.24 (9.9–18.2)	20.5 ± 7.81 ** (16.0–25.1)	17.3 ± 6.37 (13.9–20.5)	19.0 ± 5.17 (16.4–21.7)	13.559 ## (.319)	0.158 (0.005)	4.451 # (0.133)
Intact PTH (pg·mL^{-1})	36.6 ± 9.00 (31.4–41.8)	42.6 ± 8.73 * (37.6–47.7)	36.5 ± 10.18 (31.2–41.7)	38.9 ± 8.85 (34.4–43.5)	4.447 # (0.133)	0.498 (0.017)	0.800 (0.027)
OPG (pmol·L^{-1})	5.7 ± 0.80 (5.2–6.1)	5.1 ± 1.26 (4.4–5.8)	5.6 ± 1.26 (5.0–6.3)	5.3 ± 1.65 (4.4–6.1)	3.911 (0.119)	0.021 (0.001)	0.173 (0.006)
RANKL (pmol·L^{-1})	286.9 ± 178.95 (183.6–390.3)	277.8 ± 186.06 (170.3–325.2)	199.6 ± 108.34 (143.9–255.3)	224.5 ± 124.01 (160.7–288.2)	0.225 (0.008)	1.868 (0.061)	1.062 (0.035)
OPN (ng·mL^{-1})	63.2 ± 31.97 (44.7–81.6)	50.1 ± 37.46 * (28.5–71.8)	51.2 ± 15.56 (43.2–59.2)	47.8 ± 20.78 (37.1–58.5)	5.480 # (0.159)	0.622 (0.021)	1.867 (0.060)
Osteocalcin (ng·mL^{-1})	6.8 ± 1.46 (6.0–7.7)	7.3 ± 1.29 (6.6–8.1)	6.9 ± 1.69 (6.0–7.8)	6.2 ± 1.50 * (5.5–7.0)	0.132 (0.005)	1.068 (0.036)	10.514 ## (0.266)
CTX (ng·mL^{-1})	0.24 ± 0.10 (0.19–0.30)	0.28 ± 0.09 (0.23–0.34)	0.26 ± 0.16 (0.18–0.35)	0.31 ± 0.14 * (0.23–0.38)	8.768 ## (0.232)	0.296 (0.010)	0.018 (0.001)
Calcium (mg·dL^{-1})	9.7 ± 0.46 (9.5–10.0)	9.5 ± 0.40 (9.3–9.8)	9.8 ± 0.29 (9.7–10.0)	9.5 ± 0.29 ** (9.4–9.7)	7.986 ## (0.216)	0.204 (0.007)	0.442 (0.015)

Values are expressed as mean ± SD. 95% CI: 95% confidence interval, HWE: high-impact weight-bearing exercise, CON: control, PTH: parathyroid hormone, OPG: osteoprotegerin, RANKL: receptor activator of nuclear factor kB ligand, OPN: osteopontin, CTX: C-terminal telopeptide of type 1 collagen. Significant interaction or main effect, # $p < 0.05$, ## $p < 0.01$. Significant difference between pre- and post-tests, * $p < 0.05$, ** $p < 0.01$.

4. Discussion

The present study examined the effects of four months of HWE on BMD and bone metabolic markers in middle-aged premenopausal women. Our main findings showed that a significant decrease in OC and an increase in CTX were found only in the CON group while these values did not change in the HWE group. However, four months of HWE were not sufficient to improve BMD in middle-aged premenopausal women.

Substantial empirical evidence has shown that resistance and step exercise have several benefits, which work as non-pharmacological interventions for the improvement of bone health in children/adolescents, adulthood, and the elderly [31,43]. However, the effects of high-impact exercise on BMD in middle-aged pre-menopausal women remain unknown [36]. The present study showed no significant effects on femur, lumbar, and forearm BMD after four-month of high-impact weight-bearing exercise. The International and National Osteoporosis Foundation, and other organizations recommend weight-bearing exercises to prevent osteopenia and osteoporosis [44]. There are different types of body weight-bearing exercises including high-impact exercises such as running and jumping as well as low-impact exercises such as body weight training, water aerobics, and walking [44]. It has been recently reported that trochanter and femoral neck BMD were significantly improved after high-impact weight-bearing exercise in pre-menopausal women [30]. Additionally, high-impact weight-bearing and resistance training either in combination or alone, induced gains in BMD by 1–2% at the femoral neck and lumbar spine with a minimal effect on other body sites in pre-menopausal and post-menopausal women [45]. Similar results in other studies have found that high-impact exercise for 12 months (3 times/week) resulted in a significant improvement in femoral neck BMD by 0.6–1.1% in pre-menopausal women [46,47]. Although the present study did not show a significant change, there was a tendency where the femur BMD increased following four months of HWE (0.47%) without any improvement on other sites of the body. Foster and Armstrong [48] reported that a bone remodeling cycle takes about 3–4 months and a minimum of 6–8 months is required for the bone to reach a new, measurable steady-state bone mass. Therefore, the absence of the significant improvement in BMD is likely due to the insufficient duration of an exercise intervention to promote bone formation in the present study. In fact, combined-impact exercise protocols lasting more than six months (duration: 30–60 min; frequency: ≥3 days/week) have been recommended for greater bone health benefits [49]. Moreover, adults might benefit from high-impact exercises, but previous studies have suggested that its effect might occur to a lesser extent than in children or adolescents [50]. In this study, the effect of four-months of high-impact weight-bearing exercise appeared to be none or small only in particular sites such as femur BMD in middle-aged premenopausal women.

Biochemical bone metabolic markers indicate changes in bone metabolism more quickly than changes in BMD, which are commonly used to monitor osteoporosis [51]. Additionally, bone metabolic markers could be used to evaluate the antiresorptive agents in the clinical diagnosis of osteoporosis and osteopenia [52]. One intended therapeutic aim of the antiresorptive therapy is to decrease levels of bone metabolic markers below the average reference range for pre-menopausal women [53]. Bone metabolic markers provide important information such as the rate of bone remodeling by changing bone formation and resorption, and the evaluation of these markers has been used in previous intervention studies to identify the effectiveness of exercise [54–56]. The results of our study showed that serum 25-(OH) D (60.22%, $p < 0.01$), and intact PTH (23.86%, $p < 0.05$) were increased significantly in HWE between pre- and post-tests, whereas OPN (-20.45%, $p < 0.05$) was decreased significantly in HWE between pre- and post-tests. Furthermore, OC (-7.89%, $p < 0.05$) and calcium (-2.99%, $p < 0.01$) were decreased significantly in CON between pre- and post-tests, whereas CTX (30.94%, $p < 0.05$) was increased significantly in CON between pre- and post-tests. However, no significant interaction effects were found on other markers including intact PTH, OPG, RANKL, and OPN.

Vitamin D plays a critical role in promoting the intestinal absorption of phosphate and calcium [57], and participating in regular physical activity is a well-known stimulator of serum 25-(OH) D [58]. In accordance with our results, Josse et al. [55] reported that the serum 25-(OH) D increased significantly following 12 weeks of resistance training in young women, but the level of PTH was not significantly changed. It is an interesting result in the present study where the HWE group increased both vitamin D and PTH level after four-months of exercise intervention. Generally, serum calcium level is mediated by vitamin D and PTH [59] and the changes in these levels may increase or decrease the mineralization of bone. It is assumed that an increase in PTH level may help to maintain serum calcium level. In particular, our participants were healthy and had no bone-related disease, thus it is possible that PTH is increased for calcium homeostasis. Moghadasi and Siavashpour [56] reported that resistance circuit training for 12 weeks significantly increased PTH in healthy and sedentary young women, which agrees with the present result. Authors assumed that this increase in PTH after resistance training may promote anabolic activities in bone metabolism. However, it is difficult to explain the direct relations or physiological mechanism between the variables in the present study and conflicting results have been observed in previous studies. Pilch et al. [60] reported that Nordic walking training for six weeks significantly decreased serum 25-(OH) D in post-menopausal women and Evans et al. [54] reported that a recruit training program for four-months significantly decreased serum 25-(OH) D in men, whereas these values remained at baseline levels in women. Vitamin D is an important factor for bone health, and its deficiency leads to osteoporosis and CVD in adults [61,62]. Moreover, physically inactive individuals have two times lower vitamin D levels than active adults [63]. Although it is difficult to determine the direct relations between HWE and increased serum 25-(OH) D, several studies support our results that increase in physical activity is an effective manner to maintain optimal vitamin D level in later life [64,65]. In this study, the serum 25-(OH) D increased from an inadequate level (12–20 ng·mL^{-1}) to a sufficient level (≥ 20 ng·mL^{-1}) in HWE.

Bone turnover markers provide information on important biochemical indicators such as bone resorption and bone formation in managing osteoporosis [66]. A significant association between bone turnover markers and the risk of fractures has been identified for females and males [67]. Mohr et al. [68] reported that soccer training for 15 weeks significantly increased plasma OC (37 ± 15%) and CTX (42 ± 18%) in middle-aged premenopausal women. A significant increase in OC has also been observed in untrained young women following sixteen weeks of exercise intervention [69]. Additionally, exercise training caused augmentation in resting plasma OC and CTX in elderly sedentary men with no resistance training [70]. However, CTX has been shown to increase shortly or immediately after impact exercise [26]. Thus, impact exercise may have a high potential to improve bone health in the general population. Therefore, the above intervention studies and our study results indicate that impact exercise describes a feasible intervention modality in middle-aged premenopausal women.

Previous studies by Ferrucci et al. [71] and Fuller et al. [72] emphasized that changes in pro-inflammatory and anti-inflammatory cytokines have profound implications on age-related bone loss. OPN acts through binding to integrin β-3, leading to a decrease in the cytoplasmic calcium concentration associated with osteoclast activation [10]. Humphries et al. [38] reported that participants who underwent whole-body vibration with or without the combination of resistance training for 16 weeks showed a significant decrease in OPN in young healthy women, which is consistent with the present findings. Thus, exercise training induces changes in bone metabolism faster than actual changes in BMD in middle-aged premenopausal women. Therefore, it is important to monitor and stimulate bone metabolic markers to prevent osteoporosis before menopause in women, especially when considering a higher prevalence of osteoporosis after menopause.

5. Limitation of the study

In this study, there are some limitations that need to be considered. Although the present study is well designed with the randomized controlled trials, the relatively short-term intervention period (four-months) may be a limit to confirming the longitudinal effects of high-impact weight-bearing exercise on BMD in middle-aged premenopausal women. However, the positive changes in bone metabolic markers such as OC and vitamin D may provide a potential benefit on bone health. In future study, a longer period of exercise intervention (more than six months) is needed to examine how changed bone metabolic markers are linked to the BMD changes.

6. Conclusions

The present study revealed that four months of HWE is not sufficient to improve BMD and bone metabolic markers, but this exercise program may prevent the age-associated changes in bone turnover markers in middle aged premenopausal women.

Author Contributions: Conception and study design, S.-W.K. and J.-K.S.; Statistical analysis, S.-W.K. and J.-K.S.; Investigation, S.-W.K.; Data interpretation, S.-W.K., J.-K.S., M.-W.S., and H.-C.J.; Writing-original draft preparation, S.-W.K.; Writing-review and editing, H.-C.J., and J.-K.S.; Supervision, J.-K.S. All authors have read and approved the final manuscript.

Funding: This work was supported by the Ministry of Education of the Republic of Korea and the National Research Foundation of Korea (NRF-2019S1A5A2A01049721).

Institutional Review Board Statement: The study was conducted according to the guidelines of the Declaration of Helsinki, and approved by the Institutional Review Board of Kyung Hee University (KHGIRB-19-226).

Informed Consent Statement: Informed consent was obtained from all subjects involved in the study.

Conflicts of Interest: The authors declare no conflict of interest.

References

1. Hamilton, M.T.; Hamilton, D.G.; Zderic, T.W. Role of low energy expenditure and sitting in obesity, metabolic syndrome, type 2 diabetes, and cardiovascular disease. *Diabetes* **2007**, *56*, 2655–2667. [CrossRef]
2. Reginster, J.Y.; Burlet, N. Osteoporosis: A still increasing prevalence. *Bone* **2006**, *38*, S4–S9. [CrossRef] [PubMed]
3. Sweet, M.G.; Sweet, J.M.; Jeremiah, M.P.; Galazka, S.S. Diagnosis and treatment of osteoporosis. *Am. Fam. Physician* **2009**, *79*, 193–200. [PubMed]

4. Tarride, J.E.; Hopkins, R.B.; Leslie, W.D.; Morin, S.; Adachi, J.D.; Papaioannou, A.; Bessette, L.; Brown, J.P.; Goeree, R. The burden of illness of osteoporosis in Canada. *Osteoporos. Int.* **2012**, *23*, 2591–2600. [CrossRef] [PubMed]
5. Kanis, J.A.; Cooper, C.; Rizzoli, R.; Reginster, J.Y. European guidance for the diagnosis and management of osteoporosis in postmenopausal women. *Osteoporos. Int.* **2019**, *30*, 3–44. [CrossRef]
6. Singer, A.; Exuzides, A.; Spangler, L.; O'Malley, C.; Colby, C.; Johnston, K.; Agodoa, I.; Baker, J.; Kagan, R. Burden of illness for osteoporotic fractures compared with other serious diseases among postmenopausal women in the United States. *Mayo Clin. Proc.* **2015**, *90*, 53–62. [CrossRef]
7. Burch, J.; Rice, S.; Yang, H.; Neilson, A.; Stirk, L.; Francis, R.; Holloway, P.; Selby, P.; Craig, D. Systematic review of the use of bone turnover markers for monitoring the response to osteoporosis treatment: The secondary prevention of fractures, and primary prevention of fractures in high-risk groups. *Health Technol. Assess.* **2014**, *18*, 1–180. [CrossRef]
8. Sambrook, P.; Cooper, C. Osteoporosis. *Lancet* **2006**, *367*, 2010–2018. [CrossRef]
9. Cummings, S.R.; Melton, L.J. Epidemiology and outcomes of osteoporotic fractures. *Lancet* **2002**, *359*, 1761–1767. [CrossRef]
10. Lampropoulos, C.E.; Papaioannou, I.; D'Cruz, D.P. Osteoporosis—A risk factor for cardiovascular disease? *Nat. Rev. Rheumatol.* **2012**, *8*, 587–598. [CrossRef]
11. Greenblatt, M.B.; Tsai, J.N.; Wein, M.N. Bone Turnover Markers in the Diagnosis and Monitoring of Metabolic Bone Disease. *Clin. Chem.* **2017**, *63*, 464–474. [CrossRef] [PubMed]
12. Shetty, S.; Kapoor, N.; Bondu, J.D.; Thomas, N.; Paul, T.V. Bone turnover markers: Emerging tool in the management of osteoporosis. *Indian J. Endocrinol. Metab.* **2016**, *20*, 846–852. [CrossRef] [PubMed]
13. Vasikaran, S.; Eastell, R.; Bruyère, O.; Foldes, A.J.; Garnero, P.; Griesmacher, A.; McClung, M.; Morris, H.A.; Silverman, S.; Trenti, T.; et al. Markers of bone turnover for the prediction of fracture risk and monitoring of osteoporosis treatment: A need for international reference standards. *Osteoporos. Int.* **2011**, *22*, 391–420. [CrossRef] [PubMed]
14. McCarty, M.F.; DiNicolantonio, J.J. The molecular biology and pathophysiology of vascular calcification. *Postgrad. Med.* **2014**, *126*, 54–64. [CrossRef] [PubMed]
15. Osako, M.K.; Nakagami, H.; Koibuchi, N.; Shimizu, H.; Nakagami, F.; Koriyama, H.; Shimamura, M.; Miyake, T.; Rakugi, H.; Morishita, R. Estrogen inhibits vascular calcification via vascular RANKL system: Common mechanism of osteoporosis and vascular calcification. *Circ. Res.* **2010**, *107*, 466–475. [CrossRef]
16. Lello, S.; Capozzi, A.; Scambia, G. Osteoporosis and cardiovascular disease: An update. *Gynecol. Endocrinol.* **2015**, *31*, 590–594. [CrossRef]
17. Ooms, M.E.; Lips, P.; Roos, J.C.; van der Vijgh, W.J.; Popp-Snijders, C.; Bezemer, P.D.; Bouter, L.M. Vitamin D status and sex hormone binding globulin: Determinants of bone turnover and bone mineral density in elderly women. *J. Bone Min. Res.* **1995**, *10*, 1177–1184. [CrossRef]
18. Kamineni, V.; Latha, A.P.; Ramathulasi, K. Association between serum 25-hydroxyvitamin D levels and bone mineral density in normal postmenopausal women. *J. Midlife Health* **2016**, *7*, 163–168. [CrossRef]
19. Ross, A.C.; Manson, J.E.; Abrams, S.A.; Aloia, J.F.; Brannon, P.M.; Clinton, S.K.; Durazo-Arvizu, R.A.; Gallagher, J.C.; Gallo, R.L.; Jones, G.; et al. The 2011 report on dietary reference intakes for calcium and vitamin D from the Institute of Medicine: What clinicians need to know. *J. Clin. Endocrinol. Metab.* **2011**, *96*, 53–58. [CrossRef]
20. Fisher, A.; Goh, S.; Srikusalanukul, W.; Davis, M. Elevated serum PTH is independently associated with poor outcomes in older patients with hip fracture and vitamin D inadequacy. *Calcif. Tissue Int.* **2009**, *85*, 301–309. [CrossRef]
21. Hao, L.; Carson, J.L.; Schlussel, Y.; Noveck, H.; Shapses, S.A. Vitamin D deficiency is associated with reduced mobility after hip fracture surgery: A prospective study. *Am. J. Clin. Nutr.* **2020**, *112*, 613–618. [CrossRef] [PubMed]
22. Liu, M.; Yao, X.; Zhu, Z. Associations between serum calcium, 25(OH)D level and bone mineral density in older adults. *J. Orthop. Surg. Res.* **2019**, *14*, 458. [CrossRef]
23. Reid, I.R.; Birstow, S.M.; Bolland, M.J. Calcium and Cardiovascular Disease. *Endocrinol. Metab. (Seoul)* **2017**, *32*, 339–349. [CrossRef] [PubMed]
24. Rohrmann, S.; Garmo, H.; Malmström, H.; Hammar, N.; Jungner, I.; Walldius, G.; Van Hemelrijck, M. Association between serum calcium concentration and risk of incident and fatal cardiovascular disease in the prospective AMORIS study. *Atherosclerosis* **2016**, *251*, 85–93. [CrossRef] [PubMed]
25. Larsson, S.C.; Burgess, S.; Michaëlsson, K. Association of Genetic Variants Related to Serum Calcium Levels with Coronary Artery Disease and Myocardial Infarction. *JAMA* **2017**, *318*, 371–380. [CrossRef]
26. Mezil, Y.A.; Allison, D.; Kish, K.; Ditor, D.; Ward, W.E.; Tsiani, E.; Klentrou, P. Response of Bone Turnover Markers and Cytokines to High-Intensity Low-Impact Exercise. *Med. Sci. Sports Exerc.* **2015**, *47*, 1495–1502. [CrossRef] [PubMed]
27. Kohrt, W.M.; Barry, D.W.; Schwartz, R.S. Muscle forces or gravity: What predominates mechanical loading on bone? *Med. Sci. Sports Exerc.* **2009**, *41*, 2050–2055. [CrossRef]
28. Kohrt, W.M.; Bloomfield, S.A.; Little, K.D.; Nelson, M.E.; Yingling, V.R. American College of Sports Medicine Position Stand: Physical activity and bone health. *Med. Sci. Sports Exerc.* **2004**, *36*, 1985–1996. [CrossRef]
29. Babatunde, O.O.; Forsyth, J.J.; Gidlow, C.J. A meta-analysis of brief high-impact exercises for enhancing bone health in pre-menopausal women. *Osteoporos. Int.* **2012**, *23*, 109–119. [CrossRef]
30. Zhao, R.; Zhao, M.; Zhang, L. Efficiency of jumping exercise in improving bone mineral density among premenopausal women: A meta-analysis. *Sports Med.* **2014**, *44*, 1393–1402. [CrossRef]

31. Martyn-St James, M.; Carroll, S. A meta-analysis of impact exercise on postmenopausal bone loss: The case for mixed loading exercise programmes. *Br. J. Sports Med.* **2009**, *43*, 898–908. [CrossRef] [PubMed]
32. Nikander, R.; Sievanen, H.; Heinonen, A.; Daly, R.M.; Uusi-Rasi, K.; Kannus, P. Targeted exercise against osteoporosis: A systematic review and meta-analysis for optimising bone strength throughout life. *BMC Med.* **2010**, *8*, 47. [CrossRef] [PubMed]
33. Polidoulis, I.; Beyene, J.; Cheung, A.M. The effect of exercise on pQCT parameters of bone structure and strength in postmenopausal women—A systematic review and meta-analysis of randomized controlled trials. *Osteoporos. Int.* **2012**, *23*, 39–51. [CrossRef] [PubMed]
34. Marques, E.A.; Mota, J.; Carvalho, J. Exercise effects on bone mineral density in older adults: A meta-analysis of randomized controlled trials. *Age* **2012**, *34*, 1493–1515. [CrossRef] [PubMed]
35. Kelley, G.A.; Kelley, K.S.; Kohrt, W.M. Effects of ground and joint reaction force exercise on lumbar spine and femoral neck bone mineral density in postmenopausal women: A meta-analysis of randomized controlled trials. *BMC Musculoskelet. Disord.* **2012**, *13*, 177. [CrossRef] [PubMed]
36. Greenway, K.G.; Walkley, J.W.; Rich, P.A. Impact exercise and bone density in premenopausal women with below average bone density for age. *Eur. J. Appl. Physiol.* **2015**, *115*, 2457–2469. [CrossRef] [PubMed]
37. Yuan, Y.; Chen, X.; Zhang, L.; Wu, J.; Guo, J.; Zou, D.; Chen, B.; Sun, Z.; Shen, C.; Zou, J. The roles of exercise in bone remodeling and in prevention and treatment of osteoporosis. *Prog. Biophys. Mol. Biol.* **2016**, *122*, 122–130. [CrossRef]
38. Humphries, B.; Fenning, A.; Dugan, E.; Guinane, J.; MacRae, K. Whole-body vibration effects on bone mineral density in women with or without resistance training. *Aviat. Space Environ. Med.* **2009**, *80*, 1025–1031. [CrossRef]
39. Scott, J.P.; Sale, C.; Greeves, J.P.; Casey, A.; Dutton, J.; Fraser, W.D. The role of exercise intensity in the bone metabolic response to an acute bout of weight-bearing exercise. *J. Appl. Physiol.* **2011**, *110*, 423–432. [CrossRef]
40. Lester, M.E.; Urso, M.L.; Evans, R.K.; Pierce, J.R.; Spiering, B.A.; Maresh, C.M.; Hatfield, D.L.; Kraemer, W.J.; Nindl, B.C. Influence of exercise mode and osteogenic index on bone biomarker responses during short-term physical training. *Bone* **2009**, *45*, 768–776. [CrossRef]
41. Kim, S.W.; Jung, S.W.; Seo, M.W.; Park, H.Y.; Song, J.K. Effects of bone-specific physical activity on body composition, bone mineral density, and health-related physical fitness in middle-aged women. *J. Exerc. Nutr. Biochem.* **2019**, *23*, 36–42. [CrossRef] [PubMed]
42. Cohen, J. *Statistical Power Analysis for the Behavioral Sciences*; Academic Press: Cambridge, MA, USA, 2013.
43. Manske, S.L.; Lorincz, C.R.; Zernicke, R.F. Bone health: Part 2, physical activity. *Sports Health* **2009**, *1*, 341–346. [CrossRef] [PubMed]
44. Troy, K.L.; Mancuso, M.E.; Butler, T.A.; Johnson, J.E. Exercise Early and Often: Effects of Physical Activity and Exercise on Women's Bone Health. *Int. J. Environ. Res. Public Health* **2018**, *15*, 878. [CrossRef] [PubMed]
45. Sanudo, B.; de Hoyo, M.; Del Pozo-Cruz, J.; Carrasco, L.; Del Pozo-Cruz, B.; Tejero, S.; Firth, E. A systematic review of the exercise effect on bone health: The importance of assessing mechanical loading in perimenopausal and postmenopausal women. *Menopause* **2017**, *24*, 1208–1216. [CrossRef]
46. Vainionpaa, A.; Korpelainen, R.; Leppaluoto, J.; Jamsa, T. Effects of high-impact exercise on bone mineral density: A randomized controlled trial in premenopausal women. *Osteoporos. Int.* **2005**, *16*, 191–197. [CrossRef]
47. Niu, K.; Ahola, R.; Guo, H.; Korpelainen, R.; Uchimaru, J.; Vainionpaa, A.; Sato, K.; Sakai, A.; Salo, S.; Kishimoto, K.; et al. Effect of office-based brief high-impact exercise on bone mineral density in healthy premenopausal women: The Sendai Bone Health Concept Study. *J. Bone Miner. Metab.* **2010**, *28*, 568–577. [CrossRef]
48. Foster, C.; Armstrong, M. What types of physical activities are effective in developing muscle and bone strength and balance. *J. Frailty Sarcopenia Falls* **2018**, *3*, 58–65. [CrossRef]
49. Xu, J.; Lombardi, G.; Jiao, W.; Banfi, G. Effects of Exercise on Bone Status in Female Subjects, from Young Girls to Postmenopausal Women: An Overview of Systematic Reviews and Meta-Analyses. *Sports Med.* **2016**, *46*, 1165–1182. [CrossRef]
50. Santos, L.; Elliott-Sale, K.J.; Sale, C. Exercise and bone health across the lifespan. *Biogerontology* **2017**, *18*, 931–946. [CrossRef]
51. Delmas, P.D.; Hardy, P.; Garnero, P.; Dain, M. Monitoring individual response to hormone replacement therapy with bone markers. *Bone* **2000**, *26*, 553–560. [CrossRef]
52. de Papp, A.E.; Bone, H.G.; Caulfield, M.P.; Kagan, R.; Buinewicz, A.; Chen, E.; Rosenberg, E.; Reitz, R.E. A cross-sectional study of bone turnover markers in healthy premenopausal women. *Bone* **2007**, *40*, 1222–1230. [CrossRef] [PubMed]
53. Srivastava, A.K.; Vliet, E.L.; Lewiecki, E.M.; Maricic, M.; Abdelmalek, A.; Gluck, O.; Baylink, D.J. Clinical use of serum and urine bone markers in the management of osteoporosis. *Curr. Med. Res. Opin.* **2005**, *21*, 1015–1026. [CrossRef] [PubMed]
54. Evans, R.K.; Antczak, A.J.; Lester, M.; Yanovich, R.; Israeli, E.; Moran, D.S. Effects of a 4-month recruit training program on markers of bone metabolism. *Med. Sci. Sports Exerc.* **2008**, *40*, S660–S670. [CrossRef] [PubMed]
55. Josse, A.R.; Tang, J.E.; Tarnopolsky, M.A.; Phillips, S.M. Body composition and strength changes in women with milk and resistance exercise. *Med. Sci. Sports Exerc.* **2010**, *42*, 1122–1130. [CrossRef]
56. Moghadasi, M.; Siavashpour, S. The effect of 12 weeks of resistance training on hormones of bone formation in young sedentary women. *Eur. J. Appl. Physiol.* **2013**, *113*, 25–32. [CrossRef]
57. Pilch, W.; Tota, L.; Sadowska-Krepa, E.; Piotrowska, A.; Kepinska, M.; Palka, T.; Maszczyk, A. The Effect of a 12-Week Health Training Program on Selected Anthropometric and Biochemical Variables in Middle-Aged Women. *Biomed. Res. Int.* **2017**, *2017*, 9569513. [CrossRef]

58. Scragg, R.; Camargo, C.A., Jr. Frequency of leisure-time physical activity and serum 25-hydroxyvitamin D levels in the US population: Results from the Third National Health and Nutrition Examination Survey. *Am. J. Epidemiol.* **2008**, *168*, 577–586. [CrossRef] [PubMed]
59. Dawson-Hughes, B.; Heaney, R.P.; Holick, M.F.; Lips, P.; Meunier, P.J.; Vieth, R. Estimates of optimal vitamin D status. *Osteoporos. Int.* **2005**, *16*, 713–716. [CrossRef]
60. Pilch, W.; Tyka, A.; Cebula, A.; Sliwicka, E.; Pilaczynska-Szczesniak, L.; Tyka, A. Effects of a 6-week Nordic walking training on changes in 25(OH)D blood concentration in women aged over 55. *J. Sports Med. Phys. Fit.* **2017**, *57*, 124–129. [CrossRef]
61. Judd, S.E.; Tangpricha, V. Vitamin D deficiency and risk for cardiovascular disease. *Am. J. Med. Sci.* **2009**, *338*, 40–44. [CrossRef]
62. Holick, M.F. The vitamin D deficiency pandemic: Approaches for diagnosis, treatment and prevention. *Rev. Endocr. Metab. Disord.* **2017**, *18*, 153–165. [CrossRef] [PubMed]
63. Liu, X.; Baylin, A.; Levy, P.D. Vitamin D deficiency and insufficiency among US adults: Prevalence, predictors and clinical implications. *Br. J. Nutr.* **2018**, *119*, 928–936. [CrossRef] [PubMed]
64. Orces, C.H. Association between leisure-time aerobic physical activity and vitamin D concentrations among US older adults: The NHANES 2007-2012. *Aging Clin. Exp. Res.* **2019**, *31*, 685–693. [CrossRef] [PubMed]
65. Ten Haaf, D.S.M.; Balvers, M.G.J.; Timmers, S.; Eijsvogels, T.M.H.; Hopman, M.T.E.; Klein Gunnewiek, J.M.T. Determinants of vitamin D status in physically active elderly in the Netherlands. *Eur. J. Nutr.* **2019**, *58*, 3121–3128. [CrossRef] [PubMed]
66. Kerschan-Schindl, K.; Föger-Samwald, U.; Pietschmann, P. Bone Turnover Markers. In *Principles of Bone and Joint Research*; Springer: Berlin/Heidelberg, Germany, 2017; pp. 55–66. [CrossRef]
67. Johansson, H.; Odén, A.; Kanis, J.A.; McCloskey, E.V.; Morris, H.A.; Cooper, C.; Vasikaran, S. A meta-analysis of reference markers of bone turnover for prediction of fracture. *Calcif. Tissue Int.* **2014**, *94*, 560–567. [CrossRef] [PubMed]
68. Mohr, M.; Helge, E.W.; Petersen, L.F.; Lindenskov, A.; Weihe, P.; Mortensen, J.; Jørgensen, N.R.; Krustrup, P. Effects of soccer vs swim training on bone formation in sedentary middle-aged women. *Eur. J. Appl. Physiol.* **2015**, *115*, 2671–2679. [CrossRef] [PubMed]
69. Jackman, S.R.; Scott, S.; Randers, M.B.; Orntoft, C.; Blackwell, J.; Zar, A.; Helge, E.W.; Mohr, M.; Krustrup, P. Musculoskeletal health profile for elite female footballers versus untrained young women before and after 16 weeks of football training. *J. Sports Sci.* **2013**, *31*, 1468–1474. [CrossRef]
70. Helge, E.W.; Andersen, T.R.; Schmidt, J.F.; Jørgensen, N.R.; Hornstrup, T.; Krustrup, P.; Bangsbo, J. Recreational football improves bone mineral density and bone turnover marker profile in elderly men. *Scand. J. Med. Sci. Sports* **2014**, *24* (Suppl. 1), 98–104. [CrossRef] [PubMed]
71. Ferrucci, L.; Corsi, A.; Lauretani, F.; Bandinelli, S.; Bartali, B.; Taub, D.D.; Guralnik, J.M.; Longo, D.L. The origins of age-related proinflammatory state. *Blood* **2005**, *105*, 2294–2299. [CrossRef] [PubMed]
72. Fuller, K.; Murphy, C.; Kirstein, B.; Fox, S.W.; Chambers, T.J. TNFalpha potently activates osteoclasts, through a direct action independent of and strongly synergistic with RANKL. *Endocrinology* **2002**, *143*, 1108–1118. [CrossRef] [PubMed]

Review

Physical Activity and Redox Balance in the Elderly: Signal Transduction Mechanisms

Daniela Galli [1,†], Cecilia Carubbi [1,†], Elena Masselli [1,2], Mauro Vaccarezza [3,4], Valentina Presta [1], Giulia Pozzi [1], Luca Ambrosini [1], Giuliana Gobbi [1,*], Marco Vitale [1,2,*] and Prisco Mirandola [1]

1. Anatomy Unit, Department of Medicine and Surgery, University of Parma, Via Gramsci 14, 43126 Parma, Italy; daniela.galli@unipr.it (D.G.); cecilia.carubbi@unipr.it (C.C.); elena.masselli@unipr.it (E.M.); valentina.presta@unipr.it (V.P.); giulia.pozzi@unipr.it (G.P.); luca.ambrosini@unipr.it (L.A.); prisco.mirandola@unipr.it (P.M.)
2. University Hospital of Parma, AOU-PR, Via Gramsci 14, 43126 Parma, Italy
3. Curtin Health Innovation Research Institute, Curtin University, Kent St., Bentley 6102, Australia; mauro.vaccarezza@curtin.edu.au
4. Curtin Medical School, Faculty of Health Sciences, Curtin University, Kent St., Bentley 6102, Australia
* Correspondence: giuliana.gobbi@unipr.it (G.G.); marco.vitale@unipr.it (M.V.)
† Daniela Galli and Cecilia Carubbi contributed equally to this work.

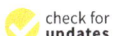

Citation: Galli, D.; Carubbi, C.; Masselli, E.; Vaccarezza, M.; Presta, V.; Pozzi, G.; Ambrosini, L.; Gobbi, G.; Vitale, M.; Mirandola, P. Physical Activity and Redox Balance in the Elderly: Signal Transduction Mechanisms. *Appl. Sci.* 2021, *11*, 2228. https://doi.org/10.3390/app11052228

Academic Editor: Mark King

Received: 9 February 2021
Accepted: 26 February 2021
Published: 3 March 2021

Publisher's Note: MDPI stays neutral with regard to jurisdictional claims in published maps and institutional affiliations.

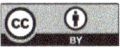

Copyright: © 2021 by the authors. Licensee MDPI, Basel, Switzerland. This article is an open access article distributed under the terms and conditions of the Creative Commons Attribution (CC BY) license (https://creativecommons.org/licenses/by/4.0/).

Abstract: Reactive Oxygen Species (ROS) are molecules naturally produced by cells. If their levels are too high, the cellular antioxidant machinery intervenes to bring back their quantity to physiological conditions. Since aging often induces malfunctioning in this machinery, ROS are considered an effective cause of age-associated diseases. Exercise stimulates ROS production on one side, and the antioxidant systems on the other side. The effects of exercise on oxidative stress markers have been shown in blood, vascular tissue, brain, cardiac and skeletal muscle, both in young and aged people. However, the intensity and volume of exercise and the individual subject characteristics are important to envisage future strategies to adequately personalize the balance of the oxidant/antioxidant environment. Here, we reviewed the literature that deals with the effects of physical activity on redox balance in young and aged people, with insights into the molecular mechanisms involved. Although many molecular pathways are involved, we are still far from a comprehensive view of the mechanisms that stand behind the effects of physical activity during aging. Although we believe that future precision medicine will be able to transform exercise administration from wellness to targeted prevention, as yet we admit that the topic is still in its infancy.

Keywords: ROS; physical activity; signal transduction; aging

1. Introduction

In 2018, the World Health Organization proposed healthy aging as "creating the environments and opportunities that enable people to be and do what they value throughout their lives". In western countries, aged people are numerous, and the pathologies associated with aging are widely studied. Besides pathogens, excessive Reactive Oxygen Species (ROS) can be considered as an effective cause of age-associated diseases [1].

ROS (i.e., hydrogen peroxide, nitric oxide radicals, hypochlorite) are molecules naturally produced in several metabolic cell processes. However, if their levels are above the physiologic threshold, they cause oxidative stress and cell damage. In fact, if ROS are too high, the cellular antioxidant machinery rises to bring their levels back below the threshold [2]. Thus, to promote healthy aging, adequate interventions should constrain ROS in their physiological boundaries and prevent their deleterious effects [3].

Physical activity is a double-edged sword in terms of oxidant/antioxidant balance, and whenever sport is practised for health—which should be the most common condition—it should be programmed on a personal basis and on the basis of validated evidence. Data in this field are quite contradictory, often making difficult their translation into practical settings, particularly for the elderly, where the effects of aging on the oxidant/antioxidant balance intersect those of exercise. In fact, during exercise, ROS are produced in at least two biochemical pathways: (1) the mitochondrial electron transport chain; and (2) the system of xanthine oxidase that is responsible in the formation of peroxynitrite. With the aim of contrasting ROS effects, all tissues use their reserve of antioxidants, vitamins and glutathione [2,4].

Keeping in mind that oxidative stress is lower in fertile women because of oestrogen protection [5], a high quantity of ROS is generally induced by exercise that provokes modifications of antioxidant activity, both in cardiac and skeletal muscle [6]. Interestingly, it seems that both aerobic and anaerobic training stimulate the antioxidant system with respect to what happens in untrained subjects. Thus, it seems there are no specific exercise effects on redox balance. Moreover, the activation of antioxidant capacity is the same between the rest conditions of the three groups (aerobically, anaerobically and untrained people), suggesting that the antioxidant system is activated only transiently by exercise [6]. From a molecular point of view, DNA analysis of oxidative damage has shown that immediately after exercise, regardless of intensity, there are no signs of oxidative damage. Additionally, acute or extended moderate exercise does not induce DNA damage. Instead, it seems to be associated with decreased levels of oxidation. Finally, extended intense exercise increase DNA modifications [7].

More recently, studies performed in hypoxic conditions have shown that low–moderate exercise exerts a positive influence to protect against altitude/hypoxia-induced oxidative stress, while higher-intensity exercise increases oxidative stress [8]. These observations should be considered for training adaptations in athletes, to hypoxic or high-altitude conditions.

Finally, moderate exercise has been shown to be important to reduce the risks of cardiovascular diseases. In fact, acute cardiovascular exercise increases the oxidative stress, while regularly performed cardiovascular exercise increases the antioxidant capacity, of the cells [9]. Thus, it seems that the body's antioxidant responses are proportional to exercise intensity, but too-high-intensity exercise produces inflammation and cell damage, both in young and elderly subjects. On the other hand, de Sousa et al. (2017) [10] showed that, independently of intensity, volume, type of exercise and population, physical exercise always has an antioxidant effect. In conclusion, moderate-intensity exercise should be the right compromise to balance oxidant effects.

Interestingly, different scenarios are present in athletes with different levels of ability: while in elite athletes, physical exercise is not enough to maintain the oxidant/antioxidant balance, making an anti-oxidant supplementation necessary, in amateur and master athletes, oxidant/antioxidant activity is kept balanced by exercise, protecting the muscle from damage [11].

Of note, physical exercise also shows positive effects on the redox environment in non-muscular systems such as the cerebral [12,13] and vascular [14] systems. In fact, de Sousa et al. (2019) [12] studied the effect of exercise volume on antioxidant enzyme levels in various brain regions. They found that 30–60 min of exercise increased Catalase (CAT) activity, while 8 weeks of training increased Superoxide Dismutase (SOD). More than 8 weeks of training increased both ROS and antioxidant activity. Thus, four to eight weeks of moderate exercise promote a healthy balance of antioxidant enzymes in the rodent brain. Recently, Pinho et al. (2019) [13] reviewed the effects of resistance training to counteract oxidative stress in the brain. In particular, they showed evidence that Insulin Growth Factor-1 (IGF-1) in muscle activates the Protein Kinase B (Akt) signalling pathway at brain level. However, further investigations are necessary, since some observations are only speculative.

In 2016 Park et al. [14] studied the positive effects of exercise on redox balance in vessels. They found that arteries from trained mice presented higher levels of antioxidant markers such as: (i) Peroxisome Proliferative Activated Receptor-coactivator-1 (PPARgamma), (ii) Cytochrome-C Oxidase Subunit IV isoform 1 (COX4I1), and (iii) Isocitrate Dehydrogenase 2 (Idh-2). Moreover, the trained mice showed higher respiratory capacity and improved oxidant/antioxidant balance compared to untrained mice. These results sustain the hypothesis that physical activity can be vasculo-protective. Unfortunately, further studies are necessary.

The aim of this review is to unravel the relationship between redox balance, physical activity and aging, analysing what is known of the involved molecular pathways. It has therefore been organized into five sections: (1) Introduction, (2) Physical activity and redox balance in the young; (3) Physical activity and redox balance in the elderly; (4) Insights into signal transduction; and (5) Conclusions.

Figure 1 reports the diagram of the process that we apply to select papers to review.

PRISMA 2009 Flow Diagram

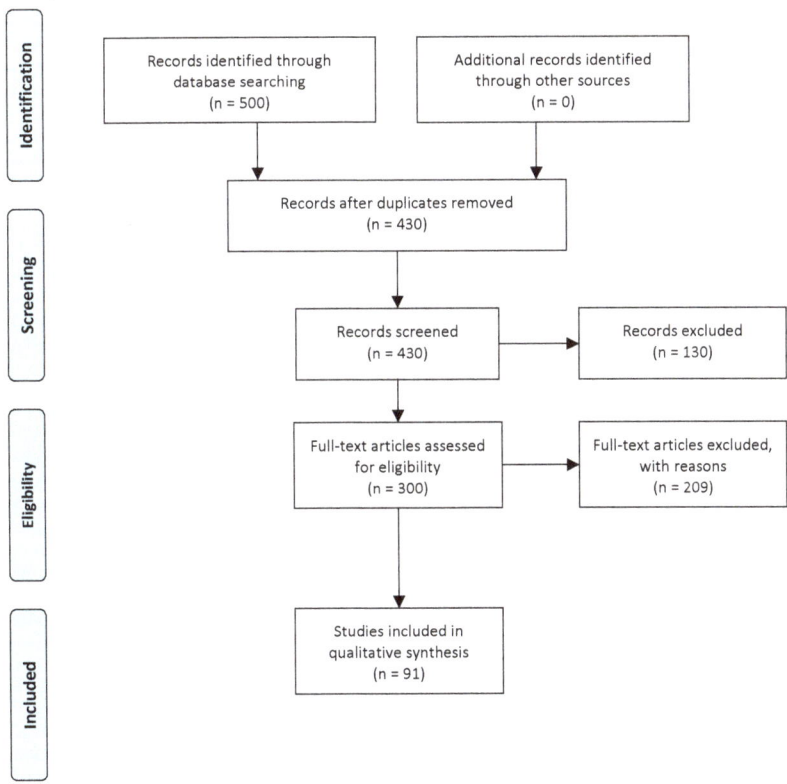

Figure 1. Flow diagram according to Prisma 2009 guidelines. A total of 500 records were identified for this study in three online databases (Pubmed, Scopus, Web of Science) using this search expression: "Redox AND Balance AND Physical activity OR Exercise AND Age AND Signal transduction". After removing duplicates, we found 430 articles, and after first screening, 130 were excluded. 300 full-text articles were assessed for eligibility, and 209 were excluded because results were partially redundant. Finally, 91 studies were included in qualitative synthesis. We did not use any date limit.

2. Physical Activity and Redox Balance in the Young and Adults

In young people, the majority of papers correlated obesity with oxidative stress. In fact, obesity is often associated with high levels of free fatty acids. This increases the levels of

NADH that generate high oxidative stress. In obese young subjects (males of 20–26 years), ROS levels are significantly higher than in non-obese, while (SOD) antioxidant activity is significantly lower [15]. After training (aerobic: 40 min treadmill, three times/week for 8 weeks; 70% Heart Rate reserve), ROS decreases and SOD increases. Interestingly, the authors also found a significant increase in Brain-Derived Neurotrophic Factor (BDNF), but not in Glial-cell-line-Derived Neurotrophic Factor (GDNF) or in Nerve Growth Factor (NGF) after aerobic training. At the same time, blood markers of blood-brain barrier (BBB) damage decreased. Notably, BDNF is lower in obese subjects, compared to non-obese. In non-obese subjects, the authors did not find significant changes in the levels of neurotrophines. Finally, Di Liegro et al. (2019) [16] reviewed the effect of physical activity on brain health. They found that BDNF is produced in the periphery of the nervous system in a physical-activity-dependent manner.

A very recent review [17] showed that overweight/obesity does not affect exercise lipid-oxidation systems, suggesting that physical activity could have a positive effect, not directly on lipid oxidation, but on blood-brain barrier damage. Interestingly, three months of Crossfit training increased BDNF level in active men [18]. In particular, they observed improvements in endurance performance (expressed by VO_{2max}) and the levels of plasma antioxidant markers such as SOD, glutathione reductase (GSH), Uric Acid (Uric Acid), the ferric reducing ability of plasma and BDNF. Altogether, these data suggest that physical activity exerts a positive effect on brain health, both reducing damages that can occur to the blood-brain barrier and increasing the levels of the antioxidant BDNF.

Besides physical activity, antioxidant supplementation is widely distributed to counteract oxidative stress. In fact, the antioxidant effect of polyphenolic compounds is related to the inhibition/inactivation of several pathways such as the Nuclear-factor kappa light-chain enhancer pathway of activated B cells (Nf-kB), and the kappa kinase/c-Jun amino-terminal kinase pathway (IKK/JNK), that are involved in oxidation [19]. Moreover, polyphenolic molecules inhibit the activity of the enzymes responsible for ROS production, such as cyclooxygenase, lipoxygenase and xanthine oxidase. Of note, the effects of polyphenols can affect the activation of antioxidant pathways by exercise. For example, Cavarretta et al. (2018) [20] studied the effect of cocoa polyphenols in elite football players practising intense physical exercise. After 30 days of chocolate intake, the elite football players showed a significant decrease in their levels of muscle-damage markers such as Creatin Kinase (CK), Lactate dehydrogenase (LDH) and Myoglobin and an increased antioxidant power, suggesting that polyphenols positively modulated redox balance and reduced muscle tissue injury in elite football players.

On the other hand, activation of antioxidant mechanisms in Glucose-6-Phosphate Dehydrogenase (G6PDH) patients (adults, 33–43 years old), with the Alpha-Lipoic Acid (ALA) supplementation, increases the antioxidant defence without modifying the effects of exercise. In fact, administration of ALA (600 mg/day) or placebo for 4 weeks did not affect their performance with 45 min of treadmill, at 70–75% VO_{2max} and then 90% until exhaustion [21]. Thus, administration of compounds like polyphenols seems to reinforce the antioxidant effect of exercise.

Additionally, some authors have checked the possibility that training level could be associated with different effects on oxidative stress. For example, in adolescent swimmers, it has been shown that high-intensity exercise modifies redox balance without inducing prolonged oxidative stress [22]. Similarly, ultra-marathon swimming did not induce oxidative stress in well-trained swimmers [23], suggesting that well-trained swimmers are able to regulate redox balance. These observations could be important in scheduling training programs for ultra-marathon swimmers.

These results, however, apparently depend on sport intensity. In fact, in amateur women gymnasts, low–moderate-intensity training increases total antioxidant activity after 48 h [24]. Instead, 48 h' recovery after high-intensity training is not enough to restore redox balance. A modest ROS increase is necessary for normal force generation, while higher ROS levels induce damage in a dose- and time-dependent manner [25]. Thus, a diet rich in antioxidants and sessions of low–moderate intensity training should be recommended to amateur gymnasts after high-intensity training [24].

Interestingly, antioxidant supplementation produces divergent results on exercise performance. For example, vitamin C and E supplementation and resistance activity induce a decrease in protein ubiquitination [26]. Moreover, vitamin supplementation reduces the phosphorylation of p38 Mitogen-Activated Protein Kinase (p38MAPK), of Extracellular signal-Regulated protein Kinases 1 and 2 (ERK1/2), and of p70S6 kinase [26,27]. Similarly, in rats trained with aerobic exercise, the antioxidant vitamin C blunts exercise-induced adaptations such as mitochondrial biogenesis and degradation of worn-out mitochondrial proteins [28].

Thus, the combination of antioxidant and exercise can induce contrasting effects, suggesting that further investigations are required on this subject.

3. Physical Activity and Redox Balance in the Adult and the Elderly

Aging is associated with a decrease in the activity of anti-oxidant systems, while exercise reduces the levels of oxidative stress markers, thus activating the antioxidant enzymes [29], suggesting that the greater the physical exercise, the smaller the effects of aging. Although this hypothesis could be very intriguing, it is generally supposed that low–moderate physical activity induces adaptations that increase resistance to oxidative stress, since exercise training decreases the risk for several diseases associated with oxidative stress. Many studies have been published on this topic, but conflicting results have been reported, likely due to different parameters and measurement methods used: many groups have reported protective effects of exercise on antioxidant systems, while others have reported negative effects of training.

What is commonly accepted is that markers of oxidative stress are significantly lower in trained subjects with respect to untrained ones, similar to the conditions observed in young people. For example, 8 weeks of walking does not induce oxidative stress in aged subjects [30]. In fact, Low-Density Lipoprotein (LDL) oxidation and nitration levels are not affected by walking. Instead, LDL nitration is modified by acute moderate activity. Thus, it seems important to practice intense exercise to stimulate antioxidant enzymes, rather than low–moderate activity. This condition appears also after acute oxidative challenge. In fact, fit aged subjects show lower oxidative stress than unfit age-matched subjects at baseline conditions and after an acute oxidative challenge such as forearm ischemia-reperfusion [29]. However, this is not due to lower levels of circulating antioxidant molecules. Moreover, reduced oxidative damage that has been shown in fit individuals cannot be attributed to physiological parameters like adiposity or High-Density Lipoprotein (HDL). Instead, it is likely related to differences in antioxidant enzyme activity. Thus, to be physically fit appears an effective strategy for fighting age-related oxidative damage [29].

In 2016, Done and Traustadottir [31] showed that sedentary middle-aged adults could increase their resistance to oxidative stress (forearm Ischemia Reperfusion (IR)) through whole-body aerobic training (45-min sessions three times per week, with an intensity of 70–85% maximal heart rate). In fact, the level of the oxidative marker F2-isoprostanes was significantly decreased after exercise, but not at the baseline pre-IR [31].

Age-related dysfunctions of redox balance also determine endothelial alterations that have been associated with cardiovascular disease. Ten days of treadmill training (1 h at 70% of VO_{2max}) significantly increase flow-mediated dilation of arteries and Vascular Endothelial Growth Factor Receptor-positive (KDR+) circulating cells, while not affecting the level of SOD mRNA, intracellular nitric oxide (NO), ROS, endothelial Nitric Oxide Synthase (eNOS), NADPH oxidase 2 and neutrophil cytosolic factor 1 in healthy older adult subjects. Thus, these data suggest that short-term aerobic training can reduce risk factors for cardiovascular disease [32].

As for young subjects, the effect of antioxidant molecules, alone or in combination with exercise, has been tested for muscle physiology and function. For muscle tissue, a good antioxidant has not been found yet, although the effect of plant extract and molecules like resveratrol and vitamins have been investigated [33–37]. For example, a waste-water polyphenolic mixture (LACHI MIX HT) containing hydroxytirosol (HT), gallic acid and homovanillic acid induced functional amelioration in the skeletal muscles of 27-month-old rats [33]. Moreover, a decrease of oxidative stress marker levels was observed [33]. The resveratrol had been used, with positive effects, in 18-month-old mice in combination with exercise for 4 weeks [34]. In particular, decreases in blood lactate, free fatty-acid levels, and gastrocnemius-muscle lipid peroxidation were observed, as well as an increase in the activity of antioxidant enzymes such as SOD and catalase [34]. Interestingly, the up-regulation of peroxisome proliferator-activated receptor gamma coactivator-1α (PGC-1α) mRNA was also observed [34], suggesting the involvement of mitochondrial biogenesis and function. Similar effects have been obtained with plant (Rhus Coriaria) extract in human myoblasts, where Najjaret et al. (2017) [36] observed an increase of the antioxidant enzymes SOD2 and catalase, together with increased viability and adhesion of human myoblasts. Finally, oral ingestion of ascorbic acid increases muscle blood flow and oxygen consumption in older adults practising rhythmic handgrip exercises [37]. Antioxidant supplements have been tested for the treatments of sarcopenia which is a muscle disease known to be associated with the oxidant/antioxidant balance in the elderly. Specifically, sarcopenia is a condition characterized by the progressive loss of muscle mass and function, a decrease in number of motor units, and wasting of muscle fibres. Among the complex biological mechanisms associated with sarcopenia, there is a pronounced imbalance between oxidant and antioxidant species. As yet, it is not clear if antioxidant supplements have a protective effect against the development of this disease [38]. On the other hand, physical exercise could have a role in counteracting this disease, because at a low–moderate intensity, it stimulates antioxidant pathways [39].

Of note, resistance exercise increases satellite cell number, and reverses muscle atrophy in aging by increasing the number of fast fibres that are reduced in the elderly [40,41]. For example, cycles of 12 weeks of resistance training, 12 weeks of de-training and 12 weeks of re-training induce amelioration of physiological and cellular parameters of muscle in aged men [42]. The training increases power and strength in knee-extension exercises, and reduces the number of both 2a and 2x fast fibres. The de-training induces a modest loss of power and strength. Finally, 12 weeks of re-training produce a significant increase in type-II fibre hypertrophy, satellite cell number and myonuclei [42]. On the other hand, 12 weeks of aerobic training in sedentary healthy subjects increase the cross-sectional area of both type-I and type-II fibres, while satellite activation and nuclei addition are found only in slow type-I fibres, suggesting that a differential regulation concerning myonuclear condition occurs [43]. Since the slow fibres have a higher oxidative content than do fast type-II fibres, resistance training could represent a better training method to counteract aging effects on muscle mass and function, but this point is still under debate. As the increase of antioxidant species was observed in many studies, and the reduction of oxidant species (malondyaldehyde) was observed in type-II diabetic patients performing moderate aerobic exercise three times/week [44], with no changes in the control group, it suggests that there is a specific effect of exercise in diabetic patients on lipid peroxidation levels and on the susceptibility of DNA to oxidative damage.

Although it is not directly influenced by physical activity, nervous tissue has the highest metabolic rates in the organism [45] and this elevated oxygen consumption promotes ROS generation, making the nervous tissue more susceptible to developing oxidative stress [45]. Moreover, antioxidant levels are lower in the brain than in other parts of the body, due to the low permeability of the blood-brain barrier to most endogenous antioxidant molecules [45]. It is well known that aging and neurodegenerative diseases show increased levels of ROS and reduction of BNDF and NGF: oxidative stress modulates the activity of neurotrophins that then become unable to save neurons from cell death and to promote neuroplasticity [46].

Lifestyle strongly influences the oxidative stress state, and as a consequence, it could directly affect the developmental and clinical aspects of neurodegenerative disease. It has been reported that diets rich in antioxidants may delay the development of neurodegenerative disease [46]. Polyphenols show potential positive effects against Alzheimer's Disease (AD), preventing ROS accumulation in brain tissue and clearing neurofibrillary tangles. For instance, curcumin can upregulate anti-tau BAG2, generating a putative beneficial factor against AD-associated tauopathy [47].

Several different physical-activity interventions in the elderly affected by degenerative diseases have been reported. However, the conclusions of the different extensive and systematic analyses reported in several reviews are not always optimistic [48].

Trials suffer from a small number of enrolled subjects, different and short follow-up times, and great differences in type, frequency, intensity and duration of physical-activity protocols. Moreover, one's sedentary status is defined and measured differently. Finally, many different cognitive tests and a plethora of fitness assays are used, making comparison more difficult.

4. Insights into Signal Transduction

The role of physical activity as an antioxidant to counteract the negative effects of aging and chronic disease has been widely studied, and we summarize below the main results obtained so far. First, it is worth noting, however, that we are still far from a structured comprehensive view of this complex topic. Besides, in this field, several studies have been done in the mouse model, and the translation to humans is far away.

Several different signalling pathways have been implicated in the control of redox balance by physical activity, also depending on the analysed organs or systems.

4.1. Plasma and Adipose Tissue

Increased oxidative stress is related to abnormal activation of the renin-angiotensin-aldosterone system [49]. Resistance exercise increases the level of Triacylglycerol Lipase Activity (TGLA), the level of plasma glycerol and the level of oxidative stress in obese with respect to lean subjects [49,50]. This is associated with higher levels of serum non-esterified fatty acid and increased lipolysis in adipose tissue [50]. The relationship between exercise and obesity is under study in a clinical trial (current controlled trials, ISRCTN95488515). In particular, they are investigating the effects of endurance and high-intensity intermittent endurance exercise on plasma concentrations of glycerol, Atrial Natriuretic Peptide (ANP) and Brain Natriuretic Peptide (BNP). In fact, ANP and BNP are potent lipolytic agents. The results of this trial will be useful for optimizing training protocols for the prevention and treatment of obesity [51].

Contrasting results have been obtained on the role of exercise on plasma levels of cytokines [52–54]. For example, triathlon competitions like Ironman or Half Ironman significantly increase the levels of oxidative stress markers, Interleukin-6 (IL-6), Interleukin-1 (IL-1) and Tumour Necrosis Factor alpha (TNF-alpha). However, the training hours spent before the competitions were inversely correlated with the level of IL-6 found, suggesting that only IL-6 is related to the time of training [52]. In aged subjects affected by rheumatoid arthritis, 10 weeks of a walking-based high-intensity interval training (HIIT) increased ROS production, but there were no significant changes in the levels of inflammatory markers such as IL-1, IL-6, TNF-alpha and Interleukin-10 (IL-10) [53]. On the other hand, a study performed in post-menopausal women observed a significant decrease in IL-2, IL-4, IL-6 and TNF-alpha levels, both after 3 months of aerobic training (60–70% of maximal heart rate on treadmill, with low speed and without inclination) and after 3 months of resistance training with better results in terms of BMI and quality-of-life in subjects performing aerobic training [54]. In contrast, a single short bout of resistance exercise in healthy untrained men increased catecholamines, Epidermal Growth Factor (EGF), IL-2 and TNF-alpha, with the levels of IL-1α, IL-1β, IL-6, IL-8 and IL-10 maintained constant levels [55]. Additionally, Accattato et al. (2017) [49] observed that a single bout of physical activity does not induce changes in plasma cytokine levels. Instead, they observed a decrease of EGF and an increase of the antioxidant enzyme Glutathione Reductase (GR).

Eccentric exercise of the elbow flexors does not induce significant change in plasma cytokine levels, even in the presence of significant muscle damage as demonstrated by the increase in Creatine Kinase (CK) activity and myoglobin [56]. In any case, a transient increase in oxidative stress and cytokines is considered relevant for improvements induced by regular exercise, in a process called mitohormesis, because mitochondria are necessary for energy production and associated with oxidative stress induction [57]. All these data suggest that, since the role of cytokines in response to oxidative stress and exercise has not been definitively clarified, the aerobic, resistance, endurance and strength training sessions should be carefully set up within physical-activity programs for adults and elderly people in order to avoid undesirable effects in inflammation-signalling pathways.

4.2. Nervous System

In the nervous system, ROS are involved in neurogenesis, proliferation and differentiation of neuronal stem cells; however, if the ROS concentrations exceed threshold levels, it can lead to neurodegeneration [58]. Physical activity increases neurogenesis by inducing neurotrophic factors. Moreover, it protects DNA from damage by stimulating antioxidant systems [58]. A recent review by Vilela et al. (2020) [59] summarizes the effects of physical exercise on brain synaptic plasticity and memory through different pathways. In particular, studies performed in rat hippocampi suggest that aerobic training induces N-Methyl-D-Aspartate phosphorylate (pNMDA) and Postsynaptic Density protein 95 (PSD-95) activity, which increases memory. Instead, the strength training ameliorates the results of memory tests by upregulating Protein Kinase C alpha (PKC-alpha) and the cytokines IL-1 and TNF-alpha. Moreover, aerobic exercise ameliorates spatial memory through BDNF signalling [60]. Interestingly, in older adults affected by mild subcortical ischaemic vascular cognitive impairment, 6 months of aerobic exercise on the treadmill improved efficiency of the affected brain areas [60].

Feter et al. (2019) [61] investigated how different training models affect memory and redox balance. Resistance training induced a significant increase in lipid peroxidation and ROS levels, compared to the sedentary group. The moderate-intensity continuous-training group and physical-activity (running wheel) group showed a higher level of the antioxidant enzyme catalase, compared to the sedentary group. Moreover, the moderate-intensity continuous-training group showed better recognition memory, suggesting that performing physical activity, with a moderate but continuous intensity, could represent a non-pharmacological strategy to counteract the symptoms of Alzheimer's disease. Of note, the role of physical activity as a strategy for counteracting Alzheimer's Disease (AD) has been reviewed elsewhere [62]. In particular, although the pathogenesis of this disease has been clarified, the exact mechanisms are still under study. The role of physical activity seems to be correlated with microRNA alterations associated with impaired autophagy. This process is mediated by the Phosphatidyl Inositol 3-Kinase (PI3Kinase)/Akt-mammalian Target Of Rapamycin (mTOR) signalling pathway [62]. In detail, physical activity, through mTOR signalling activation, downregulates the production of abnormal micro-RNAs such as miR-130a, miR106b and miRlet7c, and stimulates neurogenesis, synaptic plasticity and memory, although the exact mechanism is still vague. The mTOR activation leads to dysfunctional autophagy, and consequently, to Tau hyperphosphorylation, β-amyloid (Aβ) accumulation and neurofibrillary tangles that are characteristics of Alzheimer's disease [62]. Discovering how physical activity can exert this effect in the central nervous system and interfere with the abnormal synthesis of miRNAs in AD pathogenesis is an intriguing challenge that requires further investigation.

4.3. Liver

Nuclear factor erythroid-2-related factor 2 (Nrf2) and its antioxidant responsive elements play a prominent role in the reaction to oxidative stress. Acute aerobic exercise activates nuclear Nrf2 independently of exercise intensity, while higher-intensity physical activity increases the levels of oxidative stress and antioxidant enzymes [63]. Interestingly, a bout of moderate-intensity stationary cycling up-regulates Nrf2 in young, but not in older people. Nrf2 is involved in redox-balance modifications induced by exercise, but the underlying mechanisms are still unclear [64]. Of note, both aerobic and resistance training, although with different molecular pathways, converge on activation of the mitochondrial biogenesis through Nrf2. Although Nrf2 is ubiquitously expressed, the effects of physical activity and redox balance on Nrf2 have been well characterized in the liver. In mice, sulphorane exerts a protective role against liver damage induced by acute exercise. In particular, sulphorane reduces inflammatory cytokines like IL-1beta, IL-6 and TNF-alpha increased by exercise, and upregulates the expression of the antioxidant enzymes catalase, SOD1 and glutathione peroxidase (GPx1) through the activation of the Nrf2/Heme Oxygenase (HO1) signal-transduction pathway [65]. Moreover, it has been shown that 6 weeks of aerobic training increase triglycerides, free fatty acids and blood glucose in Nrf2-*null* mice, showing that Nrf2 is involved in training-induced adaptations of glucose homeostasis. Moreover, the levels of oxidative stress markers in the liver and in adipose tissue are increased, with respect to the control group, in Nrf2-*null* mice [66].

4.4. Skeletal and Cardiac Muscle

The importance of Nrf2 has also been evidenced in muscle. In fact, Huang et al. (2019) [67] showed that the level of Nrf2 mRNA in skeletal muscle decreases with aging, and concomitantly, a frailty phenotype arises. Muscle function and mass are similar in young wild-type and young Nrf2-*null* mice. In middle-aged and old Nrf2-*null* mice, muscle function significantly decreases with enhancement of frailty in old Nrf2-*null* mice [67]. This phenotype hinges on a decrease of mitochondrial biogenesis and alteration of mitochondrial morphology in skeletal muscle. In skeletal muscle, other pathways also seem to be involved in redox-balance signalling. In fact, skeletal muscle is a primary source of ROS during exercise, because during muscle contraction, there is a massive production of superoxide radical (O_2^-) [67]. In rats, a combination of antioxidants (such as resveratrol) and exercise significantly increases muscle mass and grip strength in sarcopenic old mice, and reduces abnormal sarcomere length [68]. Concomitantly, the authors observed a significant increase in the levels of the phosphorylated form of 5' AMP-activated protein Kinase (pAMPK) and of Sirtuin1 (Sirt1), suggesting the involvement of the AMPK/Sirt1 pathway [68]. This last pathway is also involved in AdipoRon function that is used to reduce oxidative stress and inflammation in dystrophic mice [69]. AdipoRon increases the levels of pAMPK that reduces NF-Kb and increases the dystrophin analogue utrophin [69]. AdipoRon also increases muscle strength and endurance, leading to better physical performance [69]. The antioxidant and antiaging effects of resveratrol have been studied also in the kidney [70]. In particular, the authors suggest that resveratrol can activate both Nrf2 and AMPK/sirtuin1 pathways in the kidney, to counteract the pathologic aging effect in this organ. In fact, transfection with Nrf2 and SIRT1 siRNAs in HK2 cells blocks the antioxidant effect of resveratrol [70].

The Akt signal-transduction pathway has been evidenced in skeletal muscle, in association with exercise and redox balance. For example, in mice, swimming exercise reduces ROS, and prevents high-fat diet-induced insulin resistance through the decrease of NAPDH oxidase 4 (Nox4), as well as the increase of Akt signal transduction in skeletal muscle [71].

Akt signalling is also required for the correct regulation of muscle stem-cell (MuSCs) homeostasis during aging. In fact, Lukjanenko et al. (2019) [72] found WNT1-Inducible Signalling Pathway Protein 1 (WISP1) as a fibro-adipogenic progenitor protein that is strongly downregulated during aging. This protein is important for muscle regeneration and the asymmetric division of muscle stem cells through Akt signalling. In fact, systemic treatment of aged mice with WISP1 restores the proliferation and differentiation of aged muscle stem cells [72].

Peroxisome Proliferator-Activated Receptor gamma (PPAR-gamma) and Peroxisome proliferator-activated receptor Gamma Coactivator-1 alpha (PGC1-alpha) have been proposed as important players in muscle remodelling induced by exercise through Mitogen-

Activated Protein Kinases (MAPKinases), and are also correlated with redox balance. In particular, p38 MAPKinase activates PPAR-gamma. Sirt1, in turn, depending on physical exercise, activates PGC1-alpha [73]. PGC1-alpha is implicated in aging-associated mitochondrial diseases dysregulating ROS production and mitochondrial network structure in skeletal muscle, during aging and exercise training. PGC1-alpha is also activated by ROS through NF-kB, AMPK, and finally, by nitric oxide (NO) produced during muscle contraction [73,74]. PGC1-alpha-*null* aged mice show lower running endurance, higher mitochondrial damage, increased ROS and higher oxidative stress than do young mice. Exercise training increases maximal respiratory capacity, both in PGC1-alpha-*null* and wild-type mice. Instead, the rescue of mitochondrial homeostasis occurs in a PGC1-alpha-dependent manner [74].

Regarding cardiac muscle, aerobic exercise training on the treadmill ameliorates myocardial infarction symptoms. In fact, TNF-alpha, NADPH-oxidase activity and p38 phosphorylation are diminished in infarcted trained mice, with respect to infarcted sham-trained mice [75]. The positive effect of exercise is produced also by increasing the antioxidant defence through neuronal Nitric-Oxide Synthase (nNOS) [76]. In fact, cardiac-specific overexpression of this enzyme mimics the effect of exercise on maximal oxygen capacity, while aerobic activity increases cardiac dysfunctions in nNOS-*null* mice, confirming the protective effect of this enzyme.

Interestingly, Hao et al. (2014) [77] showed that exercise is a powerful instrument for protecting the heart from ischemia, and that the molecular mechanism at the base of this phenomenon involves Protein Kinase Cε. Specifically, Sprague-Dawley rats underwent exhaustive aerobic exercise on the treadmill, to induce myocardial injury [77]. In such exhaustive conditions, PKCε translocated to the intercalated disks of the heart. The exercise pre-conditioning increased the level of the phosphorylated/activated isoform of PKCε in the cytoplasmic membrane, suggesting that PKCε is involved in the signal transduction for heart protection induced by pre-conditioning [77].

Finally, Díaz-Ruíz et al. (2019) [78] evidenced a role for redox signalling in ischemic post-conditioning protection through PKCε and Erk1/2, which indirectly regulate Nrf2 activation. In fact, the authors showed that PKCε and Erk1/2 are activated in a redox-dependent manner. It was also shown that neither the PI3K inhibitor nor the Erk1/2 inhibitor reduces Nrf2 activation, suggesting that these kinases have other direct targets [78]. Notably, Buelna-Chontal et al. (2014) [79] found that Nrf2 activation is dependent on PKC in post-conditioned hearts. In fact, the use of PKC inhibitors reduces the level of Nrf2 phosphorylation and the activity of antioxidant proteins that are regulated by Nrf2 [79].

The PKC family includes 12 isozymes divided into conventional (alpha, beta and gamma), novel (delta, epsilon, eta and theta) and atypical (zeta and iota). PKCε belongs to the novel group which is activated by the conventional signalling of Ca^{2+} and diacylglycerol. In particular, the receptor, once activated, hydrolyses Phosphatidyl-Inositol-4,5-bisPhosphate (PIP_2), generating Inositol trisPhosphate (IP_3, responsible for Ca^{2+} mobilization) and diacylglycerol which, as the second messenger, triggers PKC-kinase function, leading to phosphorylation and activation of other trans-membrane or intra-cellular proteins. PKCs are generally considered as oncoproteins. However, many different roles have been proposed for PKC proteins in cell physiology. For example, PKCε is involved in many processes that maintain cell homeostasis and proliferation in several tissues such as the vessels, blood, heart and skeletal muscle [80–85]. For example, PKCε is differently expressed in blood cells suggesting multiple roles for this PKC isoform [84]. Moreover, Martini et al. [85] evidenced that PKCε controls the migration of centrosome during mitotic spindle assembly. Recently, D'Amico and Lennartz (2018) [86] showed a role in vesicle formation for PKCε. They demonstrated that PKCε is linked to the Golgi apparatus through the interaction between the Golgi's lipids and the regulatory domain of the kinase. Moreover, the mechanism seems to be independent of the kinase activity of PKCε, although it requires the binding of PKCε to actin and cytoskeleton for budding and fission of the vesicles [86]. Finally, PKCε is important for autophagy in the breast-cancer cell line [87]. In fact, PKCε siRNA induces a significant decrease in autophagy by reducing the levels of Raptor and Rictor that are required to form mammalian Target Of Rapamycin Complex-1 (mTORC-1) and -2 (mTORC-2), which are important regulators of autophagy [87]. On the other hand, autophagy is important to counteract aging, although this process declines in the elderly. Exercise and diet downregulate mTORC-1, that acts as a negative player in autophagy and stimulates autophagy in several other tissues [88]. Moreover, mTORC-1 induces muscle atrophy in the elderly, while mTOR is essential for muscle hypertrophy. Most likely, a mechanism that involves Akt and mTORC1 is important in sarcopenia, although the definition of a clear signalling pathway is still under study [89]. Based on these considerations, we could speculate that PKCε is involved in exercise protection during the aging process.

Additionally, ROS can affect Ca^{2+} signalling at the level of channels, pumps and exchangers [90]. Alterations in ROS signalling can modify Ca^{2+} communication system, likely contributing to disease onset. In the heart, for example, Zima and Blatter [91] showed that the ROS produced during reperfusion of cardiac ischemic injury can affect ischemia-related Ca(2+) overload. More recently, Cabassi and Miragoli [92] reviewed the important role of local environment (namely ROS and Ca^{2+}) in mitochondrial re-organization and fusion in failing cardiomyocytes. In particular, a correct interplay between Ca^{2+} and ROS is important to avoid intracellular Ca^{2+} increase during diastole that leads to cardiac arrhythmia [92]. The relevance of interaction between Ca^{2+} signalling and ROS has also been described in skeletal muscle aging [40]. In fact, the increase of ROS in skeletal muscle can alter the Ca^{2+} signalling pathway that is necessary for the fibre contraction, leading to a decrease in muscle strength. Interestingly, physical activity can help to contrast strength loss by reducing ROS [40].

Finally, Peroxiredoxins (PRDXs) are important antioxidant enzymes that remove H_2O_2 to reduce oxidative stress. PRDXs are responsible for the discarding of 90% of cellular peroxides, they are ubiquitous and function as regulators of local H_2O_2 concentrations [93,94]. There are more than 3500 sequences of Peroxiredoxins, and these have been divided into six subfamilies with different expression levels in mammals, plants, yeasts and bacteria [95]. Considering the conservation of phylogenetic rhythms, the fact that PRDX proteins autoregulate independently from the transcriptional circadian clock and the highly conserved structures of these proteins, many researchers are now studying the links between aging, circadian rhythms and redox systems [96].

PRDX-3-*null* mice present a significant reduction in physical strength (measured by swimming performance), compared to their wild-type littermates at the age of ten months [97]. Moreover, PRDX-3-*null* mice show a higher number of apoptotic cells in the brain, higher expression of Nrf2 and a lower level of mitochondrial DNA (mDNA) at the age of ten months, when compared to wild-type, suggesting that the lack of PRDX-3 increases oxidative stress and mitochondrial impairment, which are characteristic of the aging process [97]. To study redox-enzyme concentrations after different types of exercise, a group of active men (mean age 28 years old) performed moderate-intensity exercise with one bout of High-Intensity Interval Exercise (HIIE) or an eccentric resistance exercise [98]. PRDX-4 (Peroxiredoxin-4) and SOD3 increased after High-Intensity Interval Exercise (HIIE), while Thioredoxin Reductase (TRX-R) decreased. Notably, resistance exercise did not determine any significant changes in redox enzymes, but induced skeletal muscle damages. Altogether, these results suggest that PRDX-4 and SOD3 could be considered as biomarkers of oxidative stress [98]. Interestingly, HIIE showed similar effects of endurance exercise in muscle mitochondria, independently from the total workload, suggesting that exercise prescription could be accommodated into individual prescriptions, generating comparable molecular effects [99].

Although the exact mechanism is not yet clear, it has been proposed that PRDX translates oxidative stress signalling by the activation of MAPKinases [100].

Figure 2 provides a schematic representation of the pathways involved in the effects of physical activity and redox balance to counteract aging. In plasma or serum, the proposed markers of oxidative stress are the increase of PRDX-4 and SOD3, while the level of EGF should decrease, given the above studies. Cytokines are inflammation markers, and contrasting results have been obtained in association with physical activity. In neural cells, PI3K/Akt/mTor seems to have a prominent role, especially in the treatment of Alzheimer's Disease. The Nrf2 pathway is central in the liver, but it also is an important effector in heart and skeletal muscle where many players have been evidenced, such as MAPKinases (p38 and Erk1/2), Akt and PPARγ/PGC1α. Finally, in adipose tissue, there are emerging results on the role of physical activity and redox balance to increase the levels of BDNF and ANF (lipolytic agents) in the elaboration of protocols to contrast obesity.

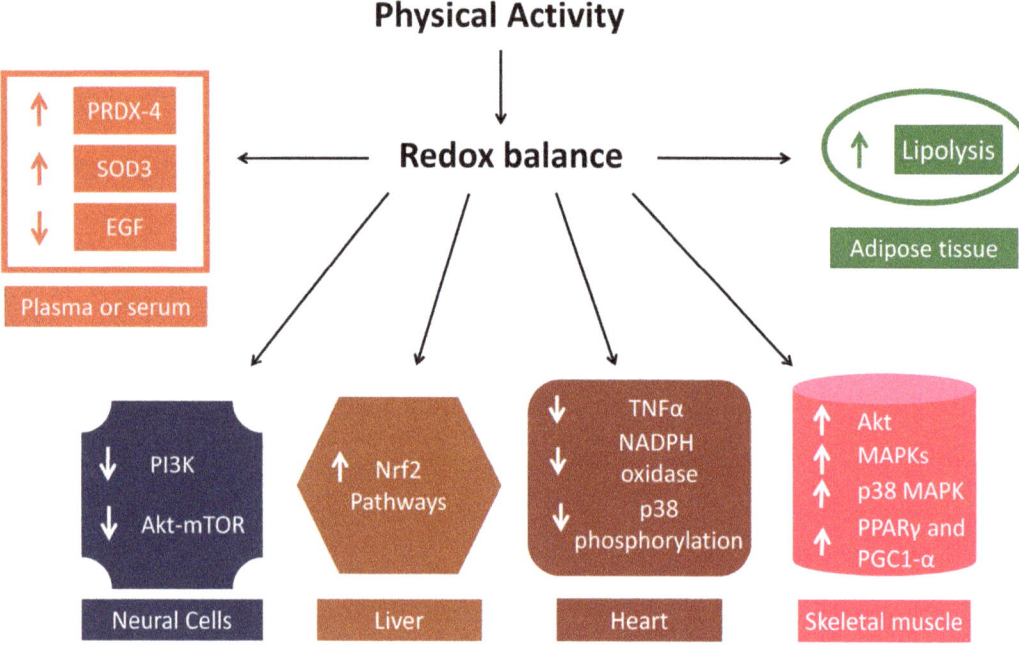

Figure 2. Schematic representation of the molecular pathways involved in redox regulation by physical activity.

In plasma and serum, the effect of physical activity on redox balance is exerted through the increase of SOD3 and PRDX-4 and the decrease of EGF; in neural cells, a decrease of PI3Kinase/Akt-mTOR is observed; in liver cells, Nrf2 pathways are activated; in the heart, the effect of physical activity is associated with a decrease of TNF-alpha and NADPH oxidase, and p38 phosphorylation; in skeletal muscle, Akt, MAPKinases, PPARgamma, PGC-1 alpha and Nrf2 are up-regulated; in adipose tissue, lipolysis is activated by physical activity.

5. Conclusions and Perspectives

Redox balance is very important for cell life. As with other cell processes, oxidant/antioxidant balance is affected by aging, with a decrease in the efficiency of antioxidant systems. To counteract this effect of aging, antioxidant foods have been shown to be useful. Physical activity, as well, has been involved in the regulation of redox balance in several tissues such as skeletal muscle, cardiac muscle, liver, as well as neural cells. Although there are several pieces of evidence of the involvement of different signalling pathways, a comprehensive view of the molecular players, modulated by physical activity, that are able to counteract the effects of ageing on redox balance, is still lacking.

The trivial perception that reactive species of oxygen are exclusively detrimental molecules, is definitively substituted with mounting evidence that exercise-induced perturbation of redox balance is the upstream signal for the activation of transcription factors and the induction of gene expression associated with exercise effects involving total body adaptation to training. However, the same signalling should be analysed on the specific tissue and organ, as well as in terms of age, fragility state and comorbidities.

At the moment, although we believe that future precision medicine will be able to transform exercise administration from generic wellness to targeted prevention, we must admit that the topic is still in its infancy.

Author Contributions: D.G., C.C., E.M. contributed to the bibliographic research, writing of the manuscript and produced the figures. M.V. (Mauro Vaccarezza), V.P., G.P., L.A. reviewed the manuscript. M.V. (Marco Vitale) reviewed the manuscript and supervised the work. G.G. and P.M. conceived the original idea and supervised the work. All authors have read and agreed to the published version of the manuscript.

Funding: D.G.: C.C.: M.V. (Marco Vitale), G.G. were supported by Fondi Locali per la Ricerca 2019—Quota Prodotti di Ricerca—Parma University. P.M. was supported by "Programmi di ricerca di Rilevante Interesse Nazionale"—Italian Ministry of Education, University and Research (MIUR-PRIN) 2017 grant entitled "ACTLIFE: IS ACTIVE LIFE STYLE ENOUGH FOR HEALTH AND WELLBEING?" codice 2017RS5M44_004.

Institutional Review Board Statement: Not applicable.

Informed Consent Statement: Not applicable.

Data Availability Statement: Not applicable.

Acknowledgments: We are grateful to Cristina Micheloni, Luciana Cerasuolo and Vincenzo Alberto Piero Palermo for technical support. We thank Devahuti Chaliha for English proofreading.

Conflicts of Interest: The authors declare no conflict of interest.

Abbreviations

SOD3	Superoxide Dismutase 3
PRDX-4	Peroxiredoxin-4
EGF	Epidermal Growth Factor
PI3Kinase	Phosphatidyl Inositol 3 Kinase
Akt	Protein Kinase B
mTOR	mammalian Target Of Rapamycin
Nrf2	Nuclear factor erythroid-2-related factor 2
TNF-alpha	Tumour Necrosis Factor alpha
NADPH	Nicotinamide Adenine Dinucleotide Phosphate
MAPKinase	Mitogen-Activated Protein Kinase
PPAR-gamma	Peroxisome Proliferator-Activated Receptor gamma
PGC-1-alpha	Peroxisome proliferator-activated receptor Gamma Coactivator 1 alpha

References

1. World Health Organization (WHO). Available online: https://www.who.int/news-room/q-a-detail/ageing-healthy-ageing-and-functional-ability (accessed on 30 October 2020).
2. Ji, L.L.; Leeuwenburgh, C.; Leichtweis, S.; Gore, M.; Fiebig, R.; Hollander, J.; Bejma, J. Oxidative stress and aging. Role of exercise and its influences on antioxidant systems. *Ann. N. Y. Acad. Sci.* **1998**, *854*, 102–117. [CrossRef]
3. Viña, J.; Olaso-Gonzalez, G.; Arc-Chagnaud, C.; De la Rosa, A.; Gomez-Cabrera, M.C. Modulating Oxidant Levels to Promote Healthy Aging. *Antioxid. Redox Signal.* **2020**. [CrossRef]
4. Ji, L.L. Antioxidants and oxidative stress in exercise. *Proc. Soc. Exp. Biol. Med.* **1999**, *222*, 283–292. [CrossRef] [PubMed]
5. Massafra, C.; Gioia, D.; De Felice, C.; Picciolini, E.; De Leo, V.; Bonifazi, M.; Bernabei, A. Effects of estrogens and androgens on erythrocyte antioxidant superoxide dismutase, catalase and glutathione peroxidase activities during the menstrual cycle. *J. Endocrinol.* **2000**, *167*, 447–452. [CrossRef] [PubMed]

6. Park, S.Y.; Kwak, Y.S. Impact of aerobic and anaerobic exercise training on oxidative stress and antioxidant defense in athletes. *J. Exerc. Rehabil.* **2016**, *12*, 113–117. [CrossRef] [PubMed]
7. Poulsen, H.E.; Weimann, A.; Loft, S. Methods to detect DNA damage by free radicals: Relation to exercise. *Proc. Nutr. Soc.* **1999**, *58*, 1007–1014. [CrossRef] [PubMed]
8. Debevec, T.; Millet, G.P.; Pialoux, V. Hypoxia-Induced Oxidative Stress Modulation with Physical Activity. *Front. Physiol.* **2017**, *8*, 84. [CrossRef]
9. Tofas, T.; Draganidis, D.; Deli, C.K.; Georgakouli, K.; Fatouros, I.G.; Jamurtas, A.Z. Exercise-Induced Regulation of Redox Status in Cardiovascular Diseases: The Role of Exercise Training and Detraining. *Antioxidants* **2019**, *9*, 13. [CrossRef]
10. de Sousa, C.V.; Sales, M.M.; Rosa, T.S.; Lewis, J.E.; de Andrade, R.V.; Simões, H.G. The Antioxidant Effect of Exercise: A Systematic Review and Meta-Analysis. *Sports Med.* **2017**, *47*, 277–293. [CrossRef]
11. Nocella, C.; Cammisotto, V.; Pigozzi, F.; Borrione, P.; Fossati, C.; D'Amico, A.; Cangemi, R.; Peruzzi, M.; Gobbi, G.; Ettorre, E.; et al. Impairment between Oxidant and Antioxidant Systems: Short- and Long-term Implications for Athletes' Health. *Nutrients* **2019**, *11*, 1353. [CrossRef] [PubMed]
12. de Souza, R.F.; de Moraes, S.R.A.; Augusto, R.L.; de Freitas Zanona, A.; Matos, D.; Aidar, F.J.; da Silveira Andrade-da-Costa, B.L. Endurance training on rodent brain antioxidant capacity: A meta-analysis. *Neurosci. Res.* **2019**, *145*, 1–9. [CrossRef] [PubMed]
13. Pinho, R.A.; Aguiar, A.S., Jr.; Radák, Z. Effects of Resistance Exercise on Cerebral Redox Regulation and Cognition: An Interplay between Muscle and Brain. *Antioxidants* **2019**, *8*, 529. [CrossRef]
14. Park, S.Y.; Rossman, M.J.; Gifford, J.R.; Bharath, L.P.; Bauersachs, J.; Richardson, R.S.; Abel, E.D.; Symons, J.D.; Riehle, C. Exercise training improves vascular mitochondrial function. *Am. J. Physiol. Heart Circ. Physiol.* **2016**, *310*, H821–H829. [CrossRef] [PubMed]
15. Roh, H.T.; So, W.Y. The effects of aerobic exercise training on oxidant-antioxidant balance, neurotrophic factor levels, and blood-brain barrier function in obese and non-obese men. *J. Sport Health Sci.* **2017**, *6*, 447–453. [CrossRef]
16. Di Liegro, C.M.; Schiera, G.; Proia, P.; Di Liegro, I. Physical Activity and Brain Health. *Genes* **2019**, *10*, 720. [CrossRef]
17. Arad, A.D.; Basile, A.J.; Albu, J.; DiMenna, F.J. No Influence of Overweight/Obesity on Exercise Lipid Oxidation. *Int. J. Mol. Sci.* **2020**, *21*, 1614. [CrossRef]
18. Sadowska-Krępa, E.; Kłapcińska, B.; Pokora, I.; Domaszewski, P.; Kempa, K.; Podgórski, T. Effects of Six-Week Ginkgo biloba Supplementation on Aerobic Performance, Blood Pro/Antioxidant Balance, and Serum Brain-Derived Neurotrophic Factor in Physically Active Men. *Nutrients* **2017**, *9*, 803. [CrossRef]
19. Yahfoufi, N.; Alsadi, N.; Jambi, M.; Matar, C. The Immunomodulatory and Anti-Inflammatory Role of Polyphenols. *Nutrients* **2018**, *10*, 1618. [CrossRef]
20. Cavarretta, E.; Peruzzi, M.; Del Vescovo, R.; Di Pilla, F.; Gobbi, G.; Serdoz, A.; Ferrara, R.; Schirone, L.; Sciarretta, S.; Nocella, C.; et al. Dark Chocolate Intake Positively Modulates Redox Status and Markers of Muscular Damage in Elite Football Athletes: A Randomized Controlled Study. *Oxidative Med. Cell Longev.* **2018**, *2018*, 4061901. [CrossRef]
21. Georgakouli, K.; Fatouros, I.G.; Fragkos, A.; Tzatzakis, T.; Deli, C.K.; Papanikolaou, K.; Koutedakis, Y.; Jamurtas, A.Z. Exercise and Redox Status Responses Following Alpha-Lipoic Acid Supplementation in G6PD Deficient Individuals. *Antioxidants* **2018**, *7*, 162. [CrossRef]
22. Kabasakalis, A.; Kyparos, A.; Tsalis, G.; Loupos, D.; Pavlidou, A.; Kouretas, D.; Kabasakalis, A.; Tsalis, G.; Zafrana, E.; Loupos, D.; et al. Effects of endurance and high-intensity swimming exercise on the redox status of adolescent male and female swimmers. *J. Sports Sci.* **2014**, *32*, 747–756. [CrossRef]
23. Kabasakalis, A.; Kyparos, A.; Tsalis, G.; Loupos, D.; Pavlidou, A.; Kouretas, D. Blood oxidative stress markers after ultramarathon swimming. *J. Strength Cond. Res.* **2011**, *25*, 805–811. [CrossRef]
24. Bellafiore, M.; Bianco, A.; Battaglia, G.; Naccari, M.S.; Caramazza, G.; Padulo, J.; Chamari, K.; Paoli, A.; Palma, A. Training session intensity affects plasma redox status in amateur rhythmic gymnasts. *J. Sport Health Sci.* **2019**, *8*, 561–566. [CrossRef]
25. Powers, S.K.; Jackson, M.J. Exercise-induced oxidative stress: Cellular mechanisms and impact on muscle force production. *Physiol. Rev.* **2008**, *88*, 1243–1276. [CrossRef] [PubMed]
26. Wolff, C.; Musci, R.; Whedbee, M. Vitamin supplementation and resistance exercise-induced muscle hypertrophy: Shifting the redox balance scale? *J. Physiol.* **2015**, *593*, 2991–2992. [CrossRef] [PubMed]
27. Paulsen, G.; Hamarsland, H.; Cumming, K.T.; Johansen, R.E.; Hulmi, J.J.; Borsheim, E.; Wiig, H.; Garthe, I.; Raastad, T. Vitamin C and E supplementation alters protein signalling after a strength training session, but not muscle growth during 10 weeks of training. *J. Physiol.* **2014**, *592*, 5391–5408. [CrossRef]
28. Bruns, D.R.; Ehrlicher, S.E.; Khademi, S.; Biela, L.M.; Peelor, F.F.; Miller, B.F.; Hamilton, K.L. Differential effects of vitamin C or protandim on skeletal muscle adaptation to exercise. *J. Appl. Physiol.* **2018**, *125*, 661–671. [CrossRef]
29. Traustadóttir, T.; Davies, S.S.; Su, Y.; Choi, L.; Brown-Borg, H.M.; Roberts, L.J., 2nd; Harman, S.M. Oxidative stress in older adults: Effects of physical fitness. *Age (Dordr.)* **2012**, *34*, 969–982. [CrossRef]
30. Aldred, S.; Rohalu, M. A moderate intensity exercise program did not increase the oxidative stress in older adults. *Arch. Gerontol. Geriatr.* **2011**, *53*, 350–353. [CrossRef] [PubMed]
31. Done, A.J.; Traustadóttir, T. Aerobic exercise increases resistance to oxidative stress in sedentary older middle-aged adults. A pilot study. *Age (Dordr.)* **2016**, *38*, 505–512. [CrossRef]

32. Landers-Ramos, R.Q.; Corrigan, K.J.; Guth, L.M.; Altom, C.N.; Spangenburg, E.E.; Prior, S.J.; Hagberg, J.M. Short-term exercise training improves flow-mediated dilation and circulating angiogenic cell number in older sedentary adults. *Appl. Physiol. Nutr. Metab.* **2016**, *41*, 832–841. [CrossRef] [PubMed]
33. Pierno, S.; Tricarico, D.; Liantonio, A.; Mele, A.; Digennaro, C.; Rolland, J.-F.; Bianco, G.; Villanova, L.; Merendino, A.; Camerino, G.M.; et al. An olive oil derived antioxidant mixture ameliorates the age-related decline of skeletal muscle function. *Age* **2014**, *36*, 73–88. [CrossRef]
34. Muhammad, M.H.; Allam, M.M. Resveratrol and/or exercise training counteract aging-associated decline of physical endurance in aged mice; targeting mitochondrial biogenesis and function. *J. Physiol. Sci.* **2018**, *68*, 681–688. [CrossRef] [PubMed]
35. Gliemann, L.; Nyberg, M.; Hellsten, Y. Effects of exercise training and resveratrol on vascular health in aging. *Free Radic. Biol. Med.* **2016**, *98*, 165–176. [CrossRef]
36. Najjar, F.; Rizk, F.; Carnac, G. Protective effect of Rhus coriaria fruit extracts against hydrogen peroxide-induced oxidative stress in muscle progenitors and zebrafish embryos. *PeerJ* **2017**, *5*, e4144. [CrossRef]
37. Richards, J.C.; Crecelius, A.R.; Larson, D.G.; Dinenno, F.A. Acute ascorbic acid ingestion increases skeletal muscle blood flow and oxygen consumption via local vasodilation during graded handgrip exercise in older adults. *Am. J. Physiol. Heart Circ. Physiol.* **2015**, *309*, H360–H368. [CrossRef] [PubMed]
38. Fougere, B.; van Kan, G.A.; Vellas, B.; Cesari, M. Redox Systems, Antioxidants and Sarcopenia. *Curr. Protein Pept. Sci.* **2018**, *19*, 643–648. [CrossRef]
39. Angulo, J.; El Assar, M.; Álvarez-Bustos, A.; Rodríguez-Mañas, L. Physical activity and exercise: Strategies to manage frailty. *Redox Biol.* **2020**, *35*, 101513. [CrossRef]
40. Szentesi, P.; Csernoch, L.; Dux, L.; Keller-Pintér, A. Changes in Redox Signaling in the Skeletal Muscle with Aging. *Oxid. Med. Cell Longev.* **2019**, *2019*, 4617801. [CrossRef]
41. Verdijk, L.B.; Snijders, T.; Drost, M.; Delhaas, T.; Kadi, F.; van Loon, L.J.C. Satellite cells in human skeletal muscle; from birth to old age. *Age* **2014**, *36*, 545–557. [CrossRef]
42. Blocquiaux, S.; Gorski, T.; Van Roie, E.; Ramaekers, M.; Van Thienen, R.; Nielens, H.; Delecluse, C.; De Bock, K.; Thomis, M. The effect of resistance training, detraining and retraining on muscle strength and power, myofibre size, satellite cells and myonuclei in older men [published correction appears in Exp Gerontol. *Exp. Gerontol.* **2020**, *133*, 110860. [CrossRef]
43. Fry, C.S.; Noehren, B.; Mula, J.; Ubele, M.F.; Westgate, P.M.; Kern, P.A.; Peterson, C.A. Fibre type-specific satellite cell response to aerobic training in sedentary adults. *J. Physiol.* **2014**, *592*, 2625–2635. [CrossRef]
44. Pittaluga, M.; Sgadari, A.; Dimauro, I.; Tavazzi, B.; Parisi, P.; Caporossi, D. Physical exercise and redox balance in type 2 diabetics: Effects of moderate training on biomarkers of oxidative stress and DNA damage evaluated through comet assay. *Oxid. Med. Cell Longev.* **2015**, 981242. [CrossRef]
45. Shukla, V.; Mishra, S.K.; Pant, H.C. Oxidative stress in neurodegeneration. *Adv. Pharmacol. Sci.* **2011**, *2011*, 572634. [CrossRef] [PubMed]
46. Espinet, C.; Gonzalo, H.; Fleitas, C.; Menal, M.J.; Egea, J. Oxidative stress and neurodegenerative diseases: A neurotrophic approach. *Curr. Drug Targets* **2015**, *16*, 20–30. [CrossRef] [PubMed]
47. Patil, S.P.; Tran, N.; Geekiyanage, H.; Liu, L.; Chan, C. Curcumin-induced upregulation of the anti-tau cochaperone BAG2 in primary rat cortical neurons. *Neurosci. Lett.* **2013**, *554*, 121–125. [CrossRef]
48. Jia, R.X.; Liang, J.H.; Xu, Y.; Wang, Y.Q. Effects of physical activity and exercise on the cognitive function of patients with Alzheimer disease: A meta-analysis. *BMC Geriatr.* **2019**, *19*, 181. [CrossRef]
49. Accattato, F.; Greco, M.; Pullano, S.A.; Carè, I.; Fiorillo, A.S.; Pujia, A.; Montalcini, T.; Foti, D.P.; Brunetti, A.; Gulletta, E. Effects of acute physical exercise on oxidative stress and inflammatory status in young, sedentary obese subjects. *PLoS ONE* **2017**, *12*, e0178900. [CrossRef] [PubMed]
50. Chatzinikolaou, A.; Fatouros, I.; Petridou, A.; Jamurtas, A.; Avloniti, A.; Douroudos, I.; Mastorakos, G.; Lazaropoulou, C.; Papassotiriou, I.; Tournis, S.; et al. Adipose tissue lipolysis is upregulated in lean and obese men during acute resistance exercise. *Diabetes Care* **2008**, *31*, 1397–1399. [CrossRef]
51. Karner-Rezek, K.; Knechtle, B.; Fenzl, M.; Gredig, J.; Rosemann, T. Does continuous endurance exercise in water elicit a higher release of ANP and BNP and a higher plasma concentration of FFAs in pre-obese and obese men than high intensity intermittent endurance exercise?‹study protocol for a randomized controlled trial. *Trials* **2013**, *14*, 328. [CrossRef]
52. Mrakic-Sposta, S.; Gussoni, M.; Vezzoli, A.; Dellanoce, C.; Comassi, M.; Giardini, G.; Bruno, R.M.; Montorsi, M.; Corciu, A.; Greco, F.; et al. Acute Effects of Triathlon Race on Oxidative Stress Biomarkers. *Oxid. Med. Cell Longev.* **2020**, *2020*, 3062807. [CrossRef]
53. Bartlett, D.B.; Willis, L.H.; Slentz, C.A.; Hoselton, A.; Kelly, L.; Huebner, J.L.; Kraus, V.B.; Moss, J.; Muehlbauer, M.J.; Spielmann, G.; et al. Ten weeks of high-intensity interval walk training is associated with reduced disease activity and improved innate immune function in older adults with rheumatoid arthritis: A pilot study. *Arthritis Res. Ther.* **2018**, *20*, 127. [CrossRef] [PubMed]
54. Abd El-Kader, S.M.; Al-Jiffri, O.H. Impact of aerobic versus resisted exercise training on systemic inflammation biomarkers and quality of Life among obese post-menopausal women. *Afr. Health Sci.* **2019**, *19*, 2881–2891. [CrossRef] [PubMed]

55. Fatouros, I.; Chatzinikolaou, A.; Paltoglou, G.; Petridou, A.; Avloniti, A.; Jamurtas, A.; Goussetis, E.; Mitrakou, A.; Mougios, V.; Lazaropoulou, C.; et al. Acute resistance exercise results in catecholaminergic rather than hypothalamic-pituitary-adrenal axis stimulation during exercise in young men. *Stress* **2010**, *13*, 461–468. [CrossRef]
56. Hirose, L.; Nosaka, K.; Newton, M.; Laveder, A.; Kano, M.; Peake, J.; Suzuki, K. Changes in inflammatory mediators following eccentric exercise of the elbow flexors. *Exerc. Immunol. Rev.* **2004**, *10*, 75–90. [PubMed]
57. Ost, M.; Coleman, V.; Kasch, J.; Klaus, S. Regulation of myokine expression: Role of exercise and cellular stress. *Free Radic. Biol. Med.* **2016**, *98*, 78–89. [CrossRef]
58. Radak, Z.; Suzuki, K.; Higuchi, M.; Balogh, L.; Boldogh, I.; Koltai, E. Physical exercise, reactive oxygen species and neuroprotection. *Free Radic. Biol. Med.* **2016**, *98*, 187–196. [CrossRef]
59. Vilela, T.C.; de Andrade, V.M.; Radak, Z.; de Pinho, R.A. The role of exercise in brain DNA damage. *Neural Regen Res.* **2020**, *15*, 1981–1985. [CrossRef]
60. Hsu, C.L.; Best, J.R.; Davis, J.C.; Nagamatsu, L.S.; Wang, S.; Boyd, L.A.; Hsiung, G.R.; Voss, M.W.; Eng, J.J.; Liu-Ambrose, T. Aerobic exercise promotes executive functions and impacts functional neural activity among older adults with vascular cognitive impairment. *Br. J. Sports Med.* **2018**, *52*, 184–191. [CrossRef]
61. Feter, N.; Spanevello, R.M.; Soares, M.S.P.; Spohr, L.; Pedra, N.S.; Bona, N.P.; Freitas, M.P.; Gonzales, N.G.; Ito, L.G.M.S.; Stefanello, F.M.; et al. How does physical activity and different models of exercise training affect oxidative parameters and memory? *Physiol. Behav.* **2019**, *201*, 42–52. [CrossRef]
62. Kou, X.; Chen, D.; Chen, N. Physical Activity Alleviates Cognitive Dysfunction of Alzheimer's Disease through Regulating the mTOR Signaling Pathway. *Int. J. Mol. Sci.* **2019**, *20*, 1591. [CrossRef]
63. Done, A.J.; Newell, M.J.; Traustadóttir, T. Effect of exercise intensity on Nrf2 signalling in young men. *Free Radic. Res.* **2017**, *51*, 646–655. [CrossRef] [PubMed]
64. Vargas-Mendoza, N.; Morales-González, Á.; Madrigal-Santillán, E.O.; Madrigal-Bujaidar, E.; Álvarez-González, I.; García-Melo, L.F.; Anguiano-Robledo, L.; Fregoso-Aguilar, T.; Morales-Gonzalez, J.A. Antioxidant and Adaptative Response Mediated by Nrf2 during Physical Exercise. *Antioxidants* **2019**, *8*, 196. [CrossRef]
65. Ruhee, R.T.; Ma, S.; Suzuki, K. Protective Effects of Sulforaphane on Exercise-Induced Organ Damage via Inducing Antioxidant Defense Responses. *Antioxidants* **2020**, *9*, 136. [CrossRef]
66. Merry, T.L.; MacRae, C.; Pham, T.; Hedges, C.P.; Ristow, M. Deficiency in ROS-sensing nuclear factor erythroid 2-like 2 causes altered glucose and lipid homeostasis following exercise training. *Am. J. Physiol. Cell Physiol.* **2020**, *318*, C337–C345. [CrossRef]
67. Huang, D.-D.; Fan, S.-D.; Chen, X.-Y.; Yan, X.-L.; Zhang, X.-Z.; Ma, B.-W.; Yu, D.-Y.; Xiao, W.-Y.; Zhuang, C.-L.; Yu, Z. Nrf2 deficiency exacerbates frailty and sarcopenia by impairing skeletal muscle mitochondrial biogenesis and dynamics in an age-dependent manner. *Exp. Gerontol.* **2019**, *119*, 61–73. [CrossRef] [PubMed]
68. Liao, Z.Y.; Chen, J.L.; Xiao, M.H. The effect of exercise, resveratrol or their combination on sarcopenia in aged rats via regulation of AMPK/Sirt 1 pathway. *Exp. Gerontol.* **2017**, *98*, 177–183.
69. Abou-Samra, M.; Selvais, C.M.; Boursereau, R.; Lecompte, S.; Noel, L.; Brichard, S.M. AdipoRon, a new therapeutic prospect for Duchenne muscular dystrophy. *J. Cachexia Sarcopenia Muscle* **2020**, *11*, 518–533. [CrossRef]
70. Kim, E.N.; Lim, J.H.; Kim, M.Y.; Ban, T.H.; Jang, I.A.; Yoon, H.E.; Park, C.W.; Chang, Y.S.; Choi, B.S. Resveratrol, an Nrf2 activator, ameliorates aging-related progressive renal injury. *Aging (Albany N. Y.)* **2018**, *10*, 83–99. [CrossRef] [PubMed]
71. Qi, J.; Luo, X.; Ma, Z.; Zhang, B.; Li, S.; Duan, X.; Yang, B.; Zhang, J. Swimming Exercise Protects against Insulin Resistance via Regulating Oxidative Stress through Nox4 and AKT Signaling in High-Fat Diet-Fed Mice. *J. Diabetes Res.* **2020**, *2020*, 2521590. [CrossRef]
72. Lukjanenko, L.; Karaz, S.; Stuelsatz, P.; Gurriaran-Rodriguez, U.; Michaud, J.; Dammone, G.; Sizzano, F.; Mashinchian, O.; Ancel, S.; Migliavacca, E.; et al. Aging Disrupts Muscle Stem Cell Function by Impairing Matricellular WISP1 Secretion from Fibro-Adipogenic Progenitors. *Cell Stem Cell* **2019**, *24*, 433–446.e7. [CrossRef]
73. Ferraro, E.; Giammarioli, A.M.; Chiandotto, S.; Spoletini, I.; Rosano, G. Exercise-induced skeletal muscle remodeling and metabolic adaptation: Redox signaling and role of autophagy. *Antioxid. Redox Signal.* **2014**, *21*, 154–176. [CrossRef]
74. Halling, J.F.; Jessen, H.; Nøhr-Meldgaard, J.; Buch, B.T.; Christensen, N.M.; Gudiksen, A.; Ringholm, S.; Neufer, P.D.; Prats, C.; Pilegaard, H. PGC-1α regulates mitochondrial properties beyond biogenesis with aging and exercise training. *Am. J. Physiol Endocrinol. Metab.* **2019**, *317*, E513–E525. [CrossRef]
75. Cunha, T.F.; Bechara, L.R.; Bacurau, A.V.; Jannig, P.R.; Voltarelli, V.A.; Dourado, P.M.; Vasconcelos, A.R.; Scavone, C.; Ferreira, J.C.; Brum, P.C. Exercise training decreases NADPH oxidase activity and restores skeletal muscle mass in heart failure rats. *J. Appl. Physiol.* **2017**, *122*, 817–827. [CrossRef] [PubMed]
76. Roof, S.R.; Ho, H.-T.; Little, S.C.; Ostler, J.E.; Brundage, E.A.; Periasamy, M.; Villamena, F.A.; Györke, S.; Biesiadecki, B.J.; Heymes, C.; et al. Obligatory role of neuronal nitric oxide synthase in the heart's antioxidant adaptation with exercise. *J. Mol. Cell Cardiol.* **2015**, *81*, 54–61. [CrossRef] [PubMed]
77. Hao, Z.; Pan, S.S.; Shen, Y.J.; Ge, J. Exercise preconditioning-induced early and late phase of cardioprotection is associated with protein kinase C epsilon translocation. *Circ. J.* **2014**, *78*, 1636–1645. [CrossRef] [PubMed]
78. Díaz-Ruíz, J.L.; Macías-López, A.; Alcalá-Vargas, F.; Guevara-Chávez, J.G.; Mejía-Uribe, A.; Silva-Palacios, A.; Zúñiga-Muñoz, A.; Zazueta, C.; Buelna-Chontal, M. Redox signaling in ischemic postconditioning protection involves PKCε and Erk1/2 pathways and converges indirectly in Nrf2 activation. *Cell Signal.* **2019**, *64*, 109417. [CrossRef]

79. Buelna-Chontal, M.; Guevara-Chávez, J.G.; Silva-Palacios, A.; Medina-Campos, O.N.; Pedraza-Chaverri, J.; Zazueta, C. Nrf2-regulated antioxidant response is activated by protein kinase C in postconditioned rat hearts. *Free Radic. Biol. Med.* **2014**, *74*, 145–156. [CrossRef] [PubMed]
80. Carubbi, C.; Masselli, E.; Nouvenne, A.; Russo, D.; Galli, D.; Mirandola, P.; Gobbi, G.; Vitale, M. Laboratory diagnostics of inherited platelet disorders. *Clin. Chem. Lab. Med.* **2014**, *52*, 1091–1106. [CrossRef] [PubMed]
81. Di Marcantonio, D.; Galli, D.; Carubbi, C.; Gobbi, G.; Queirolo, V.; Martini, S.; Merighi, S.; Vaccarezza, M.; Maffulli, N.; Sykes, S.M.; et al. PKCε as a novel promoter of skeletal muscle differentiation and regeneration. *Exp. Cell Res.* **2015**, *339*, 10–19. [CrossRef]
82. Galli, D.; Carubbi, C.; Masselli, E.; Corradi, D.; Dei Cas, A.; Nouvenne, A.; Bucci, G.; Arcari, M.L.; Mirandola, P.; Vitale, M.; et al. PKCε is a negative regulator of PVAT-derived vessel formation. *Exp. Cell Res.* **2015**, *330*, 277–286. [CrossRef] [PubMed]
83. Masselli, E.; Carubbi, C.; Gobbi, G.; Mirandola, P.; Galli, D.; Martini, S.; Bonomini, S.; Crugnola, M.; Craviotto, L.; Aversa, F.; et al. Protein kinase Cε inhibition restores megakaryocytic differentiation of hematopoietic progenitors from primary myelofibrosis patients. *Leukemia* **2015**, *29*, 2192–2201. [CrossRef] [PubMed]
84. Bassini, A.; Zauli, G.; Migliaccio, G.; Migliaccio, A.R.; Pascuccio, M.; Pierpaoli, S.; Guidotti, L.; Capitani, S.; Vitale, M. Lineage-restricted expression of protein kinase C isoforms in hematopoiesis. *Blood* **1999**, *93*, 1178–1188. [CrossRef]
85. Martini, S.; Soliman, T.; Gobbi, G.; Mirandola, P.; Carubbi, C.; Masselli, E.; Pozzi, G.; Parker, P.J.; Vitale, M. PKCε Controls Mitotic Progression by Regulating Centrosome Migration and Mitotic Spindle Assembly. *Mol. Cancer Res.* **2018**, *16*, 3–15. [CrossRef]
86. D'Amico, A.E.; Lennartz, M.R. Protein Kinase C-epsilon in Membrane Delivery during Phagocytosis. *J. Immunol. Sci.* **2018**, *2*, 26–32. [CrossRef]
87. Basu, A. Regulation of Autophagy by Protein Kinase C-ε in Breast Cancer Cells. *Int. J. Mol. Sci.* **2020**, *21*, 4247. [CrossRef]
88. Escobar, K.A.; Cole, N.H.; Mermier, C.M.; VanDusseldorp, T.A. Autophagy and aging: Maintaining the proteome through exercise and caloric restriction. *Aging Cell* **2019**, *18*, e12876. [CrossRef]
89. Tan, K.T.; Ang, S.J.; Tsai, S.Y. Sarcopenia: Tilting the Balance of Protein Homeostasis. *Proteomics* **2020**, *20*, e1800411. [CrossRef]
90. Görlach, A.; Bertram, K.; Hudecova, S.; Krizanova, O. Calcium and ROS: A mutual interplay. *Redox Biol.* **2015**, *6*, 260–271. [CrossRef] [PubMed]
91. Zima, A.V.; Blatter, L.A. Redox regulation of cardiac calcium channels and transporters. *Cardiovasc. Res.* **2006**, *71*, 310–321. [CrossRef] [PubMed]
92. Cabassi, A.; Miragoli, M. Altered Mitochondrial Metabolism and Mechanosensation in the Failing Heart: Focus on Intracellular Calcium Signaling. *Int. J. Mol. Sci.* **2017**, *18*, 1487. [CrossRef]
93. Rhee, S.G. Overview on Peroxiredoxin. *Mol. Cells* **2016**, *39*, 1–5. [CrossRef]
94. Bolduc, J.A.; Collins, J.A.; Loeser, R.F. Reactive oxygen species, aging and articular cartilage homeostasis. *Free Radic. Biol. Med.* **2019**, *132*, 73–82. [CrossRef] [PubMed]
95. Nelson, K.J.; Knutson, S.T.; Soito, L.; Klomsiri, C.; Poole, L.B.; Fetrow, J.S. Analysis of the peroxiredoxin family: Using active-site structure and sequence information for global classification and residue analysis. *Proteins* **2011**, *79*, 947–964. [CrossRef]
96. Milev, N.B.; Rhee, S.G.; Reddy, A.B. Cellular Timekeeping: It's Redox o'Clock. *Cold Spring Harb. Perspect Biol.* **2018**, *10*, a027698. [CrossRef] [PubMed]
97. Zhang, Y.G.; Wang, L.; Kaifu, T.; Li, J.; Li, X.; Li, L. Featured Article: Accelerated decline of physical strength in peroxiredoxin-3 knockout mice. *Exp. Biol. Med. (Maywood)* **2016**, *241*, 1395–1400. [CrossRef]
98. Wadley, A.J.; Keane, G.; Cullen, T.; James, L.; Vautrinot, J.; Davies, M.; Hussey, B.; Hunter, D.J.; Mastana, S.; Holliday, A.; et al. Characterization of extracellular redox enzyme concentrations in response to exercise in humans. *J. Appl. Physiol.* **2019**, *127*, 858–866. [CrossRef] [PubMed]
99. Trewin, A.J.; Parker, L.; Shaw, C.S.; Hiam, D.S.; Garnham, A.P.; Levinger, I.; McConell, G.K.; Stepto, N.K. Acute HIIE elicits similar changes in human skeletal muscle mitochondrial H_2O_2 release, respiration, and cell signaling as endurance exercise even with less work. *Am. J. Physiol. Regul. Integr. Comp. Physiol.* **2018**, *315*, R1003–R1016. [CrossRef] [PubMed]
100. Wadley, A.J.; Aldred, S.; Coles, S.J. An unexplored role for Peroxiredoxin in exercise-induced redox signalling? *Redox Biol.* **2016**, *8*, 51–58. [CrossRef] [PubMed]

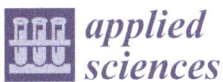

Review

Pulmonary Effects Due to Physical Exercise in Polluted Air: Evidence from Studies Conducted on Healthy Humans

Oscar F. Araneda [1,*], Franz Kosche-Cárcamo [2], Humberto Verdugo-Marchese [2] and Marcelo Tuesta [2,3]

1. Integrative Laboratory of Biomechanics and Physiology of Effort, (LIBFE, for Its Initials in Spanish), School of Kinesiology, Faculty of Medicine, Universidad de los Andes, Santiago 8320000, Chile
2. Sports Science Laboratory, Sports MD Sports Medicine Center, Viña del Mar 2520000, Chile; franzkosche@hotmail.com (F.K.-C.); drhumbertoverdugo@gmail.com (H.V.-M.); marcelo.tuesta@unab.cl (M.T.)
3. Undergraduate Program of Kinesiology, Faculty of Rehabilitation Sciences, Universidad Andres Bello, Viña del Mar 2520000, Chile
* Correspondence: ofaraneda@miuandes.cl

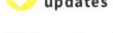

Citation: Araneda, O.F.; Kosche-Cárcamo, F.; Verdugo-Marchese, H.; Tuesta, M. Pulmonary Effects Due to Physical Exercise in Polluted Air: Evidence from Studies Conducted on Healthy Humans. *Appl. Sci.* **2021**, *11*, 2890. https://doi.org/10.3390/app11072890

Academic Editor: Daniela Galli

Received: 20 February 2021
Accepted: 18 March 2021
Published: 24 March 2021

Publisher's Note: MDPI stays neutral with regard to jurisdictional claims in published maps and institutional affiliations.

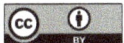

Copyright: © 2021 by the authors. Licensee MDPI, Basel, Switzerland. This article is an open access article distributed under the terms and conditions of the Creative Commons Attribution (CC BY) license (https://creativecommons.org/licenses/by/4.0/).

Abstract: Physical inactivity has caused serious effects on the health of the population, having an impact on the quality of life and the cost of healthcare for many countries. This has motivated government and private institutions to promote regular physical activity, which, paradoxically, can involve health risks when it is carried out in areas with poor air quality. This review collects information from studies conducted on healthy humans related to the pulmonary effects caused by the practice of physical activity when there is poor air quality. In addition, several challenges related to the technological and educational areas, as well as to applied and basic research, have been identified to facilitate the rational practice of exercise in poor air quality conditions.

Keywords: air pollution; physical exercise; lungs

1. Introduction

The increase in the world population and the use of polluting energy sources in the modern world have led to changes in the quality of the air we breathe. Pollutants floating in the air cause harmful effects on health, which have been extensively studied [1–3]. As a result of these studies, this type of pollution has been linked to cancer, cardiovascular disorders, acute pulmonary disorders (infections, acute bronchial obstruction), and chronic disorders (asthma, chronic obstructive pulmonary disease) [4]. According to data provided by the World Health Organization in 2018, about 90% of people are exposed to polluted air, particularly in poor or developing countries on all continents, which produce a total of around seven million deaths annually at a global level [5]. Although we breathe a mixture of substances in the air, on an individual level, it has been possible to individually identify some pollutants that cause health disorders, such as tropospheric ozone (O_3), particulate matter (PM_x), carbon monoxide (CO), nitrogen oxides (NO_x), and sulfur oxides (SO_x) [6,7]. These are usually concentrated in urban centers, and are mainly, though not exclusively, caused by activities typical of human beings, such as transport, heating, cooking, and agricultural and industrial activities [8].

Our bodies come into contact with atmospheric pollutants through the wide area of exposure of the lung tissue, making this organ particularly susceptible to damage from the components of the air we breathe, such as particulate matter, cigarette smoke, various gases, and pollen [9,10]. Consequently, this interaction will cause alterations in the functionality of this organ. The amount of polluting substances that reach the lungs during exercise will depend on both their concentration in the air and the magnitude of the pulmonary physiological phenomena typical of physical effort: bronchodilation, increased ventilation, mouth breathing, and increased diffusing capacity. This implies that, during exercise, a higher load of tissue pollutants will be observed [11], which impacts deeper lung areas and may even be associated with a greater passage of these substances into the bloodstream, as in the case of gases and ultrafine particulate matter (Figure 1).

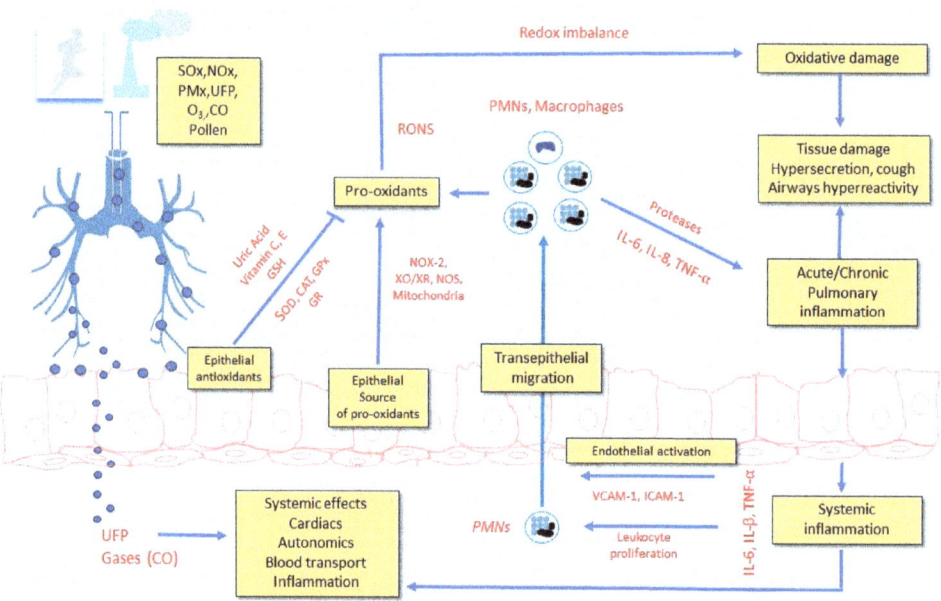

Figure 1. Systemic and localized effects at the lung level generated by air pollutants. SO_x = sulphur oxides; NO_x = nitrogen oxides; PM_x = particulate matter; UFP = ultrafine particles; SOD = superoxide dismutase; CAT = catalase; GP_x = glutathione peroxidase; GR = glutathione reductase; GSH = reduced glutathione RONS = reactive oxygen and nitrogen free radicals; NOX-2 = NADPH oxidase type 2; XO = xanthine oxidase; XR = xanthine reductase; NOS = nitric oxide synthase; PMNs = polymorphonuclear leukocytes. VCAM-1 = vascular cell adhesion molecule 1; ICAM-1 = intercellular adhesion molecule 1.

In consideration of the processes described, for some years now, the question has been what the pulmonary effects due to physical exercise in areas with poor air quality are, in the short and long term, both in healthy people and in those suffering from pathologies [12–15]. The issue is becoming relevant nowadays, since, in many countries with poor air quality, increased participation in outdoor sports activities, such as massive urban races and the use of bicycles, have been observed. In addition, there is little information about the effects and potential risks for the exposed population, as well as future measures to help to reduce exposure for both people who exercise and healthcare professionals. To address this matter, the interaction mechanisms and effects resulting from the contact between the air and lung tissue are presented in this study. In addition, some challenges in the field of research are described, and recommendations for the safe practice of physical exercise under these conditions are made. The papers used for this narrative review were original or review manuscripts, in which an exercise protocol under laboratory or field conditions was carried out, including the study of pulmonary function parameters, in the presence of air pollutants in healthy humans. The papers were mainly taken from the PubMed search engine, and there was no limitation regarding the year of publication.

2. Alteration of Ventilatory Function and Appearance/Exacerbation of Respiratory Symptoms during Physical Exercise with Polluted Air: Short- and Medium-Term Effects

By doing physical exercise in an environment with polluted air, increased airway resistance is induced. Initially, this was described in protocols that set O_3 at different concentrations [16–19]. Thus, in these studies, it is a common result to find lower values than those expected in forced expiratory volume in the first second (FEV_1), forced vital capacity (FVC), and forced mid-expiratory flow rate (FEF_{25-75}) [19,20]. Regarding the pollutant particles in suspension, particulate material less than 10 microns (PM_{10}) promotes the establishment of chronic lung function problems, mainly associated with decreased FEV_1 [21]. Likewise, $PM_{2.5}$ (<2.5 microns) has been related to a drop in FEV_1 and FVC in subjects who lived in the vicinity of a highway [22]. Physical exercise increases these effects as their intensity and duration increase as a consequence of the increased work of breathing. Minute ventilation, together with greater exposure to the pollutant, will determine their inhaled load in the airways [16,23,24]. Several authors have observed that, during moderate and maximum exercise in an environment contaminated with O_3, there are more symptoms, such as dyspnea, respiratory distress, and a feeling of tightness in the chest, which quickly lead to the cessation of exercise [25–28]. Several authors have shown an alteration in lung function parameters (FEV_1, FVC, and FEF_{25-75}) in both healthy trained and untrained subjects exposed to high concentrations of O_3 while performing physical exercise [15], with some of them even experiencing the effects a few hours after exercising [29]. Abnormal respiratory symptoms have also been observed after one hour of exercise and one hour of rest in an environment contaminated with PM_{10} and $PM_{2.5}$, however, no spirometric changes were found [21]. In another study, Brant et al. [30] observed decreased mucociliary clearance, decreased pH in the expired air, and increased symptoms of respiratory distress in motorcyclists who were chronically exposed to NO_2 during heavy traffic for 5–8 h a day, five days a week. Likewise, the practice of aerobic exercise in the open air at an average $PM_{2.5}$ concentration of 65.1 µg/m^3 over a period of five days also altered mucociliary clearance [31]. Yet, the study conducted by Kubesch et al. (2015) demonstrated improvements in lung function with physical exercise in a highly polluted environment; however, an acute pulmonary inflammatory effect was also observed [32]. Other studies on healthy subjects who performed strenuous long-duration exercise (between ~2–5 h) in a polluted environment ($PM_{2.5}$ and O_3) did not show deleterious effects on lung function parameters [33,34]. This should be interpreted with caution, since the systematization of this behavior, which constantly promotes an oxidative/inflammatory lung environment, could mean permanent lung damage in the future. Children are especially sensitive to contact with atmospheric pollutants, which leads to a higher rate of school absenteeism and an increase in high and low airway infections [35], and alters lung function, thereby increasing the probability of death [36]. Infant lungs show an incomplete respiratory tree where the pulmonary epithelium is being formed, which has been associated with greater permeability of this structure. Similarly, some studies have suggested that long-term exposure to air pollutants could potentially affect children's lung development [37–39]. Modification of lung function in children who are active in polluted air has been associated with high concentrations of O_3 [40], MP_{10}, NO_x, and CO [41]. McConell et al. [42] demonstrated that there was an association between the prevalence of asthma in children and prolonged and intense exercise done outdoors with high levels of O_3. In the case of adults, moderate exercise increases the amount of particulate material entering the lungs by 4.5 times versus resting [12], where similar results are expected for the other environmental pollutants. One group of subjects who can be particularly affected by polluted air is the group of amateur long-distance athletes (e.g., marathons, cross-country cycling). Thus, a group of cyclists exercised in open-top field chambers for dispensing O_3, showing a decrease in FEV_1 after moderate exercise for sixty minutes [24]. Furthermore, a group of cyclists in competition (75 min) increased their respiratory symptoms (wheezing, dyspnea) after inhaling a mixture of pollutants. Respiratory distress and spirometric alterations were correlated with the concentration of O_3 [43]. Korrick et al. [44] found a decrease in FEV_1 and FVC in subjects who took prolonged walks in an environment with low levels of O_3 and particulate matter, demonstrating that the changes in lung function were caused by exercise, even with low levels of pollutants. Gong et al. [45] conducted an intermittent exercise protocol (two hours) in healthy subjects and subjects with asthma using an environmental test chamber with ultrafine particulate matter seven to eight times higher than average air levels in unpolluted areas. Thus, a decrease in arterial oxygen saturation and FEV_1 was observed the day after the test, with no differences between healthy subjects and subjects with asthma. A total of 23 studies evaluated the effect of O_3 on the decline of FEV_1, which were carried out under standardized conditions in a test chamber. Here, relationship models were observed in various conditions of O_3 concentration, exposure time, and minute ventilation; in addition, the thresholds for the appearance of the broncho-constrictor phenomenon were attained [46]. Kim et al. [47] observed a decline in FEV_1 in an exercise protocol at 0.06 ppm O_3 and stable ventilation of 35 L/min in six cycles of 50 min. The obstructive modification caused by O_3 is the result of a bronchoconstrictive response induced by a vagal reflex activated by irritation [48]. The release of acetylcholine (parasympathetic response) will increase the activation of the submucosal glands, leading to greater release of mucus [49]. The results found in relation to NO_2 on lung function have been variable; Bauer et al. [50] and Strand et al. [51] demonstrated a broncho-constrictor effect in asthmatics. Likewise, Kulstrunk and Bohini (1992) observed decreased FEV_1 after a maximal exercise test (~8 min) with high NO_2 levels was performed by healthy subjects [52]. However, Jorres et al. [53] did not observe any changes in FEV_1 after exercising for 1.5 h with 3 h of exposure to 1 ppm of NO_2. In relation to CO, due to its high diffusion capacity in the alveolar capillary membrane and its great affinity with carboxyhemoglobin (COHb), systemic effects have mainly been recognized in healthy subjects who exercise. Due to COHb, there will be less availability of hemoglobin to bind oxygen (hypoxemia), thus altering the transport capacity of this gas to active muscles [54] and limiting energy production and physical effort. Decreased physical performance in healthy subjects due to CO exposure alone was observed with maximum intensity exercise [55], but not when it was performed at submaximal intensity and a lower concentration of this gas [56].

All previously mentioned studies describe the short- and medium-term effects of exposure to air pollutants, with little evidence to clarify the long-term effects. However, subjects exposed for years to outdoor jobs on the streets, but who did not exert great physical effort, showed a decreased ability to perform physical work, as well as a decreased maximum voluntary ventilation (MVV) [57].

3. Lung Inflammation and Oxidative Stress Due to Exercise in Polluted Air

In the lung region, there is a complex microenvironment where the interaction of the cells of this organ (pneumocytes, endothelial cells, alveolar macrophages) and inflammatory cells (various types of leukocytes) from the bloodstream takes place. Due to the gas exchange function between the lungs and the environment, this tissue organization is constantly exposed to the action of pollutants present in the air. The interaction between lung tissue and air pollutants largely depends on the physical and chemical characteristics of the latter. In this way, some air pollutants will cause direct damage at the cellular level (O_3, SO_x, NO_x), others will be deposited in the airway (particulate matter), and some will diffuse through the alveolus capillary membrane into the bloodstream (ultrafine particulate matter and gases), as shown in Figure 1.

Lung inflammation and oxidative stress play an essential role in altering lung function with exposure to O_3, especially when exercising [58]. In this sense, the low solubility of O_3 in water suggests that the main interaction of this molecule will be with the surface of the epithelium, and, in particular, with the epithelial lining fluid. This contact will promote reactions with thiol groups (-SH), antioxidants (glutathione, ascorbic acid), and macromolecules (lipids, proteins, carbohydrates), among others found in the epithelial fluid, promoting an oxidative/inflammatory environment. A higher number of molecules that are attracted due to the increased ventilatory flow induced by exercise will enhance these effects, especially for long-duration exercises (e.g., marathons). A study conducted by Kinney et al. [59] observed increases in lung inflammation markers with low levels of O_3 in the air during moderate exercise in a group of amateur runners. The predominance of this phenomenon occurred during the spring and summer seasons in comparison to the winter season. Both seasons are characterized by a higher production/concentration of ozone in the environment due to a higher level of ultraviolet radiation. The effect of the time of exposure to O_3 was also addressed by Aris et al. [60], who observed an increase in polymorphonuclear leukocytes (PMNs or neutrophils) 18 h after exposing healthy subjects and athletes to 0.20 ppm of O_3 during 4 h of moderate exercise. A study conducted by Gomes et al. (2011) showed a lung inflammatory/oxidative effect in subjects who ran 8 km in a hot environment (31 °C) with increased levels of O_3, but this was not the case in a cold environment (20 °C); nevertheless, no changes in lung function were observed in any environment [61]. This suggests that O_3 has a high capacity to promote inflammation and damage in the respiratory epithelium, affecting lung function, even more so when intense and long-term exercise is done. Other environmental factors, such as ambient temperature, must also be considered.

In the case of particulate matter, exposure to larger particles, such as PM_{10}, has also shown lung inflammatory effects [62,63]. However, the main target structures of the smallest particles ($PM_{2.5}$ and UFPs) will be the pulmonary vascular and cardiovascular components [64,65]. Some inflammatory responses against contamination are the infiltration of PMNs and macrophages that release proteases with degradative and pro-oxidant activity, favoring cell damage [9,11,66]. Depending on the degree of exposure, this phenomenon can occur on multiple occasions, and can even become a chronic process [39], similar to that seen in subjects who smoke [67]. In this way, it is necessary to detail these processes when exercising during exposure to a polluted environment. Ghio et al. [68] observed an increase in PMNs in the bronchial and alveolar fractions of bronchoalveolar lavage (BAL) after 1 h of intermittent light exercise in an environment with PM_{10} (23.1–311 µg/m^3) and $PM_{2.5}$ (47.2–206.7 µg/m^3). Larsson et al. [69], 14 h later, observed increases in alveolar macrophages and lymphocytes in BAL after one hour of light exercise in an environment with PM_{10} and $PM_{2.5}$. In asthmatics, Pietropaoli et al. [70] found increased macrophages in induced sputum when they performed two hours of intermittent exercise in an environment with ultrafine particulate matter (10 µg/m^3), unlike healthy subjects (10, 25, and 50 µg/m^3). A recent study highlighted the effect of outdoor endurance training as an immune protection factor against exposure to particulate matter by controlling lung inflammation in this group, but not in exposed sedentary subjects [71]. This reinforces the importance of controlling air quality, the type of exercise, and the level of physical condition in order to take advantage of its benefits and thus avoid the deleterious effects of pollution. Cavalcante de Sá et al. [31] observed higher pH values in the exhaled condensed air of athletes who ran (45 min/day for five days) in an unpolluted environment versus athletes who ran in a polluted environment with high $PM_{2.5}$. Some studies have focused on the pro-inflammatory effects of NO_2 [56,72,73]. Jorres et al. [53] found increases in pro-inflammatory mediators in BAL in asthmatics, but not in healthy subjects, after 1.5 h of exercising and 3 h of exposure to NO_2 (1 ppm). Devlin et al. [74] showed that light/moderate exercise for two hours at a concentration of 2 ppm of NO_2 increased the levels of PMNs, IL–6, and IL–8 in BAL after 24 h. The action of pro-oxidants released directly by PMNs or produced secondarily from reactions involving metals contained in particulate matter are a challenge for enzymatic (catalase, superoxide dismutase, and glutathione peroxidase) and non-enzymatic (glutathione, vitamins C, vitamin E, and uric acid) lung antioxidant defenses. If they are overcome by pro-oxidants, an imbalance called oxidative stress is established, causing damage to structural molecules, in which lipoperoxidation is the most studied phenomenon. The association between oxidative damage and the modification of lung function has previously been described and confirmed by observing the negative correlations between plasma lipoperoxidation and glutathione, each with

FEV$_1$, as well as the positive correlations between the activity of the enzyme glutathione peroxidase and FEV$_1$ [75]. Therefore, it is possible to think of a potential benefit on lung function in subjects exposed to polluted air [76–78] with the consumption of antioxidants in the diet (β-carotene, vitamins C and E), for example, through the consumption of fresh fruits and vegetables [79].

4. Recommendations to Consider When Prescribing Exercise in Areas with Low Air Quality

Our biological design requires us to perform physical activity to stay healthy. Thus, the study of physical exercise has been the concern of researchers from the most diverse disciplines of knowledge. In this regard, one of the most relevant results, which is derived from research in this area, indicates that low levels of physical activity are associated with obesity, metabolic diseases, cancer, cardiovascular diseases, stress, anxiety, and depression [80–83]. In addition, low levels of physical activity have an impact on the quality of life of the population [84,85], and may be the cause of economic losses [86]. Hence, countries should promote exercise, but they should also be responsible for ensuring that it is done in a safe environment. Exercising with polluted air will be a problem for the foreseeable future, particularly since the concentration of pollutants in the air in many cities in developing countries will continue to be high. Hence, it is important for health personnel and the general population to be aware of the effects of pollution on the lungs, and to know both the guidelines regarding potential preventive measures and the status of issues that are not yet resolved in the research arena. In relation to prevention matters, one of the first pillars of the exercise/polluted air interaction consists of efforts to reduce air pollution. Firstly, we must think that the result of a high concentration of pollutants is a multifactorial outcome, thus, it depends on geographical factors (location and design of urban centers), environmental factors (temperature, humidity, luminosity), and derivatives of human activity (population growth, energy matrix used in industry/means of transport). Regarding these determinants, there are few factors that can be changed in the short term; however, both state and private organizations can devise plans for the re-evaluation of air quality and emission standards. At the same time, programs of general environmental education focused on air quality can be created. One measure with a direct impact on those who exercise under these conditions is to reduce the load of pollutants they are exposed to. To address this objective, it is necessary to favor access to air quality information by establishing monitoring points in cities where there are none, and by increasing their number in cities where they already exist. In addition, it will be advantageous to increase the number of mobile stations at training points and during sporting events, such as massive urban races. Along this line, there is a challenge for technological innovation in order to reduce the size and costs of the monitoring units, or, ideally, for them to be individual devices. The information obtained from the monitoring should also be integrated into applications for smartphones that can suggest routes with better air quality at the time of exercising. In the same direction, the development of new technologies focused on physical measures to reduce the entry of pollutants into the airway is pending [87]. In this regard, the greater social tolerance to the use of masks in times of the COVID-19 pandemic must be an advantage [88]. Finally, the identification of pollutants that are typical of indoor sporting environments should be improved by promoting measures to transform them into healthy environments and by using technology for the development and installation of filters in these places [89].

Regarding the biological phenomena of this problem, from our review, we conclude that it is necessary to increase the number of studies conducted on humans in relation to the acute effect of exposure to polluted air, and particularly in relation to chronic changes, where the information is practically nil. Likewise, the most solid information on biological effects refers to the action of individual pollutants, and progress must be made in the study of the interaction between pollutants and the influence of environmental conditions, such as humidity and temperature. The above objective is essential to optimize current models of inhalation load exposure [90,91] and the recommendations arising from it in the future.

Another pending task in research is to improve and establish biological monitoring, which should be done by optimizing non-invasive methods (spirometric tests, analysis of expired air, and sputum analysis) and in ideal conditions carried out by the users themselves. One of the objectives of this biological monitoring is the monitoring of at-risk populations (patients with chronic lung diseases, professional athletes, urban long-distance runners or cyclists) and to carry out preventive interventions in these populations. Once these groups have been identified, targeted environmental education programs should be carried out. Another relevant aspect both for this group and for the general population is to optimize exercise planning and to be flexible regarding the time and place it will be done and its intensity, balancing this programming with the health objectives of the general population and competitive athletes. Finally, from the studies regarding the damage mechanisms, the dietary and pharmacological recommendations are alternative solutions, among which the maintenance of a healthy diet with an important content of antioxidants (fruits and vegetables) is noted, as well as the search for new strategies to complement these substances, since evidence has not shown any effectiveness in lung diseases [92]. From the perspective of pharmacological agents, the production and administration of anti-inflammatory agents focused on airway epithelial damage should be studied (a summary of the topics discussed in this chapter is presented in Figure 2).

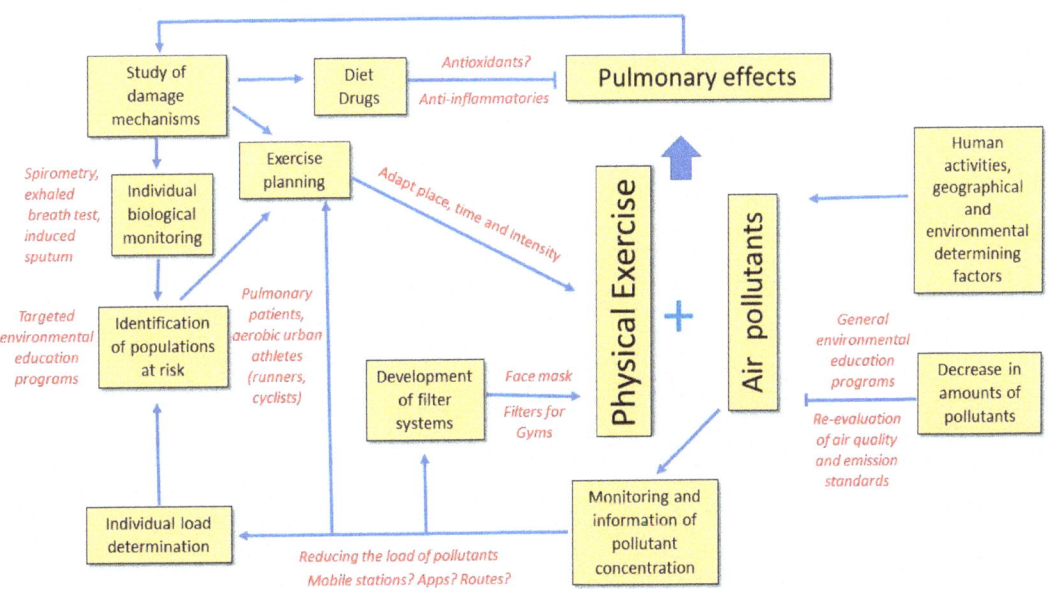

Figure 2. Overview of future goals and strategies to optimize the performance of exercise in polluted conditions.

Author Contributions: O.F.A., H.V.-M., F.K.-C., and M.T. worked on the design, methodology, and drafting of the manuscript. All authors have read and agreed to the published version of the manuscript.

Funding: This research received no external funding.

Institutional Review Board Statement: Not applicable.

Informed Consent Statement: Not applicable.

Data Availability Statement: Not applicable.

Conflicts of Interest: The authors declare no conflict of interest.

References

1. Harrison, R.M.; Yin, J. Particulate matter in the atmosphere: Which particle properties are important for its effects on health? *Sci. Total Environ.* **2000**, *249*, 85–101. [CrossRef]
2. Samet, J.M.; Dominici, F.; Curriero, F.C.; Coursac, I.; Zeger, S.L. Fine Particulate Air Pollution and Mortality in 20 U.S. Cities, 1987–1994. *N. Engl. J. Med.* **2000**, *343*, 1742–1749. [CrossRef]
3. Schwartz, J. Air Pollution and Daily Mortality: A Review and Meta Analysis. *Environ. Res.* **1994**, *64*, 36–52. [CrossRef]
4. Kurt, O.K.; Zhang, J.; Pinkerton, K.E. Pulmonary health effects of air pollution. *Curr. Opin. Pulm. Med.* **2016**, *22*, 138–143. [CrossRef] [PubMed]
5. First WHO Global Conference on Air Pollution and Health, 30 October–1 November 2018. Available online: https://www.who.int/airpollution/events/conference/ (accessed on 20 January 2021).
6. Tan, X.; Han, L.; Zhang, X.; Zhou, W.; Li, W.; Qian, Y. A review of current air quality indexes and improvements under the multi-contaminant air pollution exposure. *J. Environ. Manag.* **2021**, *279*, 111681. [CrossRef] [PubMed]
7. Guarnieri, M.; Balmes, J.R. Outdoor air pollution and asthma. *Lancet* **2014**, *383*, 1581–1592. [CrossRef]
8. Guo, X.; Ren, D.; Li, C. Study on clean heating based on air pollution and energy consumption. *Environ. Sci. Pollut. Res.* **2019**, *27*, 6549–6559. [CrossRef] [PubMed]
9. Cross, C.E.; Valacchi, G.; Schock, B.; Wilson, M.; Weber, S.; Eiserich, J.; van der Vliet, A. Environmental oxidant pollutant effects on biologic systems: A focus on micronutrient antioxidant-oxidant interactions. *Am. J. Respir. Crit. Care Med.* **2002**, *166 Pt 2*, S44–S50. [CrossRef]
10. Stone, V. Environmental Air Pollution. *Am. J. Respir. Crit. Care Med.* **2000**, *162*, S44–S47. [CrossRef]
11. Daigle, C.C.; Chalupa, D.C.; Gibb, F.R.; Morrow, P.E.; Oberdörster, G.; Utell, M.J.; Frampton, M.W. Ultrafine Particle Deposition in Humans During Rest and Exercise. *Inhal. Toxicol.* **2003**, *15*, 539–552. [CrossRef]
12. Campbell, M.E.; Li, Q.; Gingrich, S.E.; Macfarlane, R.G.; Cheng, S. Should People Be Physically Active Outdoors on Smog Alert Days? *Can. J. Public Health* **2005**, *96*, 24–28. [CrossRef] [PubMed]
13. Cutrufello, P.T.; Smoliga, J.; Rundell, K.W. Small things make a big difference: Particulate matter and exercise. *Sports Med.* **2012**, *42*. [CrossRef] [PubMed]
14. Sharman, J.E. Clinicians prescribing exercise: Is air pollution a hazard? *Med. J. Aust.* **2005**, *182*, 606–607. [CrossRef]
15. Giles, L.V.; Koehle, M.S. The Health Effects of Exercising in Air Pollution. *Sports Med.* **2014**, *44*, 223–249. [CrossRef]
16. Adams, W.C. Effects of Ozone Exposure at Ambient Air Pollution Episode Levels on Exercise Performance. *Sports Med.* **1987**, *4*, 395–424. [CrossRef]
17. Adams, W.C.; Schelegle, E.S. Ozone and high ventilation effects on pulmonary function and endurance per-formance. *J. Appl. Physiol. Respir. Environ. Exerc. Physiol.* **1983**, *55*, 805–812.
18. Foxcroft, W.J.; Adams, W.C. Effects of ozone exposure on four consecutive days on work performance and VO2max. *J. Appl. Physiol.* **1986**, *61*, 960–966. [CrossRef] [PubMed]
19. Schonfeld, B.R.; Adams, W.C.; Schelegle, E.S. Duration of Enhanced Responsiveness upon Re-Exposure to Ozone. *Arch. Environ. Health Int. J.* **1989**, *44*, 229–236. [CrossRef]
20. Balmes, J.R.; Chen, L.L.; Scannell, C.; Tager, I.; Christian, D.; Hearne, P.Q.; Kelly, T.; Aris, R.M. Ozone-induced decre-ments in FEV1 and FVC do not correlate with measures of inflammation. *Am. J. Respir. Crit. Care Med.* **1996**, *153*, 904–909. [CrossRef] [PubMed]
21. Rundell, K.W. High Levels of Airborne Ultrafine and Fine Particulate Matter in Indoor Ice Arenas. *Inhal. Toxicol.* **2003**, *15*, 237–250. [CrossRef]
22. Rice, M.B.; Ljungman, P.L.; Wilker, E.H.; Dorans, K.S.; Gold, D.R.; Schwartz, J.; Koutrakis, P.; Washko, G.R.; O'Connor, G.T.; Mittleman, M.A. Long-Term Exposure to Traffic Emissions and Fine Particulate Matter and Lung Function Decline in the Framingham Heart Study. *Am. J. Respir. Crit. Care Med.* **2015**, *191*, 656–664. [CrossRef]
23. Avol, E.L.; Linn, W.S.; Venet, T.G.; Shamoo, D.A.; Hackney, J.D. Comparative respiratory effects of ozone and am-bient oxidant pollution exposure during heavy exercise. *J. Air Pollut. Control Assoc.* **1984**, *34*, 804–809. [CrossRef] [PubMed]
24. Gong, H., Jr.; Bradley, P.W.; Simmons, M.S.; Tashkin, D.P. Impaired exercise performance and pulmonary function in elite cyclists during low-level ozone exposure in a hot environment. *Am. Rev. Respir. Dis.* **1986**, *134*, 726–733. [PubMed]
25. McDonnell, W.F.; Stewart, P.W.; Smith, M.V.; Pan, W.K.; Pan, J. Ozone-induced respiratory symptoms: Expo-sure-response models and association with lung function. *Eur. Respir. J.* **1999**, *14*, 845–853. [CrossRef] [PubMed]
26. Folinsbee, L.J.; McDonnell, W.F.; Horstman, D.H. Pulmonary Function and Symptom Responses after 6.6-Hour Exposure to 0.12 ppm Ozone with Moderate Exercise. *JAPCA* **1988**, *38*, 28–35. [CrossRef]
27. Linder, J.; Herren, D.; Monn, C.; Wanner, H.U. Effect of ozone on physical performance capacity. *Int. J. Public Health* **1987**, *32*, 251–252.
28. Morales Cardona, T. Performance of athletes exercising in ozone polluted air. *Bol. Asoc. Med. Puerto Rico* **1990**, *82*, 517–522.
29. Adams, W.C. Ozone dose–response effects of varied equivalent minute ventilation rates. *J. Expo. Sci. Environ. Epidemiol.* **2000**, *10*, 217–226. [CrossRef]

30. Brant, T.C.S.; Yoshida, C.T.; Carvalho, T.D.S.; Nicola, M.L.; Martins, J.A.; Braga, L.M.; De Oliveira, R.C.; Leyton, V.; De André, C.S.; Saldiva, P.H.N.; et al. Mucociliary clearance, airway inflammation and nasal symptoms in urban motorcyclists. *Clinics* **2014**, *69*, 867–870. [CrossRef]
31. de Sa, M.C.; Nakagawa, N.K.; Saldiva de Andre, C.D.; Carvalho-Oliveira, R.; de Santana Carvalho, T.; Nicola, M.L.; de Andre, P.A.; Nascimento Saldiva, P.H.; Vaisberg, M. Aerobic exercise in polluted urban environments: Effects on airway defense mechanisms in young healthy amateur runners. *J. Breath Res.* **2016**, *10*, 046018. [CrossRef]
32. Kubesch, N.J.; De Nazelle, A.; Westerdahl, D.; Martinez, D.; Carrasco-Turigas, G.; Bouso, L.; Guerra, S.; Nieuwenhuijsen, M.J. Respiratory and inflammatory responses to short-term exposure to traffic-related air pollution with and without moderate physical activity. *Occup. Environ. Med.* **2014**, *72*, 284–293. [CrossRef] [PubMed]
33. Brauner, E.V.; Mortensen, J.; Moller, P. Effects of ambient airparticulate exposure on blood–gas barrier permeability and lung function. *Inhal. Toxicol.* **2009**, *21*, 38–47. [CrossRef] [PubMed]
34. Girardot, S.P.; Ryan, P.B.; Smith, S.M.; Davis, W.T.; Hamilton, C.B.; Obenour, R.A.; Renfro, J.R.; Tromatore, K.A.; Reed, G.D. Ozone and PM 2.5 Exposure and Acute Pulmonary Health Effects: A Study of Hikers in theGreat Smoky Mountains National Park. *Environ. Health Perspect.* **2006**, *114*, 1044–1052. [CrossRef] [PubMed]
35. Gilliland, F.D.; Berhane, K.; Rappaport, E.B.; Thomas, D.C.; Avol, E.; Gauderman, W.J.; London, S.J.; Margolis, H.G.; McConnell, R.; Islam, K.T.; et al. The effects of ambient air pollution on school absenteeism due to respiratory illnesses. *Epidemiology* **2001**, *12*, 43–54. [CrossRef] [PubMed]
36. Loomis, D.; Castillejos, M.; Gold, D.R.; McDonnell, W.; Borja-Aburto, V.H. Air Pollution and Infant Mortality in Mexico City. *Epidemiology* **1999**, *10*, 118–123. [CrossRef] [PubMed]
37. Gauderman, W.J.; Avol, E.; Gilliland, F.; Vora, H.; Thomas, D.; Berhane, K.; McConnell, R.; Kuenzli, N.; Lurmann, F.; Rappaport, E.; et al. The Effect of Air Pollution on Lung Development from 10 to 18 Years of Age. *N. Engl. J. Med.* **2004**, *351*, 1057–1067. [CrossRef] [PubMed]
38. Gauderman, W.J.; Urman, R.; Avol, E.; Berhane, K.; McConnell, R.; Rappaport, E.; Chang, R.; Lurmann, F.; Gilliland, F. Association of Improved Air Quality with Lung Development in Children. *N. Engl. J. Med.* **2015**, *372*, 905–913. [CrossRef] [PubMed]
39. Gilliland, F.D.; McConnell, R.; Peters, J.; Gong, H., Jr. A theoretical basis for investigating ambient air pollution and children's respiratory health. *Environ Health Perspect.* **1999**, *107* (Suppl. S3), 403–407. [CrossRef]
40. Braun-Fahrlander, C.; Kunzli, N.; Domenighetti, G.; Carell, C.F.; Ackermann-Liebrich, U. Acute effects of ambient ozone on respiratory function of Swiss schoolchildren after a 10-min heavy exercise. *Pediatr. Pulmonol.* **1994**, *17*, 169–177. [CrossRef] [PubMed]
41. Timonen, K.L.; Pekkanen, J.; Tiittanen, P.; Salonen, R.O. Effects of air pollution on changes in lung function induced by exercise in children with chronic respiratory symptoms. *Occup. Environ. Med.* **2002**, *59*, 129–134. [CrossRef] [PubMed]
42. McConell, G.K.; Lee-Young, R.S.; Chen, Z.-P.; Stepto, N.K.; Huynh, N.N.; Stephens, T.J.; Canny, B.J.; Kemp, B.E. Short-term exercise training in humans reduces AMPK signalling during prolonged exercise independent of muscle glycogen. *J. Physiol.* **2005**, *568*, 665–676. [CrossRef]
43. Brunekreef, B.; Hoek, G.; Breugelmans, O.; Leentvaar, M. Respiratory effects of low-level photochemical air pollution in amateur cyclists. *Am. J. Respir. Crit. Care Med.* **1994**, *150*, 962–966. [CrossRef]
44. Korrick, S.A.; Neas, L.M.; Dockery, D.W.; Gold, D.R.; Allen, G.A.; Hill, L.B.; Kimball, K.D.; Rosner, B.A.; Speizer, F.E. Effects of ozone and other pollutants on the pulmonary function of adult hikers. *Environ. Health Perspect.* **1998**, *106*, 93–99. [CrossRef]
45. Gong, H., Jr.; Linn, W.S.; Clark, K.W.; Anderson, K.R.; Sioutas, C.; Alexis, N.E.; Cascio, W.E.; Devlin, R.B. Exposures of healthy and asthmatic volunteers to concentrated ambient ultrafine particles in Los Angeles. *Inhal. Toxicol.* **2008**, *20*, 533–545. [CrossRef]
46. McDonnell, W.F.; Stewart, P.W.; Smith, M.V.; Kim, C.S.; Schelegle, E.S. Prediction of lung function response for populations exposed to a wide range of ozone conditions. *Inhal. Toxicol.* **2012**, *24*, 619–633. [CrossRef] [PubMed]
47. Kim, C.S.; Alexis, N.E.; Rappold, A.G.; Kehrl, H.; Hazucha, M.J.; Lay, J.C.; Schmitt, M.T.; Case, M.; Devlin, R.B.; Peden, D.B.; et al. Lung Function and Inflammatory Responses in Healthy Young Adults Exposed to 0.06 ppm Ozone for 6.6 Hours. *Am. J. Respir. Crit. Care Med.* **2011**, *183*, 1215–1221. [CrossRef]
48. Olsen, C.R.; Colebatch, H.J.H.; Mebel, P.E.; Nadel, J.A.; Staub, N.C. Motor control of pulmonary airways studied by nerve stimulation. *J. Appl. Physiol.* **1965**, *20*, 202–208. [CrossRef]
49. Ramnarine, S.I.; Haddad, E.B.; Khawaja, A.M.; Mak, J.C.; Rogers, D.F. On muscarinic control of neurogenic mucus secretion in ferret trachea. *J. Physiol.* **1996**, *494*, 577–586. [CrossRef] [PubMed]
50. Bauer, J.A.; Wald, J.A.; Doran, S.; Soda, D. Endogenous nitric oxide in expired air: Effects of acute exercise in humans. *Life Sci.* **1994**, *55*, 1903–1909. [CrossRef]
51. Strand, V.; Svartengren, M.; Rak, S.; Barck, C.; Bylin, G. Repeated exposure to an ambient level of NO2 enhances asthmatic response to a nonsymptomatic allergen dose. *Eur. Respir. J.* **1998**, *12*, 6–12. [CrossRef]
52. Kulstrunk, M.; Bohni, B. Comparison of lung function parameters in healthy non-smokers following exertion in urban environmental air and in air-conditioned inside air. *Schweiz. Med. Wochenschr.* **1992**, *122*, 375–381. [PubMed]
53. Jörres, R.; Nowak, D.; Grimminger, F.; Seeger, W.; Oldigs, M.; Magnussen, H. The effect of 1 ppm nitrogen dioxide on bronchoalveolar lavage cells and inflammatory mediators in normal and asthmatic subjects. *Eur. Respir. J.* **1995**, *8*, 416–424. [CrossRef] [PubMed]
54. Vogel, J.A.; Gleser, M.A. Effect of carbon monoxide on oxygen transport during exercise. *J. Appl. Physiol.* **1972**, *32*, 234–239. [CrossRef]

55. Koike, A.; Wasserman, K.; Armon, Y.; Weiler-Ravell, D. The work-rate-dependent effect of carbon monoxide on ventilatory control during exercise. *Respir. Physiol.* **1991**, *85*, 169–183. [CrossRef]
56. Turner, J.A.; McNicol, M.W. The effect of nicotine and carbon monoxide on exercise performance in normal subjects. *Respir. Med.* **1993**, *87*, 427–431. [CrossRef]
57. Volpino, P.; Tomei, F.; La Valle, C.; Tomao, E.; Rosati, M.V.; Ciarrocca, M.; De Sio, S.; Cangemi, B.; Vigliarolo, R.; Fedele, F. Respiratory and cardiovascular function at rest and during exercise testing in a healthy working population: Effects of outdoor traffic air pollution. *Occup. Med. (Lond.)* **2004**, *54*, 475–482. [CrossRef]
58. Gong, H., Jr.; Bedi, J.F.; Horvath, S.M. Inhaled albuterol does not protect against ozone toxicity in nonasthmatic athletes. *Arch. Environ. Health* **1988**, *43*, 46–53. [CrossRef] [PubMed]
59. Kinney, P.L.; Nilsen, D.; Lippmann, M.; Brescia, M.; Gordon, T.; McGovern, T.; El-Fawal, H.; Devlin, R.B.; Rom, W.N. Biomarkers of lung inflammation in recreational joggers exposed to ozone. *Am. J. Respir. Crit. Care Med.* **1996**, *154*, 1430–1435. [CrossRef] [PubMed]
60. Aris, R.M.; Christian, D.; Hearne, P.Q.; Kerr, K.; Finkbeiner, W.E.; Balmes, J.R. Ozone-induced Airway Inflammation in Human Subjects as Determined by Airway Lavage and Biopsy. *Am. Rev. Respir. Dis.* **1993**, *148*, 1363–1372. [CrossRef] [PubMed]
61. Gomes, E.C.; Stone, V.; Florida-James, G. Impact of heat and pollution on oxidative stress and CC16 secretion after 8 km run. *Graefe's Arch. Clin. Exp. Ophthalmol.* **2011**, *111*, 2089–2097. [CrossRef]
62. Alonso, J.R.; Cardellach, F.; López, S.; Casademont, J.; Miró, O. Carbon monoxide specifically inhibits cytochrome c oxidase of human mitochondrial respiratory chain. *Pharmacol. Toxicol.* **2003**, *93*, 142–146. [CrossRef]
63. Yoshizaki, K.; Brito, J.M.; Silva, L.F.; Lino-Dos-Santos-Franco, A.; Frias, D.P.; ESilva, R.C.R.; Amato-Lourenço, L.F.; Saldiva, P.H.N.; de Fátima Lopes Calvo Tibério, I.; Mauad, T.; et al. The effects of particulate matter on inflammation of respiratory system: Differences between male and female. *Sci. Total Environ.* **2017**, *586*, 284–295. [CrossRef]
64. Madureira, J.; Brancher, E.A.; Costa, C.; de Pinho, R.A.; Teixeira, J.P. Cardio-respiratory health effects of exposure to traffic-related air pollutants while exercising outdoors: A systematic review. *Environ. Res.* **2019**, *178*, 108647. [CrossRef]
65. Miller, M.R. Oxidative stress and the cardiovascular effects of air pollution. *Free Radic. Biol. Med.* **2020**, *151*, 69–87. [CrossRef] [PubMed]
66. Mudway, I.S.; Kelly, F.J. An Investigation of Inhaled Ozone Dose and the Magnitude of Airway Inflammation in Healthy Adults. *Am. J. Respir. Crit. Care Med.* **2004**, *169*, 1089–1095. [CrossRef] [PubMed]
67. Garey, K.W.; Neuhauser, M.M.; Robbins, R.A.; Danziger, L.H.; Rubinstein, I. Markers of inflammation in exhaled breath condensate of young healthy smokers. *Chest* **2004**, *125*, 22–26. [CrossRef] [PubMed]
68. Ghio, A.J.; Kim, C.; Devlin, R.B. Concentrated Ambient Air Particles Induce Mild Pulmonary Inflammation in Healthy Human Volunteers. *Am. J. Respir. Crit. Care Med.* **2000**, *162*, 981–988. [CrossRef] [PubMed]
69. Larsson, B.-M.; Sehlstedt, M.; Grunewald, J.; Sköld, C.M.; Lundin, A.; Blomberg, A.; Sandström, T.; Eklund, A.; Svartengren, M. Road tunnel air pollution induces bronchoalveolar inflammation in healthy subjects. *Eur. Respir. J.* **2007**, *29*, 699–705. [CrossRef]
70. Pietropaoli, A.P.; Frampton, M.W.; Hyde, R.W.; Morrow, P.E.; Oberdörster, G.; Cox, C.; Speers, D.M.; Frasier, L.M.; Chalupa, D.C.; Huang, L.-S.; et al. Pulmonary Function, Diffusing Capacity, and Inflammation in Healthy and Asthmatic Subjects Exposed to Ultrafine Particles. *Inhal. Toxicol.* **2004**, *16*, 59–72. [CrossRef] [PubMed]
71. Pagani, L.G.; Santos, J.M.B.; Foster, R.; Rossi, M.; Luna Junior, L.A.; Katekaru, C.M.; de Sá, M.C.; Jonckheere, A.-C.; Almeida, F.M.; Amaral, J.B.; et al. The Effect of Particulate Matter Exposure on the Inflammatory Airway Response of Street Runners and Sedentary People. *Atmosphere* **2020**, *11*, 43. [CrossRef]
72. Bartoli, M.L.; Novelli, F.; Costa, F.; Malagrinò, L.; Melosini, L.; Bacci, E.; Cianchetti, S.; Dente, F.L.; Di Franco, A.; Vagaggini, B.; et al. Malondialdehyde in Exhaled Breath Condensate as a Marker of Oxidative Stress in Different Pulmonary Diseases. *Mediat. Inflamm.* **2011**, *2011*, 1–7. [CrossRef] [PubMed]
73. Witten, A.; Solomon, C.; Abbritti, E.; Arjomandi, M.; Zhai, W.; Kleinman, M.; Balmes, J. Effects of Nitrogen Dioxide on Allergic Airway Responses in Subjects with Asthma. *J. Occup. Environ. Med.* **2005**, *47*, 1250–1259. [CrossRef] [PubMed]
74. Devlin, R.B.; Horstman, D.P.; Gerrity, T.R.; Becker, S.; Madden, M.C.; Biscardi, F.; Hatch, G.E.; Koren, H.S. Inflammatory response in humans exposed to 2.0 ppm nitrogen dioxide. *Inhal. Toxicol.* **1999**, *11*, 89–109. [CrossRef]
75. Lavie, C.J.; Ozemek, C.; Carbone, S.; Katzmarzyk, P.T.; Blair, S.N. Sedentary Behavior, Exercise, and Cardiovascular Health. *Circ. Res.* **2019**, *124*, 799–815. [CrossRef] [PubMed]
76. Hills, A.P.; Andersen, L.B.; Byrne, N.M. Physical activity and obesity in children. *Br. J. Sports Med.* **2011**, *45*, 866–870. [CrossRef] [PubMed]
77. Brown, J.C.; Winters-Stone, K.; Lee, A.; Schmitz, K.H. Cancer, Physical Activity, and Exercise. *Compr. Physiol.* **2012**, *2*, 2775–2809. [CrossRef] [PubMed]
78. Kandola, A.; Vancampfort, D.; Herring, M.; Rebar, A.; Hallgren, M.; Firth, J.; Stubbs, B. Moving to Beat Anxiety: Epidemiology and Therapeutic Issues with Physical Activity for Anxiety. *Curr. Psychiatry Rep.* **2018**, *20*, 1–9. [CrossRef] [PubMed]
79. Wu, X.Y.; Han, L.H.; Zhang, J.H.; Luo, S.; Hu, J.W.; Sun, K. The influence of physical activity, sedentary behavior on health-related quality of life among the general population of children and adolescents: A systematic review. *PLoS ONE* **2017**, *12*, e0187668. [CrossRef] [PubMed]
80. Marker, A.M.; Steele, R.G.; Noser, A.E. Physical activity and health-related quality of life in children and adolescents: A systematic review and meta-analysis. *Health Psychol.* **2018**, *37*, 893–903. [CrossRef] [PubMed]
81. Ding, D.; Lawson, K.D.; Kolbe-Alexander, T.L.; A Finkelstein, E.; Katzmarzyk, P.T.; van Mechelen, W.; Pratt, M. The economic burden of physical inactivity: A global analysis of major non-communicable diseases. *Lancet* **2016**, *388*, 1311–1324. [CrossRef]

82. Ochs-Balcom, H.M.; Grant, B.J.B.; Muti, P.; Sempos, C.T.; Freudenheim, J.L.; Browne, R.W.; Trevisan, M.; Iacoviello, L.; Cassano, P.A.; Schünemann, H.J. Oxidative Stress and Pulmonary Function in the General Population. *Am. J. Epidemiol.* **2005**, *162*, 1137–1145. [CrossRef]
83. Grievink, L.; De Waart, F.G.; Schouten, E.G.; Kok, F.J. Serum Carotenoids, α-Tocopherol, and Lung Function among Dutch Elderly. *Am. J. Respir. Crit. Care Med.* **2000**, *161*, 790–795. [CrossRef] [PubMed]
84. Hu, G.; Cassano, P.A. Antioxidant nutrients and pulmonary function: The Third National Health and Nutri-tion Examination Survey (NHANES III). *Am. J. Epidemiol.* **2000**, *151*, 975–981. [CrossRef] [PubMed]
85. Samet, J.M.; Hatch, G.E.; Horstman, D.; Steck-Scott, S.; Arab, L.; Bromberg, P.A.; Levine, M.; McDonnell, W.F.; Devlin, R.B. Effect of Antioxidant Supplementation on Ozone-Induced Lung Injury in Human Subjects. *Am. J. Respir. Crit. Care Med.* **2001**, *164*, 819–825. [CrossRef] [PubMed]
86. Schünemann, H.J.; McCann, S.; Grant, B.J.B.; Trevisan, M.; Muti, P.; Freudenheim, J.L. Lung Function in Relation to Intake of Carotenoids and Other Antioxidant Vitamins in a Population-based Study. *Am. J. Epidemiol.* **2002**, *155*, 463–471. [CrossRef] [PubMed]
87. Cherrie, J.W.; Apsley, A.; Cowie, H.; Steinle, S.; Mueller, W.; Lin, C.; Horwell, C.J.; Sleeuwenhoek, A.; Loh, M. Effec-tiveness of face masks used to protect Beijing residents against particulate air pollution. *Occup. Environ. Med.* **2018**, *75*, 446–452. [CrossRef]
88. Epstein, D.; Korytny, A.; Isenberg, Y.; Marcusohn, E.; Zukermann, R.; Bishop, B.; Minha, S.; Raz, A.; Miller, A. Return to training in the COVID-19 era: The physiological effects of face masks during exercise. *Scand. J. Med. Sci. Sports* **2021**, *31*, 70–75. [CrossRef]
89. Salonen, H.; Salthammer, T.; Morawska, L. Human exposure to air contaminants in sports environments. *Indoor Air* **2020**, *30*, 1109–1129. [CrossRef] [PubMed]
90. Pasqua, L.A.; Damasceno, M.V.; Cruz, R.; Matsuda, M.; Martins, M.G.; Lima-Silva, A.E.; Marquezini, M.; Saldiva, P.H.N.; Bertuzzi, R. Exercising in Air Pollution: The Cleanest versus Dirtiest Cities Challenge. *Int. J. Environ. Res. Public Health* **2018**, *15*, 1502. [CrossRef] [PubMed]
91. Tainio, M.; de Nazelle, A.J.; Götschi, T.; Kahlmeier, S.; Rojas-Rueda, D.; Nieuwenhuijsen, M.J.; de Sá, T.H.; Kelly, P.; Woodcock, J. Can air pollution negate the health benefits of cycling and walking? *Prev. Med.* **2016**, *87*, 233–236. [CrossRef] [PubMed]
92. Whyand, T.; Hurst, J.R.; Beckles, M.; Caplin, M.E. Pollution and respiratory disease: Can diet or supplements help? A review. *Respir. Res.* **2018**, *19*, 79. [CrossRef] [PubMed]

Article

Augmentation Index Is Inversely Associated with Skeletal Muscle Mass, Muscle Strength, and Anaerobic Power in Young Male Adults: A Preliminary Study

Dongmin Lee [1], Kyengho Byun [2,3,4], Moon-Hyon Hwang [3,4,5] and Sewon Lee [2,3,4,*]

[1] Department of Human Movement Science, Graduate School, Incheon National University, Incheon 22012, Korea; dmdm1026@gmail.com
[2] Division of Sport Science, College of Arts & Physical Education, Incheon National University, Incheon 22012, Korea; kbyun21@inu.ac.kr
[3] Sport Science Institute, College of Arts & Physical Education, Incheon National University, Incheon 22012, Korea; mhwang@inu.ac.kr
[4] Health Promotion Center, College of Arts & Physical Education, Incheon National University, Incheon 22012, Korea
[5] Division of Health & Kinesiology, College of Arts & Physical Education, Incheon National University, Incheon 22012, Korea
* Correspondence: leesew@inu.ac.kr; Tel.: +82-32-835-8572; Fax: +82-32-835-0788

Abstract: Arterial stiffness is associated with an increased risk of cardiovascular disease. Previous studies have shown that there is a negative correlation between arterial stiffness and variables such as skeletal muscle mass, muscular strength, and anaerobic power in older individuals. However, little research has been undertaken on relationships in healthy young adults. This study presents a preliminary research that investigates the association between arterial stiffness and muscular factors in healthy male college students. Twenty-three healthy young males (23.9 ± 0.5 years) participated in the study. The participants visited the laboratory, and variables including body composition, blood pressure, arterial stiffness, blood parameters, grip strength, and anaerobic power were measured. Measurements of augmentation index (AIx) and brachial-ankle pulse wave velocity (baPWV) were performed to determine arterial stiffness. There were significant positive correlations among skeletal muscle mass, muscle strength, and anaerobic power in healthy young adult males. AIx was negatively associated with a skeletal muscle mass (r = −0.785, $p < 0.01$), muscular strength (r = −0.500, $p < 0.05$), and anaerobic power (r = −0.469, $p < 0.05$), respectively. Likewise, AIx@75 corrected with a heart rate of 75 was negatively associated with skeletal muscle mass (r = −0.738, $p < 0.01$), muscular strength (r = −0.461, $p < 0.05$), and anaerobic power (r = −0.420, $p < 0.05$) respectively. However, the baPWV showed no correlation with all muscular factors. Our findings suggest that maintaining high levels of skeletal muscle mass, muscular strength, and anaerobic power from relatively young age may lower AIx.

Keywords: skeletal muscle mass; muscular strength; anaerobic power; arterial stiffness

1. Introduction

Arterial stiffness, one of the factors indicating the function of blood vessels, is a main independent risk factor that can predict cardiovascular diseases [1]. Especially, this indicator is a leading cause of myocardial infarction in male adults [2]. Stiffening of the arterial wall causes an increase in the blood pressure by reducing the storage and buffering function of the arteries as well as by increasing the rate of pulse transmission regardless of the causes [3]. Usually, arterial stiffness worsens with aging [4]. Aging leads to thickening of the lining of blood vessels by increasing the amount of collagen in the smooth muscle layer and destroying the elastin structure [5]. These alterations result in increased arterial stiffness, leading to cardiometabolic diseases such as hypertension, diabetes, and dyslipidemia [6]. Body mass index (BMI), systolic blood pressure (SBP), low-density lipoprotein cholesterol (LDL-C), and vascular dysfunction are independent risk factors for cardiovascular disease [7–9]. According to a previous study, regarding the relationships among these factors, young adults with a greater number of risk factors for cardiovascular diseases showed significantly lower dilatory capacity of the brachial artery [7]. This finding suggests that vascular function is related to the risk factors for cardiovascular disease even in the younger generation, and managing the blood vessel function from a relatively younger age may be effective in preventing future cardiovascular diseases.

Pulse wave velocity (PWV) and augmentation index (AIx) are widely used as valid methods for non-invasive measurement of arterial stiffness to evaluate the function of blood vessels in human [10–13]. AIx is estimated as the ratio of waveform reflection amplitude to central pulse pressure and has a high correlation with carotid-femoral pulse wave velocity (cf-PWV), a golden standard that can directly measure central arterial stiffness [14]. The measurement of PWV is accepted as the most reliable technology through a recent consensus statement and is the most widely used technique to assess arterial stiffness [15,16].

Recent studies have reported that physical fitness-related factors such as cardiorespiratory endurance and muscular strength are correlated with arterial stiffness [17,18]. Improving cardiorespiratory endurance with regular aerobic exercise lowers arterial stiffness and reduces the risk factors for cardiovascular diseases, consequently reducing mortality due to cardiovascular disease [19]. In addition, increasing skeletal muscle mass and muscular strength with resistance exercise has been known to prevent sarcopenia caused by aging process, and the American Heart Association recommends resistance exercise for prevention and treatment of cardiovascular diseases [17,20]. A study by Fahs et al. on 79 young male adults reported that upper body muscular strength was negatively correlated with aortic stiffness independent of cardiorespiratory capacity [21]. In addition, Ochi et al. study showed that the greater cross-sectional area of the thigh muscles in middle-aged male adults was associated with lower baPWV, suggesting that higher muscle strength and skeletal muscles may be correlated with arterial compliance [22]. It has been reported that an elevation in anaerobic power with anaerobic exercise has a positive effect on cardiovascular health as well as on the aerobic ability [23]. Moreover, improvement in anaerobic capacity with high-intensity interval training has a positive effect on releasing vasodilatory substances such as nitric oxide, suggesting improvement in anaerobic power has a positive effect on vascular function [24,25].

Taken together, anaerobic capacity such as skeletal muscle mass, muscle strength, and anaerobic power may be related to arterial stiffness. However, studies confirming this correlation among young adults are insufficient; especially, it is unclear whether there is a direct relationship between anaerobic power and arterial stiffness. Therefore, the present study aimed to investigate the correlation of skeletal muscle mass, muscular strength, and anaerobic power with arterial stiffness in physically-active healthy college young male adults.

2. Materials and Methods

2.1. Participants

Twenty-three healthy young male college students participated in the study. The exclusion criteria were specified as follows: (1) smokers; (2) high blood pressure $\geq$ 140/90 mmHg; and (3) reported history of any cardiovascular, chronic, and orthopedic disease. The participants visited the laboratory between 9:00 AM and 10:00 AM. All experimental measurements were conducted with the approval of the Institutional Review Board of Incheon National University (permission# 7007971-201904-006-01). The purpose and the procedure of the study were explained, and informed consent was obtained from all participants involved in the study prior to the experiment. The number of participations in the weekly exercise was recorded through a separate questionnaire to determine whether they participated in the exercise regularly. The weekly exercise questionnaire contained self-report of habitual physical activity combined into leisure-time and sports-time. Basic clinical characteristics of the participants were presented in Table 1.

Table 1. Basic clinical characteristics of participants.

Variables (Unit)	Mean ± SEM
Age (year)	23.9 ± 0.5
Height (cm)	176.3 ± 1.3
Weight (kg)	77.7 ± 2.0
Body fat (%)	16.6 ± 1.0
Muscle Mass (kg)	37.1 ± 4.5
Muscle Mass (kg/m^2)	11.9 ± 0.2
Hand Grip Strength (kg)	50.30 ± 0.8
Hand Grip Strength (kg/m^2)	16.2 ± 0.4
Peak Anaerobic Power (W)	918.4 ± 25.1
Average Anaerobic Power (W)	634.2 ± 20.2
Minimum Anaerobic Power (W)	395.0 ± 21.7
HR_{rest} (beats min^{-1})	60.3 ± 2.5
AIx (%)	4.0 ± 1.4
AIx@75 (%)	−3.1 ± 3.0
baPWV (cm/s)	1173.5 ± 30.4
Weekly engaged exercise times (times/week)	4.4 ± 0.2

Values express means ± SEM. AIx, augmentation index; AIx@75, augmentation index corrected for heart rate 75; baPWV, brachial-ankle pulse wave velocity; HR_{rest}, heart rate at rest.

2.2. Study Procedure

All variables were measured in the following order: body composition, blood pressure in both arms at rest, arterial stiffness including AIx and baPWV, levels of lipid and glucose profiles in circulation, muscular strength, and anaerobic power. Participants fasted for at least 8 h before the measurement and were instructed to abstain from vigorous exercises or alcohol drinking for 24 h before visiting the laboratory. The order of measurements was arranged in such a way that the previous measure did not adversely affect the next one. Measurements for all participants were conducted at similar times and same place in a similar environment with controlled temperature 23–25 °C and humidity 40–60%.

2.2.1. Measurements of Anthropometric Parameters and Cardiometabolic Risk Factors

Height was measured using an extensometer (Sanwa, South Korea), and body composition was measured using an Inbody 720 (Biospace, Seoul, South Korea) machine utilizing the bioelectric impedance analysis (BIA) method. Body weight (kg), BMI (kg/m^2), fat mass (kg), body fat (%), and fat free mass (kg) were measured and obtained from BIA method. Skeletal muscle mass corrected by height (kg/m^2) was used in this study [26,27]. Blood pressure was evaluated using Accuniq BP850 (Jawon, Seoul, South Korea). Participants measured blood pressure twice in a stable state, and the average of values was used in the analysis. For blood analysis, participants were seated in a chair and wiped their index fingers with alcohol cotton to draw whole blood. After placing the capillaries horizontally, 35 μL of whole blood was collected from index finger of each participant. Total cholesterol (Total-C), LDL-C, high-density lipoprotein cholesterol (HDL-C), triglycerides (TG), and fasting glucose (FG) were measured through Cholestech LDX system (Alere, Oslo, Norway), and hemoglobin A1c (HbA1c) was measured using Afinion AS100 Analyzer (Alere, Oslo, Norway). Anthropometric parameters and cardiometabolic risk factors of all participants were presented in Table 2.

Table 2. Anthropometric parameters and cardiometabolic risk factor of participants.

Variables (Unit)	Mean ± SEM
BMI (kg/m^2)	25.1 ± 0.6
SBP (mmHg)	119.4 ± 2.1
DBP (mmHg)	66.9 ± 2.1
Total-C (mg/dL)	174.6 ± 7.5
HDL-C (mg/dL)	54.4 ± 2.2
LDL-C (mg/dL)	98.9 ± 6.7
TG (mg/dL)	108.2 ± 10.9
FG (mg/dL)	91.4 ± 2.6
HbA1c (%)	5.3 ± 0.0

Values express means ± SEM. BMI, body mass index; DBP, diastolic blood pressure; FG, fasting glucose; HbA1c, hemoglobin A1c; HDL-C, high-density lipoprotein cholesterol; LDL-C, low-density lipoprotein cholesterol; SBP, systolic blood pressure; Total-C, total cholesterol; TG, triglycerides.

2.2.2. Brachial-Ankle Pulse Wave Velocity (baPWV)

Peripheral arterial stiffness was measured with a non-invasive method using the Omron vp-1000 plus (Omron, Tokyo, Japan). Participants waited comfortably on the experimental bed for 10 min, placed cuffs at the same position of both upper arms and ankles, and prepared measurements by attaching electrodes to the left sternum. When the participant's resting heart rate was reached to stable condition, peripheral arterial stiffness was measured twice through an automatic waveform analyzer, and the value was obtained by calculating the movement distance and pulse wave propagation time between the limb arteries based on the height.

2.2.3. Augmentation Index (AIx)

AIx was assessed using SphygmoCor Xcel system (AtCor Medical, Sydney, Australia) to measure aortic stiffness in a non-invasive way. The participants lay in bed and rested for approximately 10 min with the cuff placed on the right upper arm. Before AIx measurement, participants' systolic and diastolic blood pressure were measured, and then AIx was measured using SphygmoCor Xcel software. The sphygmoCor device represents a pulse wave value calculated in consideration of age, heart rate, and height through a gender-specific equation [28]. AIx was obtained by dividing the augmented aortic pressure by the aortic pulse pressure. The augmented aortic pressure is made when the forward pulse wave generated from the left ventricle during the systolic period overlaps with the reflected pulse wave returned from the peripheral arterial trees. Since previous studies suggested that AIx and heart rate have a linear relationship, the value corrected to a heart rate of 75 bpm was used in the study [29,30]. AIx@75 was calculated through the following mathematical formula. AIx@75 = {−0.48 × (75-HR)} + AIx [31].

2.2.4. Muscular Strength

Muscular strength was measured using hydraulic hand dynamometer (Saehan, Seoul, South Korea). Hand grip strength was measured in a vertical position with 15° flexion at the elbow. After measuring each arm twice with an interval of 1 min, a higher value was selected and used as a parameter of muscular strength in the study.

2.2.5. Anaerobic Power

Wingate test (Monark 894E model, Vansbro, Sweden) was adopted to assess the anaerobic power. The participants adjusted the position of the saddle to bend 15° after the knee was completely extended from the bicycle ergometer saddle, and the participant lightly practiced pedaling at 50 rpm for 5 min. After a sufficient warm-up practice to relax their hip coxa and femoral muscle before the Wingate test, participants started pedaling maximum speed according to their willingness. The weight load was set to 0.075 kg per body weight. During the measurement, participants were encouraged orally to perform pedaling at maximum speed and power for 30 s. In this study, the absolute and relative peak anaerobic power, mean anaerobic power, and minimum anaerobic power were calculated and used.

2.3. Statistics

Statistical analysis of all variables was performed using the SPSS version 23.0 software (SPSS Inc., Chicago, IL, USA). All measurements were presented as mean and standard error (mean ± SEM). Pearson correlation analysis was performed after the normality test of all variables. All statistical significance levels were set to $p < 0.05$.

3. Results

3.1. Correlation between Skeletal Muscle Mass, Muscular Strength, and Anaerobic Power

Pearson's correlation analysis was performed among skeletal muscle mass, muscular strength, and anaerobic power (peak power, average power, and minimum power). As expected, skeletal muscle mass adjusted by the height was positively correlated with muscular strength, peak power, average power, and minimum power (Table 3). In addition, muscular strength adjusted by the height was positively correlated with peak power, average power, and minimum power (Table 3).

Table 3. Results of Pearson's correlation analysis between skeletal muscle mass, muscular strength, and anaerobic power.

Variables	r-Value				
	Skeletal Muscle Mass	Muscular Strength	Peak Power	Average Power	Minimum Power
Skeletal muscle mass		0.849	0.625	0.563	0.468
		<0.001	0.001	0.005	0.024
Muscular strength			0.543	0.608	0.598
			0.007	0.002	0.003
Peak power				0.825	0.590
				<0.001	0.003
Average power					0.828
					<0.001
Minimum power					

Correlation coefficient is in the upper line and p value in the lower one. The correlation analysis between all measurements.

3.2. Correlation between Cardiometabolic Risk Factors and Arterial Stiffness (baPWV, AIx, AIx@75)

Pearson's correlation analysis between risk factors for cardiometabolic diseases and arterial stiffness revealed that both AIx and AIx@75 showed a negative correlation with BMI and FG and no significant correlation with SBP, diastolic blood pressure (DBP), total-C, HDL-C, LDL-C, TG, and HbA1c (Table 4). In addition, a positive correlation was observed between baPWV and DBP. However, baPWV showed no correlation with other variables, including BMI, SBP, Total-C, HDL-C, LDL-C, FG, TG, and HbA1c (Table 4).

3.3. Correlation between Muscular Variables and Arterial Stiffness (baPWV, AIx)

Correlation between muscular variables and arterial stiffness was depicted in Figure 1. Pearson's correlation analysis revealed significant negative correlation between skeletal muscle, muscle strength, anaerobic, and AIx, respectively (Figure 1A–C). Likewise, AIx@75 (Figure 1D–F) revealed significant negative correlation with muscular variables. However, skeletal muscle mass, muscle strength, and anaerobic power showed no correlation with baPWV, respectively (Figure 1G–I).

Table 4. Association between arterial stiffness (baPWV, AIx, and AIx@75) and cardiometabolic risk factors.

Variables	r-Value								
	BMI	SBP	DBP	Total-C	HDL-C	LDL-C	FG	TG	HbA1c
baPWV	0.247	0.382	0.476	−0.326	0.135	−0.309	0.235	−0.147	−0.015
	0.256	0.072	0.022	0.129	0.539	0.151	0.281	0.503	0.946
AIx	−0.636	−0.178	−0.084	−0.081	−0.151	−0.014	−0.513	−0.036	−0.068
	0.001	0.416	0.702	0.713	0.491	0.950	0.012	0.870	0.757
AIx@75	−0.557	−0.168	−0.021	−0.073	−0.119	−0.014	−0.483	−0.001	−0.022
	0.006	0.444	0.924	0.741	0.589	0.951	0.020	0.995	0.920

Correlation coefficient is in the upper line and p value in the lower one. AIx, augmentation index; AIx@75, AIx corrected for heart rate 75; BIA, bioelectrical impedance analysis; baPWV, brachial-ankle pulse wave velocity; DBP, diastolic pressure; FG, fasting glucose; HDL-C, high-density lipoprotein cholesterol; LDL-C, low-density lipoprotein cholesterol; TG, triglycerides; Total-C, total cholesterol; SBP, systolic blood pressure.

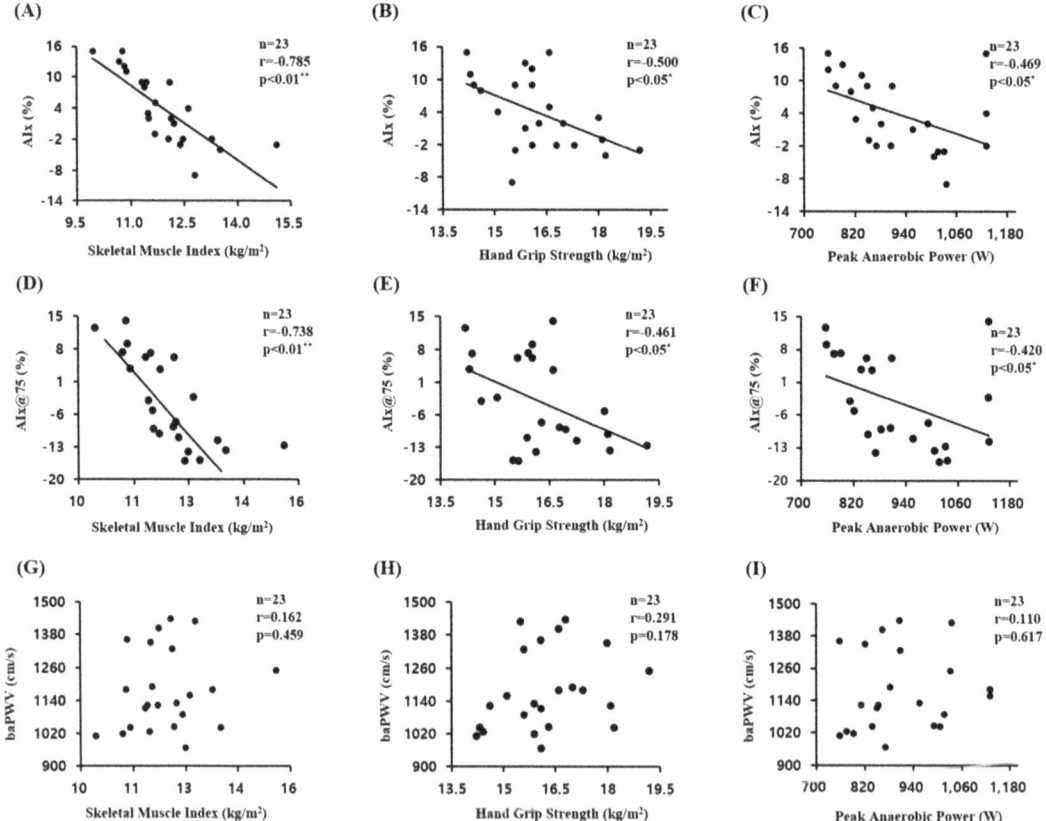

Figure 1. Associations between arterial stiffness (AIx, AIx@75, baPWV) and muscular variables (skeletal muscle mass, muscular strength, anaerobic power). Pearson's correlations between AIx and skeletal muscle index (**A**), hand grip strength (**B**), and peak anaerobic power (**C**). Pearson's correlations between AIx@75 and skeletal muscle index (**D**), hand grip strength (**E**), and peak anaerobic power (**F**). Pearson's correlations between baPWV and skeletal muscle index (**G**), hand grip strength (**H**), and peak anaerobic power (**I**). * $p < 0.05$, ** $p < 0.01$.

4. Discussion

The present study aimed to examine whether muscular variables, including skeletal muscle mass, muscular strength, and anaerobic power, are related to arterial stiffness, an independent risk factor for cardiovascular disease. The major findings of the present study were that higher skeletal muscle mass, muscular strength, and anaerobic power were associated with decreased AIx, while baPWV was not associated with these muscular variables in physically-active young male adults.

This finding is consistent with the previous study, which reported a negative correlation between muscle mass and AIx in both males and females over 65 years of age [32]. In addition, according to study by Fahs et al., it represented a negative correlation between muscle strength and cf-PWV in 79 young male adults [21]; nevertheless, whether a correlation exists between AIx as a determinant of cf-PWV and muscle strength remains unknown. However, this study presented negative correlations between muscle strength and AIx, including corrected age, height, and heart rate 75 bpm. Interestingly, anaerobic power showed a negative correlation with AIx in the present study. Anaerobic power, which is an ability to express explosive energy, is an essential element for independent daily life [23]. It is well known that anaerobic power increases with elevated muscle mass and muscular strength and is improved with anaerobic training via short-term whole-body exercise [33]. Furthermore, it was reported that anaerobic power was reduced with aging and that the anaerobic energy system declined across the aging process without alteration in aerobic capacity in trained masters athletes [34]. For the most part, previous studies have examined anaerobic power in relation to sports-related performance in athletes [35,36], however, few studies have confirmed its correlation with cardiovascular risk factors [23,37]. According to previous studies, anaerobic exercise performed along with aerobic exercise has a positive effect on enhancing cardiovascular health by improving lipid components and BMI, and it improves vascular function by promoting vasodilators such as nitric oxide through high-intensity interval training [23,24,38]. Based on the results of this study and on those of previous studies, maintaining and increasing anaerobic power to a higher level may have a positive effect on AIx.

In the present study, skeletal muscle mass, muscular strength, and anaerobic power were not correlated with baPWV. Sugawara et al. have shown that baPWV was positively correlated with aortic PWV as well as with leg PWV [15]. Particularly, they suggested that baPWV was associated with central arterial stiffness, suggesting that baPWV may reflect central arterial stiffness as well as peripheral arterial stiffness [15,39]. However, Cortez-Cooper et al. indicated that baPWV was correlated with both central and peripheral arterial stiffness, but its correlation with peripheral arterial stiffness was stronger [40]. In addition, Laurent et al. suggested that it is clinically meaningful to evaluate central arterial stiffness rather than peripheral arterial stiffness while assessing cardiovascular diseases [16]. Taken together, central arterial stiffness may be an accurate indicator for the assessment of cardiovascular risk factors in a relatively younger age group [41]. Arterial stiffness shows a high incidence in patients with hypertension, and blood pressure is an index for predicting arterial stiffness even in young adolescents. Moreover, peripheral SBP was higher than central SBP even in adolescents, suggesting that peripheral arterial stiffness is greatly affected by blood pressure even in a relatively younger age group [42]. In case of young male adults in this study, the systolic (119.4 mmHg ± 2.1) and diastolic (66.9 mmHg ± 2.0) blood pressure measurements were within the normal range. Hence, baPWV may not show significant correlation in younger individuals unlike other age groups. In addition, an increase in skeletal muscle mass and muscular strength with resistance exercise may not affect peripheral arterial stiffness in young adults. For example, a study reported that lean body mass and muscular strength significantly increased after 11 weeks of high-intensity resistance exercise, but femoral-ankle PWV reflecting peripheral arterial stiffness did not ameliorate after the exercise [43]. The current study measured grip strength, an index reflecting muscular strength, and analyzed its correlation with baPWV. BaPWV accurately reflects arterial stiffness in the lower body when compared with that in the upper body because it reflects peripheral arterial stiffness [44]. However, grip strength is better correlated with muscle mass and muscular strength of the upper extremities and is rather limited in assessing the ability of the lower extremities [45]. This fact may explain the lack of correlation between grip strength and baPWV in this study.

Several limits of this study should be mentioned to benefit future research. First, in the present study, we conducted in a small number of healthy young male adults as a preliminary research. Therefore, the results of our study cannot be generalized to female subjects and individuals of different age ranges. Second, causality between anaerobic power and arterial stiffness was not confirmed in the present study; therefore, future studies investigating the physiological relationship between these factors are warranted.

Although the present study did not suggest the exact mechanism of how skeletal muscle mass, muscular strength, and anaerobic power mutually affect the arterial stiffness, it showed that higher skeletal muscle mass and muscular strength might have a positive effect on AIx. These findings support the fact that maintaining or improving skeletal muscle mass, muscular strength, and anaerobic power to a higher level can produce a positive effect on AIx even in the young male adults.

5. Conclusions

In conclusion, higher skeletal muscle mass, muscular strength, and anaerobic power are associated with decreased AIx in young male adults. However, baPWV is not associated with these muscular parameters. These findings suggest that maintaining or improving skeletal muscle mass, muscular strength, and anaerobic power to a higher level from a young age may have a positive effect on AIx.

Author Contributions: Conceptualization, D.L. and S.L.; Formal analysis, D.L., M.-H.H.; Investigation, D.L., K.B., M.-H.H., and S.L.; Methodology, D.L., K.B., and M.-H.H.; Original manuscript draft preparation, D.L. and S.L.; Review and editing, K.B., M.-H.H., and S.L. All authors have read and agreed to the published version of the manuscript.

Funding: This research received no external funding.

Institutional Review Board Statement: All experimental measurements were conducted with the approval of the Incheon National University Institutional Review Board (Permission# 7007971-201904-006-01).

Informed Consent Statement: Informed consent was obtained from all subjects involved in the study.

Data Availability Statement: Data are not publicly available due to privacy or ethical restrictions.

Conflicts of Interest: The authors declare no conflict of interest.

References

1. Dolan, E.; Thijs, L.; Li, Y.; Atkins, N.; McCormack, P.; McClory, S.; O'Brien, E.; Staessen, J.A.; Stanton, A.V. Ambulatory arterial stiffness index as a predictor of cardiovascular mortality in the dublin outcome study. *Hypertension* **2006**, *47*, 365–370. [CrossRef]
2. Weber, T.; Auer, J.; O'Rourke, M.F.; Kvas, E.; Lassnig, E.; Berent, R.; Eber, B. Arterial stiffness, wave reflections, and the risk of coronary artery disease. *Circulation* **2004**, *109*, 184–189. [CrossRef]
3. Said, M.A.; Eppinga, R.N.; Lipsic, E.; Verweij, N.; van der Harst, P. Relationship of arterial stiffness index and pulse pressure with cardiovascular disease and mortality. *J. Am. Heart Assoc.* **2018**, *7*, e007621. [CrossRef] [PubMed]
4. Lee, H.-Y.; Oh, B.-H. Aging and arterial stiffness. *Circ. J.* **2010**, 1010120923. [CrossRef] [PubMed]
5. Sun, Z. Aging, arterial stiffness, and hypertension. *Hypertension* **2015**, *65*, 252–256. [CrossRef]
6. Lakatta, E.G. Age-associated cardiovascular changes in health: Impact on cardiovascular disease in older persons. *Heart Fail. Rev.* **2002**, *7*, 29–49. [CrossRef] [PubMed]
7. Urbina, E.M.; Kieltkya, L.; Tsai, J.; Srinivasan, S.R.; Berenson, G.S. Impact of multiple cardiovascular risk factors on brachial artery distensibility in young adults: The bogalusa heart study. *Am. J. Hypertens.* **2005**, *18*, 767–771. [CrossRef]
8. Jackson, R.; Lawes, C.M.; Bennett, D.A.; Milne, R.J.; Rodgers, A. Treatment with drugs to lower blood pressure and blood cholesterol based on an individual's absolute cardiovascular risk. *Lancet* **2005**, *365*, 434–441. [CrossRef]
9. Cook, S.; Togni, M.; Schaub, M.C.; Wenaweser, P.; Hess, O.M. High heart rate: A cardiovascular risk factor? *Eur. Heart J.* **2006**, *27*, 2387–2393. [CrossRef]

10. Nakae, I.; Matsuo, S.; Matsumoto, T.; Mitsunami, K.; Horie, M. Augmentation index and pulse wave velocity as indicators of cardiovascular stiffness. *Angiology* **2008**, *59*, 421–426. [CrossRef]
11. Higashi, H.; Okayama, H.; Saito, M.; Morioka, H.; Aono, J.; Yoshii, T.; Hiasa, G.; Sumimoto, T.; Nishimura, K.; Inoue, K. Relationship between augmentation index and left ventricular diastolic function in healthy women and men. *Am. J. Hypertens.* **2013**, *26*, 1280–1286. [CrossRef] [PubMed]
12. Takami, T.; Saito, Y. Azelnidipine plus olmesartan versus amlodipine plus olmesartan on arterial stiffness and cardiac function in hypertensive patients: A randomized trial. *Drug Des. Dev. Ther.* **2013**, *7*, 175. [CrossRef] [PubMed]
13. Ogawa, O.; Hiraoka, K.; Watanabe, T.; Kinoshita, J.; Kawasumi, M.; Yoshii, H.; Kawamori, R. Diabetic retinopathy is associated with pulse wave velocity, not with the augmentation index of pulse waveform. *Cardiovasc. Diabetol.* **2008**, *7*, 1–5. [CrossRef] [PubMed]
14. Lee, C.W.; Sung, S.H.; Chen, C.K.; Chen, I.M.; Cheng, H.M.; Yu, W.C.; Shih, C.C.; Chen, C.H. Measures of carotid–femoral pulse wave velocity and augmentation index are not reliable in patients with abdominal aortic aneurysm. *J. Hypertens.* **2013**, *31*, 1853–1860. [CrossRef] [PubMed]
15. Sugawara, J.; Hayashi, K.; Yokoi, T.; Cortez-Cooper, M.Y.; DeVan, A.; Anton, M.; Tanaka, H. Brachial–ankle pulse wave velocity: An index of central arterial stiffness? *J. Hum. Hypertens.* **2005**, *19*, 401–406. [CrossRef]
16. Laurent, S.; Cockcroft, J.; Van Bortel, L.; Boutouyrie, P.; Giannattasio, C.; Hayoz, D.; Pannier, B.; Vlachopoulos, C.; Wilkinson, I.; Struijker-Boudier, H. Expert consensus document on arterial stiffness: Methodological issues and clinical applications. *Eur. Heart J.* **2006**, *27*, 2588–2605. [CrossRef]
17. Veijalainen, A.; Tompuri, T.; Haapala, E.; Viitasalo, A.; Lintu, N.; Väistö, J.; Laitinen, T.; Lindi, V.; Lakka, T. Associations of cardiorespiratory fitness, physical activity, and adiposity with arterial stiffness in children. *Scand. J. Med. Sci. Sports* **2016**, *26*, 943–950. [CrossRef]
18. Boreham, C.A.; Ferreira, I.; Twisk, J.W.; Gallagher, A.M.; Savage, M.J.; Murray, L.J. Cardiorespiratory fitness, physical activity, and arterial stiffness: The northern ireland young hearts project. *Hypertension* **2004**, *44*, 721–726. [CrossRef]
19. Madden, K.M.; Lockhart, C.; Cuff, D.; Potter, T.F.; Meneilly, G.S. Short-term aerobic exercise reduces arterial stiffness in older adults with type 2 diabetes, hypertension, and hypercholesterolemia. *Diabetes Care* **2009**, *32*, 1531–1535. [CrossRef]
20. Haskell, W.L.; Lee, I.M.; Pate, R.R.; Powell, K.E.; Blair, S.N.; Franklin, B.A.; Macera, C.A.; Heath, G.W.; Thompson, P.D.; Bauman, A. Physical activity and public health: Updated recommendation for adults from the american college of sports medicine and the american heart association. *Med. Sci. Sports Exerc.* **2007**, *39*, 1423–1434. [CrossRef]
21. Fahs, C.; Heffernan, K.; Ranadive, S.; Jae, S.; Fernhall, B. Muscular strength is inversely associated with aortic stiffness in young men. *Med. Sci. Sports Exerc.* **2010**, *42*, 1619–1624. [CrossRef]
22. Ochi, M.; Kohara, K.; Tabara, Y.; Kido, T.; Uetani, E.; Ochi, N.; Igase, M.; Miki, T. Arterial stiffness is associated with low thigh muscle mass in middle-aged to elderly men. *Atherosclerosis* **2010**, *212*, 327–332. [CrossRef] [PubMed]
23. Patel, H.; Alkhawam, H.; Madanieh, R.; Shah, N.; Kosmas, C.E.; Vittorio, T.J. Aerobic vs anaerobic exercise training effects on the cardiovascular system. *World J. Cardiol.* **2017**, *9*, 134. [CrossRef]
24. Thomas, G.D.; Shaul, P.W.; Yuhanna, I.S.; Froehner, S.C.; Adams, M.E. Vasomodulation by skeletal muscle–derived nitric oxide requires α-syntrophin–mediated sarcolemmal localization of neuronal nitric oxide synthase. *Circ. Res.* **2003**, *92*, 554–560. [CrossRef] [PubMed]
25. Koral, J.; Oranchuk, D.J.; Herrera, R.; Millet, G.Y. Six sessions of sprint interval training improves running performance in trained athletes. *J. Strength Cond. Res.* **2018**, *32*, 617–623. [CrossRef] [PubMed]
26. Kim, T.N.; Park, M.S.; Lim, K.I.; Yang, S.J.; Yoo, H.J.; Kang, H.J.; Song, W.; Seo, J.A.; Kim, S.G.; Kim, N.H. Skeletal muscle mass to visceral fat area ratio is associated with metabolic syndrome and arterial stiffness: The korean sarcopenic obesity study (ksos). *Diabetes Res. Clin. Pract.* **2011**, *93*, 285–291. [CrossRef] [PubMed]
27. Baumgartner, R.N.; Koehler, K.M.; Gallagher, D.; Romero, L.; Heymsfield, S.B.; Ross, R.R.; Garry, P.J.; Lindeman, R.D. Epidemiology of sarcopenia among the elderly in New Mexico. *Am. J. Epidemiol.* **1998**, *147*, 755–763. [CrossRef]
28. Janner, J.H.; Godtfredsen, N.S.; Ladelund, S.; Vestbo, J.; Prescott, E. Aortic augmentation index: Reference values in a large unselected population by means of the sphygmocor device. *Am. J. Hypertens.* **2010**, *23*, 180–185. [CrossRef]
29. Fujime, M.; Tomimatsu, T.; Okaue, Y.; Koyama, S.; Kanagawa, T.; Taniguchi, T.; Kimura, T. Central aortic blood pressure and augmentation index during normal pregnancy. *Hypertens. Res.* **2012**, *35*, 633–638. [CrossRef]
30. Figueroa, A.; Kalfon, R.; Madzima, T.; Wong, A. Effects of whole-body vibration exercise training on aortic wave reflection and muscle strength in postmenopausal women with prehypertension and hypertension. *J. Hum. Hypertens.* **2014**, *28*, 118–122. [CrossRef] [PubMed]
31. Wilkinson, I.B.; MacCallum, H.; Flint, L.; Cockcroft, J.R.; Newby, D.E.; Webb, D.J. The influence of heart rate on augmentation index and central arterial pressure in humans. *J. Physiol.* **2000**, *525*(Pt. 1), 263–270. [CrossRef]
32. Lee, S.W.; Youm, Y.; Kim, C.O.; Lee, W.J.; Choi, W.; Chu, S.H.; Park, Y.-R.; Kim, H.C. Association between skeletal muscle mass and radial augmentation index in an elderly korean population. *Arch. Gerontol. Geriatr.* **2014**, *59*, 49–55. [CrossRef] [PubMed]
33. Marsh, G.D.; Paterson, D.H.; Govindasamy, D.; Cunningham, D.A. Anaerobic power of the arms and legs of young and older men. *Exp. Physiol* **1999**, *84*, 589–597. [CrossRef] [PubMed]
34. Gent, D.N.; Norton, K. Aging has greater impact on anaerobic versus aerobic power in trained masters athletes. *J. Sports Sci.* **2013**, *31*, 97–103. [CrossRef]

35. Potteiger, J.A.; Smith, D.L.; Maier, M.L.; Foster, T.S. Relationship between body composition, leg strength, anaerobic power, and on-ice skating performance in division i men's hockey athletes. *J. Strength Cond. Res.* **2010**, *24*, 1755–1762. [CrossRef] [PubMed]
36. Coppin, E.; Heath, E.M.; Bressel, E.; Wagner, D.R. Wingate anaerobic test reference values for male power athletes. *Int. J. Sports Physiol. Perform.* **2012**, *7*, 232–236. [CrossRef]
37. Bera, T.; Rajapurkar, M. Body composition, cardiovascular endurance and anaerobic power of yogic practitioner. *Indian J. Physiol. Pharmacol.* **1993**, *37*, 225. [PubMed]
38. Gitt, A.K.; Wasserman, K.; Kilkowski, C.; Kleemann, T.; Kilkowski, A.; Bangert, M.; Schneider, S.; Schwarz, A.; Senges, J. Exercise anaerobic threshold and ventilatory efficiency identify heart failure patients for high risk of early death. *Circulation* **2002**, *106*, 3079–3084. [CrossRef] [PubMed]
39. Tsuchikura, S.; Shoji, T.; Kimoto, E.; Shinohara, K.; Hatsuda, S.; Koyama, H.; Emoto, M.; Nishizawa, Y. Brachial-ankle pulse wave velocity as an index of central arterial stiffness. *J. Atheroscler. Thromb.* **2010**, *17*, 658–665. [CrossRef]
40. Cortez-Cooper, M.Y.; Supak, J.A.; Tanaka, H. A new device for automatic measurements of arterial stiffness and ankle-brachial index. *Am. J. Cardiol.* **2003**, *91*, 1519–1522. [CrossRef]
41. Safar, M.; Frohlich, E.D. *Atherosclerosis, Large Arteries and Cardiovascular Risk*; Karger Medical and Scientific Publishers: Basel, Switzerland, 2007; Volume 44.
42. O'Rourke, M.F.; Blazek, J.V.; Morreels, C.L., Jr.; Krovetz, L.J. Pressure wave transmission along the human aorta: >changes with age and in arterial degenerative disease. *Circ. Res.* **1968**, *23*, 567–579. [CrossRef] [PubMed]
43. Cortez-Cooper, M.Y.; DeVan, A.E.; Anton, M.M.; Farrar, R.P.; Beckwith, K.A.; Todd, J.S.; Tanaka, H. Effects of high intensity resistance training on arterial stiffness and wave reflection in women. *Am. J. Hypertens.* **2005**, *18*, 930–934. [CrossRef] [PubMed]
44. Watanabe, Y.; Masaki, H.; Yunoki, Y.; Tabuchi, A.; Morita, I.; Mohri, S.; Tanemoto, K. Ankle-brachial index, toe-brachial index, and pulse volume recording in healthy young adults. *Ann. Vasc. Dis.* **2015**, *8*, 227–235. [CrossRef] [PubMed]
45. Kuh, D.; Bassey, E.J.; Butterworth, S.; Hardy, R.; Wadsworth, M.E.; Musculoskeletal Study, T. Grip strength, postural control, and functional leg power in a representative cohort of british men and women: Associations with physical activity, health status, and socioeconomic conditions. *J. Gerontol. A Biol. Sci. Med. Sci.* **2005**, *60*, 224–231. [CrossRef]

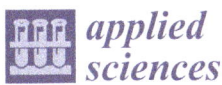

Article

The Role of Cholinesterases in Post-Exercise HRV Recovery in University Volleyball Players

José Raúl Hoyos-Flores [1,2], Blanca R. Rangel-Colmenero [2], Zeltzin N. Alonso-Ramos [2], Myriam Z. García-Dávila [2], Rosa M. Cruz-Castruita [2], José Naranjo-Orellana [3] and Germán Hernández-Cruz [2,*]

[1] Department of Academic Quality, Universidad Interamericana para el Desarrollo Campus Zacatecas, Guadalupe 98617, Mexico; jose.hoyosfl@uanl.edu.mx
[2] Faculty of Sports Organization, Universidad Autónoma de Nuevo León, San Nicolas de los Garza 66455, Mexico; blanca.rangelcl@uanl.edu.mx (B.R.R.-C.); zeltzin.alonsorms@uanl.edu.mx (Z.N.A.-R.); myriam.garciadvl@uanl.edu.mx (M.Z.G.-D.); rosa.cruzcst@uanl.edu.mx (R.M.C.-C.)
[3] Department of Sports and Computing, Universidad Pablo de Olavide, 41013 Seville, Spain; jnarore@upo.es
* Correspondence: german.hernandezcrz@uanl.edu.mx

Abstract: Some studies show interest in measuring heart rate variability (HRV) during post-exercise recovery. It is known that the parasympathetic system is relevant during this process, where one of the factors of this modulation is the interaction of acetylcholine and cholinesterases (ChE). However, the behavior of ChE and its relationship during recovery is little known; therefore, the objective of this study was to analyze the behavior of ChE and its relationship with recovery evaluated in HRV indicators in volleyball players. An exercise protocol with long-term and intermittent high-intensity phases was applied in nine volleyball players. HRV measurements were made, and blood samples were drawn to evaluate the ChE before exercise and after 24 and 48 h post-exercise. The results show a modification of the variables after exercises with respect to the baseline values (ChE: 1818.4 ± 588.75 to 2218.78 ± 1101.58; RMSSD: 42.64 ± 12.86 to 17.72 ± 12.55 ($p < 0.05$); SS: 8.76 ± 1.93 to 21.93 ± 10.05 ($p < 0.01$); S/PS Ratio: 0.32 ± 0.14 to 3.26 ± 3.28 ($p < 0.01$)), as well as recovery after 24 and 48 h with respect to postexercise (ChE: 1608.81 ± 546.88 ($p < 0.05$) and 1454.54 ± 580.45 ($p < 0.01$); RMSSD: 43.83 ± 24.50 and 46.18 ± 33.22 ($p < 0.01$); SS; 10.93 ± 5.16 and 11.86 ± 4.32 ($p < 0.01$); S/PS Ratio: 0.46 ± 0.32 and 0.50 ± 0.28 ($p < 0.01$)). ChE correlations ($p < 0.001$) were found with moderate (SS: $r = 0.465$) and large (RMSSD: $r = -0.654$; S/PS Ratio: $r = 0.666$) HRV indexes. In conclusion, ChE modifications are related to changes in HRV showing a very similar behavior in the case of the study subjects.

Keywords: cholinesterases; heart rate variability; autonomic recovery mechanisms; sympathetic–parasympathetic modulation; postexercise recovery

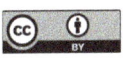

Citation: Hoyos-Flores, J.R.; Rangel-Colmenero, B.R.; Alonso-Ramos, Z.N.; García-Dávila, M.Z.; Cruz-Castruita, R.M.; Naranjo-Orellana, J.; Hernández-Cruz, G. The Role of Cholinesterases in Post-Exercise HRV Recovery in University Volleyball Players. *Appl. Sci.* **2021**, *11*, 4188. https://doi.org/10.3390/app11094188

Academic Editor: Daniela Galli

Received: 25 March 2021
Accepted: 23 April 2021
Published: 4 May 2021

Publisher's Note: MDPI stays neutral with regard to jurisdictional claims in published maps and institutional affiliations.

Copyright: © 2021 by the authors. Licensee MDPI, Basel, Switzerland. This article is an open access article distributed under the terms and conditions of the Creative Commons Attribution (CC BY) license (https://creativecommons.org/licenses/by/4.0/).

1. Introduction

Training load monitoring has become of vital importance to achieve better exercise adaptations [1,2]. Postexercise recovery plays an important role in this working load monitoring where there is great interest in the use of heart rate variability (HRV), since it is an easily accessible noninvasive tool [3–5] for monitoring the state of the autonomic nervous system (ANS) through its sympathetic and parasympathetic branches [6]. It is also useful for athlete monitoring [7,8], since it allows observing adaptations to training by measuring the fatigue and recovery state [9]. One of the most analyzed indexes of HRV is the root mean square of successive RR interval differences (RMSSD) or its natural logarithm (lnRMSSD) to reduce interindividual variations [3,10]. Recently, Naranjo Orellana et al. [11] published two new HRV indexes, the stress score (SS) and the sympathetic–parasympathetic ratio (S:PS ratio), which provide another viewpoint regarding sympathetic activity and the balance between both branches of the ANS, respectively.

215

A large number of studies have focused on measuring these variables in postexercise recovery and in determining how the duration and intensity affect them [5,12–14]. However, there is a discrepancy in the use of these results, since, as far as we know, this tool has not been considered for evaluating the internal load [15]. Recovery is a complex interaction between the sympathetic and the parasympathetic system [5,12], where the sympathetic influence is measured by the release of catecholamines and the activation of adrenergic receptors, and the parasympathetic influence is controlled by the release of acetylcholine in the vagus nerve increasing the parasympathetic tone [6]. However, during recovery, parasympathetic activity becomes relevant in returning the organism to a stable state [12,16,17]; thus, afferent vagal stimulation will lead to a reflex excitation of efferent vagal activity that inhibits sympathetic activity [6].

Parasympathetic control depends on the release of acetylcholine from the vagus nerve, which will bind to muscarinic receptors that hyperpolarize the cardiac muscle to decrease the slope of depolarization, resulting in a slowing of the heart rate [18,19]. Efferent parasympathetic control is mediated by cholinergic signaling in the sinoatrial node, which is rich in acetylcholinesterase (AChE), which hydrolyzes acetylcholine after vagal impulses [6,20,21] that will maintain the parasympathetic tone [22,23]. Several studies have analyzed the inhibition of AChE using pyridostigmine bromide to increase the parasympathetic activity, measuring it by HRV [20,24,25].

Since the cholinergic system is involved in the process of ANS modulation, its measurement could provide information on the regulation of the parasympathetic activity. However, clinical measurements of ACh are complicated [26]; therefore, cholinesterase (ChE) measurements could provide this information, as plasma total free ChE has been reported to determine the hydrolysis capacity of ACh [27] and is effective in observing cholinergic events [28]. It seems logical to think that cholinesterases (ChE), divided into the isoenzymes AChE and butyrylcholinesterase (BChE), are the enzymes that hydrolyze ACh descending into muscles after physical exercise to favor parasympathetic activity, thus increase their concentration in the blood.

However, no studies have been found regarding the behavior of ChE in postexercise situations, relating it to HRV recovery. To our knowledge, two studies measure ChE after physical exercise but without associating it with postexercise recovery. One of these [29] assessed whether gender and a physical activity session could modify the AChE and BChE values in people not exposed to pesticides, concluding that physical activity modifies ChE levels after an exercise session. The other [30] analyzed the metabolic responses of traditional clinical markers of the liver; muscle; heart; and bone function (ChE, creatine kinase, lactate dehydrogenase, alkaline phosphatase, etc.) in response to a session of aerobic medium-long distance free running in football players. The authors concluded that these markers provided valuable information on postexercise muscle conditions. However, they mention that ChE should not be used as a marker of the metabolic response, possibly because it was analyzed as a marker of liver damage in this study. We assume at a theoretical level that it could be novel to study the behavior of ChE during recovery and its possible relationship with the ANS regulation process.

We hypothesize that ChE behavior is associated with the process of ANS modulation in postexercise recovery and may be a marker of internal loading. Therefore, the objective of this study was to analyze the influence of ChE behavior on ANS modulation, as assessed across HRV indicators after a combined long-duration and intermittent high-intensity phases exercise in collegiate volleyball players.

2. Materials and Methods

2.1. Headings

This was a quasi-experimental study with an explicit–correlative scope. The study began with a medical examination of the study subjects, measures of body composition, and a stress test, followed by the application of a physical exercise intervention protocol. After the intervention, the subjects had a recovery period of 48 h concentrated in the installations, controlling rest, the intake of any supplements or drugs that could affect the results, and food. The study duration had a total of 15 days.

2.2. Subjects

A total of nine volunteer volleyball players (21.44 ± 2.07 years; 77.38 ± 6.44 kg body weight; 185.82 ± 10.71 cm height; $25.48 \pm 2.50\%$ adipose mass; $48.07 \pm 1.86\%$ muscle mass; $18.33 \pm 5.16\%$ fat mass; and 49.47 ± 6.36-mL·kg^{-1}·min^{-1} VO$_2$max) from the representative team of the Universidad Autónoma de Nuevo León were studied. Sample selection was non-probabilistic, and size was determined using the statistical package G*Power version 3.1.9 (G*Power, Heinrich-Heine, Universität Düsseldorf, Germany) with a probabilistic error of $\alpha = 0.05$, a statistical power of the probabilistic error of $1 - \beta = 0.80$, and an effect size of $d = 1.20$.

An informative meeting was held regarding the research objectives, and afterward, all the subjects signed written informed consent for their participation in the study. This study was carried out in accordance with the recommendations of the Ethics Committee of the Universidad Autónoma de Nuevo León (COBICIS-16.09/2012.01GHC), following the ethical standards of all the principles expressed in the Helsinki Declaration [31].

2.3. Procedure

The research was carried out during a training recess of the volleyball players in the winter vacation period. The assessment began with a medical history, physical examination, a blood sample and an HRV measure as a baseline (BASELINE), a body composition analysis (subjects were asked as much as possible to come with the bladder and bowel emptied) by dual X-ray densitometry (DXA (Lunar Prodigy, GE Healthcare, Madison, WI, USA)), kinanthropometry using the complete profile proposed by the International Society for the Advancement of Kinanthropometry (ISAK) [32], and a stress test. These measures were carried out during the first 12 days of the study, as shown in Figure 1.

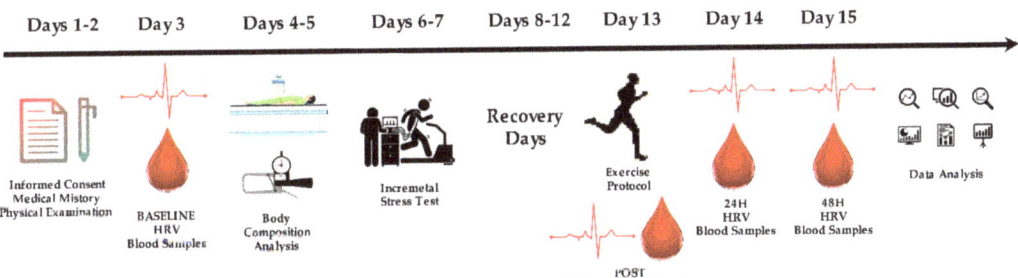

Figure 1. Experimental approach.

To determine the VO$_2$max, an incremental stress test was performed starting at 8 km·h^{-1} and increasing 0.5 km·h^{-1} every 30 s until exhaustion with a COSMED Quark PFT ergospirometer (COSMED The Metabolic Company, Rome, Italy) and a TuffTread NF4616HRT treadmill (Tuff Tread, Conroe, TX, USA). VO$_2$ was determined when a VO$_2$ concentration plateau was reached; if this plateau was not reached, the value considered was when the respiratory coefficient was greater than 1.15, and the theoretical maximum heart rate was greater than 95%. In this way, the maximum aerobic speed (MAS) was established as the starting speed of the VO$_2$ max plateau. The methodology proposed by Skinner and McLellan [33] was used to obtain the ventilatory thresholds.

Afterward, a high-intensity and long-duration intermittent exercise protocol was applied to produce elevated physiological stress. Then, blood samples were drawn, and HRV during the immediate recovery period (AFTER) and at 24 (24H) and 48 (48H) hours was measured. The subjects were concentrated in the installations of the university where they avoided stimulating food, supplements, or drugs that could alter the results. Food intake (they were given a balanced, proportional, and correct diet) and rest were controlled during the postexercise recovery process.

2.4. Blood Samples

The extraction area was sterilized to obtain the blood sample, and a puncture was made in the median cubital vein with a double-bevel needle, collecting the sample in a 4-mL tube with the anticoagulant EDTA (K2 EDTA, BD Vacutainer, Franklin Lakes, NJ, USA). Afterward, the samples were placed in a Solbat J-40 (SOLBAT S.A. de C.V., Puebla, Mexico) centrifuge at 3000 rpm for 10 min to obtain plasma. Aliquots of plasma were placed in 1.5-mL Eppendorf tubes and stored at $-20\,°C$.

2.5. Exercise Protocol

To obtain a physical demand greater than at a competition and higher physiological stress in volleyball players, a combined exercise protocol was designed based on the Loughborough Intermittent Test [34]. The aim of this protocol was to equal the physical load on athletes to avoid unequal physical loads that commonly occur in team sports during competition, depending on the time of play of the athletes. The VT2 speed percentage reached was used to determine the mean intensity of work for each block.

The protocol consisted of 6 work blocks with 3 min of passive recovery between each. The sequence of the first five blocks was 3 rounds of walking, 3 jumps over a 50-cm hurdle, 1 maximum sprint round, three trotting rounds, and 3 maximum sprint rounds; each round was continuous without recovery with a distance of 20 m and repeating each of the blocks five times. Last, the sixth block consisted of performing a round trotting and a maximum sprint round, repeating these until no more rounds could be performed.

2.6. Cholinesterases

An ELISA in 96-well microplates was used for total and overall concentration of AChE and BChE, following the protocol of the Human Acetylcholinesterase/ACHE ELISA kit (DuoSet ELISA Development System, R&D Systems, Minneapolis, MN, USA). This was done in duplicate, placing 100 µL of the standard solution and its dilutions for the calibration curve and the subjects' plasma samples. Afterward, concentration readings were performed with a Bio-Rad iMark Microplate Reader spectrophotometer (Bio-Rad Laboratories, Inc., Hercules, CA, USA) at a wavelength of 450 nm. To calculate the results, a four-parameter logistic (4PL) curve formula was used for logistic regression. For the BASAL level, two nonconsecutive measures were performed. The coefficient of determination of the linear regression of the real and the measured concentration was calculated with an $R^2 = 0.995$ and an ICC reliability = 0.998, $p < 0.001$. For the baseline measure, the determination coefficient was $R^2 = 0.878$ and the ICC reliability = 0.853 (95% CI = 0.731; 0.984); $p < 0.01$.

2.7. Heart Rate Variability

The heart signal was recorded using the Polar Team 2 system (Polar Team^2, Polar Electro OY, Kempele, Finland). Ten-minute recordings at rest lying down supine were obtained every day of the week (6:00 a.m.–8:00 a.m.). Data were transferred to the Polar ProtrainerTM software version 1.4.5 in its beat-to-beat version to extract the time series (R-R). This temporary series was exported to Kubios software version 2.2 (Kubios HRV Analysis Software, The MathWorks Inc, University of Eastern Finland, Kuopio, Finland) for filtration and analysis, obtaining the RMSSD, SD1, and SD2 parameters. Later, the SS and S:PS ratio values were obtained using the protocols proposed by Naranjo Orellana et al. [11].

2.8. Statistical Analysis

Statistical analysis was carried out using SPSS statistical software version 25 (IBM Corp., Armonk, NY, USA) with a significance level of $p < 0.05$ for all analyses. Descriptive data are presented as means and standard deviations. A normality analysis was performed with the Shapiro–Wilk test, and Friedman with a Wilcoxon post-hoc tests were used to compare means. Regarding ChE, a reliability analysis was performed using the intraclass correlation coefficient (ICC) and linear regression with a coefficient of determination (R^2). Subsequently, the data were normalized using the Z-Score to adjust for a change in intra-subject values in inter-subject samples. To observe the relationship between variables, Pearson's correlation was used, and for the interpretation of correlation magnitudes (r), the following criteria were adopted: ≤ 0.10, trivial; >0.10 to 0.30, small; >0.30 to 0.50, moderate; >0.50 to 0.70, large; >0.70 to 0.90, very large; >0.90, extremely large; and 1.0, perfect [35].

3. Results

The training load was similar for all study subjects with regards to the first five blocks. In relation to block 6, the individual workload varied a little because of the characteristics. Table 1 shows the workload performed by the participants.

Table 1. Training load of the exercise protocol.

	Variable	M	SD	CV (%)
Blocks 1–5	Total distance (m)	7500	0	0
	Mean speed (km·h^{-1})	8.7	0.8	9.1
	VT2 speed (km·h^{-1})	14.9	0.9	6.3
	VT2 (%)	58.6	6.4	10.9
Block 6	Distance (m)	546	322.2	58.9
	Mean speed (km·h^{-1})	11	0.7	6.6
	VT2 (%)	74	2.3	3.1
Total exercise protocol	Total time (min)	52.2	5	9.6
	Total distance (m)	8046.7	322.2	4

VT2: second ventilatory threshold; M: mean; SD: standard deviation; CV: coefficient of variation.

Regarding the descriptive values of ChE, the RMSSD, SS, and the S:PS ratio for the different measures, these are shown in Table 2 with the means and standard deviation.

Table 2. Descriptive analysis of the analyzed variables.

Variable		BASELINE	AFTER	24H	48H
ChE (pg/mL)	M	1818.41	2218.78	1608.81	1454.54
	SD	588.75	1101.58	546.88	580.45
RMSSD (ms)	M	12.64	17.72	43.83	46.18
	SD	12.86	12.55	24.50	33.22
SS (AU)	M	8.76	21.93	10.93	11.86
	SD	1.93	10.05	5.16	4.32
S:PS ratio (AU)	M	0.32	3.26	0.46	0.50
	SD	0.14	3.28	0.32	0.28

ChE: cholinesterase; RMSSD: root mean square of successive RR interval differences; SS: stress score; S:PS ratio: sympathetic–parasympathetic ratio; M: mean; SD: standard deviation.

Figure 2 shows the behavior of the analyzed variables, which shows that ChE, SS, and the S:PS ratio had a greater elevation in the AFTER measure compared to the BASELINE measure, with a significant change of the SS, as well as the S:PS ratio ($p < 0.01$). The RMSSD has a significant descent ($p < 0.05$) in the AFTER measure compared to the BASELINE measure. All significantly returns to baseline levels at 24H and 48H ($p < 0.01$), except for ChE, which decreases significantly more than its baseline level ($p < 0.05$ and $p < 0.01$) compared to AFTER; in the 48H measure, it continues to descend with a significant change ($p < 0.05$) compared to 24H.

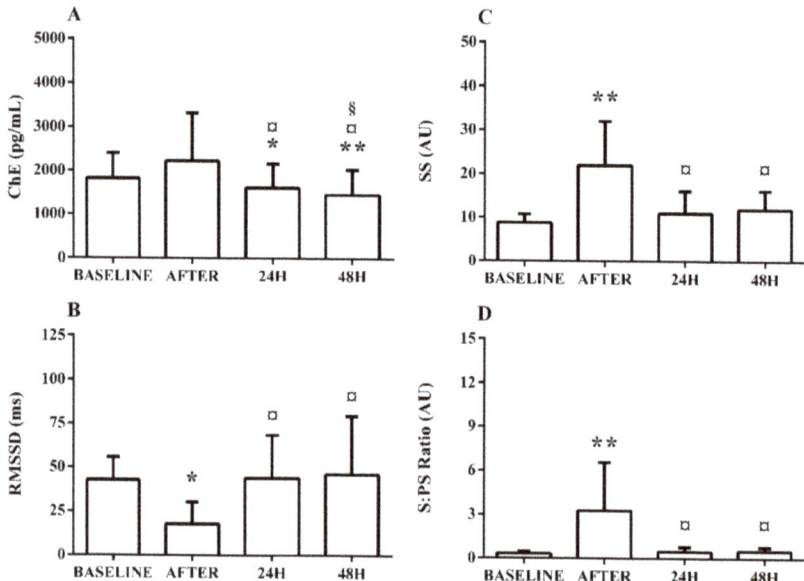

Figure 2. Changes in cholinesterases and HRV at baseline, postexercise, and 24H and 48H after recovery. (**A**) Cholinesterases, (**B**) root mean square of successive RR interval differences, (**C**) stress score, and (**D**) sympathetic/parasympathetic ratio. * $p < 0.05$, in relation to the BASELINE. ** $p < 0.01$, in relation to the BASELINE. ◻ $p < 0.01$, in relation to AFTER. § $p < 0.05$, in relation to 24H.

The relationship of the behavior between variables during the measures is shown in Table 3, where statistically significant mean and high correlations between all the variables can be seen. The correlations of ChE with the HRV indexes are presented graphically in Figure 3 by linear regressions to observe the trend line adjustment and the coefficient of determination (R^2).

Table 3. Correlation between the variables ChE, RMSSD, SS, and the S:PS ratio.

		ChE	RMSSD	SS
RMSSD	Pearson's correlation	−0.654 **		
SS	Pearson's correlation	0.465 **	−0.879 **	
S:PS ratio	Pearson's correlation	0.666 **	−0.926 **	0.942 **

** Two-tailed bilateral significance at the level $p < 0.001$. ChE: cholinesterase; RMSSD: root mean square of successive RR interval differences; SS: stress score; S:PS ratio: sympathetic–parasympathetic ratio.

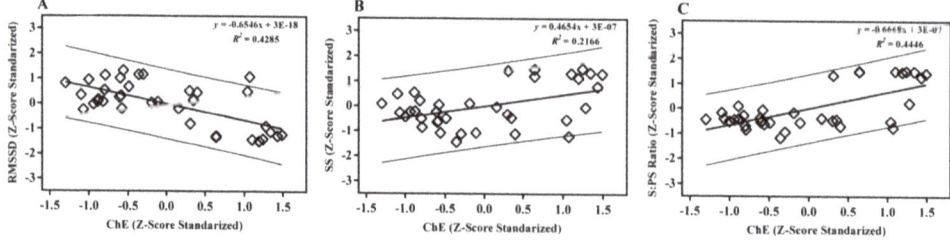

Figure 3. Correlation R^2 of the ChE with the root mean square of successive RR interval differences (**A**), the stress score (**B**), and the sympathetic/parasympathetic ratio (**C**).

4. Discussion

The main contribution of our study is that ChE shows a behavior during postexercise recovery that is similar to the RMSSD indexes, SS, and S:PS ratio of HRV; therefore, we can consider these internal load markers.

It has been described in the literature that during a postexercise recovery, the interaction of the parasympathetic and sympathetic systems is complex [5,12] and mediated mainly by parasympathetic reactivation [36,37]. This includes multiple regulations such as the descent of circulating catecholamines, blood pressure, baroreflexes, and metaboloreflexes that cause a drop in sympathetic stimulation [4,5,17] due to an efferent reflex effect of vagal stimulation [6].

This effect is regulated by cholinergic signaling in the sinoatrial node, and in a certain way, ChE are mediators of the vagal impulse by hydrolyzing ACh [6,20,21]; thus, an increase of ChE in blood indirectly reflects an increase in the rate of ACh hydrolysis leading to ACh descent [27,38,39]. Our results support this idea since. in postexercise measures, the increase of ChE widely correlated with an increase in sympathetic activity (SS and S:PS ratio) and a decrease in RMSSD (Table 3). Afterward, in the 24H and 48H measures, ChE normalized, and RMSSD returned to her initial values, as well as the SS and the S:PS ratio. These changes may be because AChE facilitates the signaling of the onset and termination of the cardioinhibitory effect by hydrolyzing ACh in the synaptic cleft in a very short time (<1 s) [4,40]. Subsequently, the parasympathetic nerve will be stimulated in the phasic mode, where released acetylcholine will hyperpolarize the sinoatrial node by binding to its muscarinic receptors decreasing the depolarization slope and thereby delaying the next sinoatrial node impulse [18,19,41] and, thus, favoring postexercise HRV recovery.

This seems to indicate that these variables evaluate the internal load regardless of the type of exercise performed since, although some authors relate the recovery with duration [4,42] or with intensity [5,43], in our results, it can be seen that the workload was very similar for all subjects (Table 1), demonstrating that the changes in response show the individual assimilation of that load. Therefore, the changes in these variables would fit into the concept of internal load. The indexes, RMSSD, SS, and S:PS ratio have been used jointly in various studies to see the behavior of the sympathetic and parasympathetic systems, both in training control and in competition, concluding that these indicators are valid and reliable for training and competence monitoring [13,44–46].

On the other hand, cholinesterase values (Table 2) are within the range of acceptable clinical values for the technique used (1278 ± 338 pg/mL), so the changes observed in this variable are not at any time abnormal or pathological values. Thus, we observed that the postexercise ChE behavior coincides with the increase reported in the study by Zimmer et al. [29]. However, this does not seem to be the case with that reported by Chamera et al. [30], as the behavior of ChE in women is very similar to our results but not so in men. This could be because the impact of the session was not sufficiently demanding to provoke high rates of ACh hydrolysis. The values of RMSSD, SS, and the S:PS ratio coincide with those presented by other authors [13,44,47], and they would be within the 25–50 percentile of the reference tables reported by Corrales et al. [47]. The behavior of HRV indices following such an exercise is similar to what has already been well-documented in the literature [13,48], where it has been reported that HRV is a reliable indicator to measure fatigue and postexercise recovery with acceptable relations [3–5,8,9,49], establishing the average values for a good state of the athlete (recovered) of RMSSD above 30–40 ms, SS below 10AU and S:PS ratio below 0.5AU [11,44,50]. In addition, acceptable relationships have been shown with other classical markers of recovery (creatine kinase, testosterone/cortisol ratio, immune/inflammatory markers, and training load) [9,13,51–53].

To support the idea of the role of ChE during recovery, in our results, the correlation of ChE with HRV indexes was observed. This could indicate the modulation effect of the pacemaker potential of the sinoatrial node by parasympathetic innervations mediated by ACh and ChE [6,12,21,36,37,54,55]. This may be explained by the fact that, when central command and mechanoreceptor feedback cease, the arterial baroreflex is reset to a lower level, increasing the parasympathetic activity and rendering it phasic [36,37,40,56,57]. Since this parasympathetic activity is controlled by the release of ACh from the efferent vagal nerve discharge, its modulation will largely depend on the ChE activity [6,20,21], supporting this idea by the association found with HRV indices, since as mentioned above, plasma ChE could provide information on cholinergic events [27,28].

4.1. Limitations

The main limitations of this study are the sample size, which has been set at this number to prioritize the homogeneity offered by being a team contemplating a statistical analysis to obtain the ideal sample size and not having the means that allow us to simultaneously contrast what happens in synaptic transmission. Nevertheless, the relationships found between the variables allow us to reasonably assume the conclusions found and to set a starting point for new studies in this direction.

4.2. Practical Applications

Our results describe the behavior of ChE and how it is associated with the recovery of parasympathetic activity postexercise, which could be of useful application in understanding—more specifically, the behavior of HRV indices following a training load similar to that of this study.

5. Conclusions

The modifications observed in ChE appear to influence the changes in sympathetic and parasympathetic activity, since they show an acceptable relationship with HRV indices, which could improve the physiological interpretation of the recovery of parasympathetic activity after a combined long-duration and intermittent high-intensity phases exercise. These findings might have relevance for specialists in the control of training areas for future research, since these results suggest that the ChE and HRV levels might be considered internal load markers.

Author Contributions: Conceptualization, J.R.H.-F., B.R.R.-C., and G.H.-C.; Methodology, J.R.H.-F., G.H.-C., R.M.C.-C., and J.N.-O.; Formal Analysis, J.R.H.-F., R.M.C.-C., and J.N.-O.; Investigation, J.R.H.-F., B.R.R.-C., Z.N.A.-R., M.Z.G.-D., and J.N.-O.; Resources, J.R.H.-F., B.R.R.-C., and G.H.-C.; Data Curation, J.R.H.-F. and M.Z.G.-D.; Project Administration, J.R.H.-F., B.R.R.-C., Z.N.A.-R., and G.H.-C.; Funding Acquisition, B.R.R.-C. and G.H.-C.; Writing—Original Draft Preparation, J.R.H.-F. and J.N.-O.; and Writing—Review and Editing, J.R.H.-F., G.H.-C., and J.N.-O. All authors have read and agreed to the published version of the manuscript.

Funding: This research was funded by Scientific and Technological Research Program (Programa de Apoyo a la Investigación Científica y Tecnológica (PAICYT)) of the Universidad Autónoma de Nuevo León, grant number CSA949-19.

Institutional Review Board Statement: The study was conducted according to the guidelines of the Declaration of Helsinki and approved by the Ethics Committee of the Universidad Autónoma de Nuevo León (COBICIS-16.09/2012.01GHC).

Informed Consent Statement: Informed consent was obtained from all subjects involved in the study.

Data Availability Statement: The raw data supporting the conclusions of this article will be made available by the authors, without undue reservation.

Acknowledgments: We thank the coach Jorge Azair and his team of athletes for their support and help in performing this research.

Conflicts of Interest: The authors declare no conflict of interest.

References

1. Bourdon, P.C.; Cardinale, M.; Murray, A.; Gastin, P.; Kellmann, M.; Varley, M.C.; Gabbett, T.J.; Coutts, A.J.; Burgess, D.J.; Gregson, W.; et al. Monitoring athlete training loads: Consensus statement. *Int. J. Sports Physiol. Perform.* **2017**, *12*, S2161–S2170. [CrossRef]

2. Halson, S.L. Monitoring training load to understand fatigue in athletes. *Sports Med.* **2014**, *44* (Suppl. 2), S139–S147. [CrossRef] [PubMed]
3. Buchheit, M. Monitoring training status with HR measures: Do all roads lead to Rome? *Front. Physiol.* **2014**, *5*, 73. [CrossRef] [PubMed]
4. Michael, S.; Graham, K.S.; Davis, G.M. Cardiac autonomic responses during exercise and post-exercise recovery using heart rate variability and systolic time intervals—A review. *Front. Physiol.* **2017**, *8*, 301. [CrossRef] [PubMed]
5. Stanley, J.; Peake, J.M.; Buchheit, M. Cardiac parasympathetic reactivation following exercise: Implications for training prescription. *Sports Med.* **2013**, *43*, 1259–1277. [CrossRef]
6. Camm, A.J.; Malik, M.; Bigger, J.T.; Breithardt, G.; Cerutti, S.; Cohen, R.J.; Coumel, P.; Fallen, E.L.; Kennedy, H.L.; Kleiger, R.E.; et al. Heart rate variability: Standards of measurement, physiological interpretation, and clinical use. Task Force of the European Society of Cardiology and the North American Society of Pacing and Electrophysiology. *Circulation* **1996**, *93*, 1043–1065.
7. Borresen, J.; Lambert, M.I. Autonomic control of heart rate during and after exercise—Measurements and implications for monitoring training status. *Sports Med.* **2008**, *38*, 633–646. [CrossRef]
8. Daanen, H.A.M.; Lamberts, R.P.; Kallen, V.L.; Jin, A.; Van Meeteren, N.L.U. A systematic review on heart-rate recovery to monitor changes in training status in athletes. *Int. J. Sports Physiol. Perform.* **2012**, *7*, 251–260. [CrossRef]
9. Wallace, L.K.; Slattery, K.M.; Coutts, A.J. A comparison of methods for quantifying training load: Relationships between modelled and actual training responses. *Eur. J. Appl. Physiol.* **2014**, *114*, 11–20. [CrossRef]
10. Plews, D.J.; Laursen, P.B.; Kilding, A.E.; Buchheit, M. Training adaptation and heart rate variability in elite endurance athletes—Opening the door to effective monitoring. *Sports Med.* **2013**, *43*, 773–781. [CrossRef]
11. Naranjo Orellana, J.; de la Cruz Torres, B.; Sarabia Cachadiña, E.; de Hoyo, M.; Domínguez Cobo, S. Two new indexes for the assessment of autonomic balance in elite soccer players. *Int. J. Sports Physiol. Perform.* **2015**, *10*, 452–457. [CrossRef]
12. Goldberger, J.J.; Le, F.K.; Lahiri, M.; Kannankeril, P.J.; Ng, J.; Kadish, A.H. Assessment of parasympathetic reactivation after exercise. *Am. J. Physiol. Heart Circ. Physiol.* **2006**, *290*, H2446–H2452. [CrossRef]
13. Miranda-Mendoza, J.; Reynoso-Sánchez, L.F.; Hoyos-Flores, J.R.; Quezada-Chacón, J.T.; Naranjo, J.; Rangel-Colmenero, B.; Hernández-Cruz, G. Stress score and LnrMSSD as internal load parameters during competition. *Rev. Int. Med. Cienc. Act. Fís. Deporte* **2020**, *20*, 21–35.
14. Saboul, D.; Balducci, P.; Millet, G.; Pialoux, V.; Hautier, C. A pilot study on quantification of training load: The use of HRV in training practice. *Eur. J. Sport Sci.* **2015**, *16*, 172–181. [CrossRef]
15. McLaren, S.J.; Macpherson, T.W.; Coutts, A.J.; Hurst, C.; Spears, I.R.; Weston, M. The relationships between internal and external measures of training load and intensity in team sports. A Meta-Analysis. *Sports Med.* **2018**, *48*, 641–658. [CrossRef]
16. Ahmadian, M.; Roshan, V.D.; Hosseinzadeh, M. Parasympathetic reactivation in children: Influence of two various modes of exercise. *Clin. Auton. Res.* **2015**, *25*, 207–212. [CrossRef]
17. Buchheit, M.; Laursen, P.B.; Ahmaidi, S. Parasympathetic reactivation after repeated sprint exercise. *Am. J. Physiol. Heart Circ. Physiol.* **2007**, *293*, H133–H141. [CrossRef]
18. Noma, A.; Trautwein, W. Relaxation of the ACh-induced potassium current in the rabbit sinoatrial node cell. *Pflug. Arch.* **1978**, *377*, 193–200. [CrossRef]
19. Osterrieder, W.; Noma, A.; Trautwein, W. On the kinetics of the potassium channel activated by acetylcholine in the S-A node of the rabbit heart. *Pflug. Arch.* **1980**, *386*, 101–109. [CrossRef]
20. Dewland, T.A.; Androne, A.S.; Lee, F.A.; Lampert, R.J.; Katz, S.D. Effect of acetylcholinesterase inhibition with pyridostigmine on cardiac parasympathetic function in sedentary adults and trained athletes. *Am. J. Physiol. Heart Circ. Physiol.* **2007**, *293*, H86–H92. [CrossRef]
21. Taylor, P. Acetylcholinesterase Agents. In *Goodman and Gilman's The Pharmacological Basis of Therapeutics*, 13th ed.; Brunton, L., Hilal-Dandan, R., Knollmann, B.C., Eds.; McGraw-Hill Education: New York, NY, USA, 2017; pp. 163–175.
22. Akselrod, S.; Gordon, D.; Madwed, J.B.; Snidman, N.C.; Shannon, D.C.; Cohen, R.J. Hemodynamic regulation: Investigation by spectral analysis. *Am. J. Physiol. Heart Circ. Physiol.* **1985**, *249*, H867–H875. [CrossRef]
23. Levy, M.N. Brief Reviews: Sympathetic-parasympathetic Interactions in the heart. *Circ. Res.* **1971**, *29*, 437–445. [CrossRef]
24. Nóbrega, A.C.L.; dos Reis, A.F.; Moraes, R.S.; Bastos, B.G.; Ferlin, E.L.; Ribeiro, J.P. Enhancement of heart rate variability by cholinergic stimulation with pyridostigmine in healthy subjects. *Clin. Auton. Res.* **2001**, *11*, 11–17. [CrossRef]
25. Zarei, A.; Foroutan, S.; Foroutan, S.; Erfanian Omidvar, A. Enhancement of Frequency Domain Indices of Heart Rate Variability by Cholinergic Stimulation with Pyridostigmine Bromide. *Iran. J. Pharm. Res.* **2011**, *10*, 889–894.
26. Soreq, H.; Seidman, S. Acetylcholinesterase—New roles for an old actor. *Nat. Rev. Neurosci.* **2001**, *2*, 294–302. [CrossRef]
27. Ofek, K.; Krabbe, K.S.; Evron, T.; Debecco, M.; Nielsen, A.R.; Brunnsgaad, H.; Yirmiya, R.; Soreq, H.; Pedersen, B.K. Cholinergic status modulations in human volunteers under acute inflammation. *J. Mol. Med.* **2007**, *85*, 1239–1251. [CrossRef]
28. Shenhar-Tsarfaty, S.; Berliner, S.; Bornstein, N.M.; Soreq, H. Cholinesterases as biomarkers for parasympathetic dysfunction and inflammation-related disease. *J. Mol. Neurosci.* **2014**, *53*, 298–305. [CrossRef]
29. Zimmer, K.R.; Lencina, C.L.; Zimmer, A.R.; Thiesen, F.V. Influence of physical exercise and gender on acetylcholinesterase and butyrylcholinesterase activity in human blood samples. *Int. J. Environ. Health Res.* **2012**, *22*, 279–286. [CrossRef] [PubMed]

30. Chamera, T.; Spieszny, M.; Klocek, T.; Kostrzewa-Nowak, D.; Nowak, R.; Lachowicz, M.; Buryta, R.; Ficek, K.; Eider, J.; Moska, W.; et al. Post-Effort Changes in Activity of Traditional Diagnostic Enzymatic Markers in Football Players' Blood. *J. Med. Biochem.* **2015**, *34*, 179–190. [CrossRef] [PubMed]
31. World Medical Association. World Medical Association Declaration of Helsinki: Ethical principles for medical research involving human subjects. *JAMA* **2013**, *310*, 2191–2194. [CrossRef] [PubMed]
32. Stewart, A.; Marfell-Jones, M.; Olds, T.; De Ridder, H. *International Standards for Anthropometric Assessment (ISAK)*; IAAS: Lower Hutt, New Zealand, 2011.
33. Skinner, J.S.; McLellan, T.H. The transition from aerobic to anaerobic metabolism. *Res. Q. Exerc. Sport* **1980**, *51*, 234–248. [CrossRef]
34. Nicholas, C.W.; Nuttall, F.E.; Williams, C. The Loughborough Intermittent Shuttle Test: A field test that simulates the activity pattern of soccer. *J. Sports Sci.* **2000**, *18*, 97–104. [CrossRef]
35. Hopkins, W.G.; Marshall, S.W.; Batterham, A.M.; Hanin, J. Progressive statistics for studies in sports medicine and exercise science. *Med. Sci. Sports Exerc.* **2009**, *41*, 3–13. [CrossRef]
36. Kannankeril, P.J.; Goldberger, J.J. Parasympathetic effects on cardiac electrophysiology during exercise and recovery. *Am. J. Physiol. Heart Circ. Physiol.* **2002**, *282*, H2091–H2098. [CrossRef]
37. Kannankeril, P.J.; Le, F.K.; Kadish, A.H.; Goldberger, J.J. Parasympathetic effects on heart rate recovery after exercise. *J. Investig. Med.* **2004**, *52*, 394–401. [CrossRef]
38. Das, U.N. Acetylcholinesterase and butyrylcholinesterase as possible markers of low-grade systemic inflammation. *Med. Sci. Monit.* **2007**, *13*, RA214–RA221.
39. Reale, M.; Costantini, E.; Di Nicola, M.; D'Angelo, C.; Franchi, S.; D'Aurora, M.; Di Bari, M.; Orlando, V.; Galizia, S.; Ruggieri, S.; et al. Butyrylcholinesterase and acetylcholinesterase polymorphisms in multiple sclerosis patients: Implication in peripheral inflammation. *Sci. Rep.* **2018**, *8*, 1319. [CrossRef]
40. Masuda, Y.; Kawamura, A. Acetylcholinesterase inhibitor (donepezil hydrochloride) reduces heart rate variability. *J. Cardiovasc. Pharmacol.* **2003**, *41*, S67–S71.
41. Jalife, J.; Slenter, V.A.; Salata, J.J.; Michaels, D.C. Dynamic vagal control of pacemaker activity in the mammalian sinoatrial node. *Circ. Res.* **1983**, *52*, 642–656. [CrossRef]
42. Seiler, S.; Haugen, O.; Kuffel, E. Autonomic recovery after exercise in trained athletes: Intensity and duration effects. *Med. Sci. Sports Exerc.* **2007**, *39*, 1366–1373. [CrossRef]
43. Casonatto, J.; Tinucci, T.; Dourado, A.C.; Polito, M. Cardiovascular and autonomic responses after exercise sessions with different intensities and durations. *Clinics* **2011**, *66*, 453–458. [CrossRef] [PubMed]
44. Naranjo, J.; La Cruz, B.; de Sarabia, E.; Hoyo, M.; de Domínguez-Cobo, S. Heart rate variability. A follow-up in elite soccer players throughout the season. *Int. J. Sports Med.* **2015**, *36*, 881–886. [CrossRef] [PubMed]
45. Nieto-Jiménez, C.; Pardos-Mainer, E.; Ruso-Álvarez, J.F.; Naranjo-Orellana, J. Training Load and HRV in a Female Athlete: A Case Study. *Rev. Int. Med. Cienc. Act. Fís. Deporte* **2020**, *20*, 321–333.
46. Proietti, R.; Di Fronso, S.; Pereira, L.A.; Bortoli, L.; Robazza, C.; Nakamura, F.Y.; Bertollo, M. Heart rate variability discriminates competitive levels in professional soccer players. *J. Strength Cond. Res.* **2017**, *31*, 1719–1725. [CrossRef]
47. Corrales, M.M.; de la Cruz Torres, B.; Garrido Esquivel, A.; Garrido Salazar, M.A.; Naranjo Orellana, J. Normal values of heart rate variability at rest in a young, healthy and active mexican population. *Health* **2012**, *4*, 377–385. [CrossRef]
48. Al Haddad, H.; Laursen, P.B.; Ahmaidi, S.; Buchheit, M. Nocturnal heart rate variability following supramaximal intermittent exercise. *Int. J. Sport Physiol. Perform.* **2009**, *4*, 435–447.
49. Schmitt, L.; Regnard, J.; Millet, G.P. Monitoring fatigue status with HRV measures in elite athletes: An avenue beyond RMSSD? *Front. Physiol.* **2015**, *6*, 343. [CrossRef]
50. Naranjo, J. *Variabilidad de la Frecuencia Cardíaca: Fundamentos y Aplicaciones a la Actividad Física y el Deporte*; Fénix Editora: Sevilla, Spain, 2018.
51. Cruz, G.H.; Orellana, J.N.; Taraco, A.R.; Colmenero, B.R. Leukocyte populations are associated with heart rate variability after a triathlon. *J. Hum. Kinet.* **2016**, *54*, 55–63. [CrossRef]
52. DeBlauw, J.A.; Crawford, D.A.; Kurtz, B.K.; Drake, N.B.; Heinrich, K.M. Evaluating the Clinical Utility of Daily Heart Rate Variability Assessment for Classifying Meaningful Change in Testosterone-to-Cortisol Ratio: A Preliminary Study. *Int. J. Exerc. Sci.* **2021**, *14*, 260–273.
53. Weippert, M.; Behrens, M.; Mau-Moeller, A.; Bruhn, S.; Behrens, K. Relationship between morning heart rate variability and creatine kinase response during intensified training in recreational endurance athletes. *Front. Physiol.* **2018**, *9*, 1267. [CrossRef]
54. Campbell, G.D.; Edwards, F.R.; Hirst, G.D.; O'Shea, J.E. Effects of vagal stimulation and applied acetylcholine on pacemaker potentials in the guinea-pig heart. *J. Physiol.* **1989**, *415*, 57–68. [CrossRef]
55. Dong, J.G. The role of heart rate variability in sports physiology. *Exp. Ther. Med.* **2016**, *11*, 1531–1536. [CrossRef]
56. Coote, J.H. Recovery of heart rate following intense dynamic exercise. *Exp. Physiol.* **2010**, *95*, 431–440. [CrossRef]
57. Pierpont, G.L.; Voth, E.J. Assessing autonomic function by analysis of heart rate recovery from exercise in healthy subjects. *Am. J. Cardiol.* **2004**, *94*, 64–68. [CrossRef]

Article

Changes in Plasma Bioactive Lipids and Inflammatory Markers during a Half-Marathon in Trained Athletes

Melania Gaggini [1], Cristina Vassalle [2,*], Fabrizia Carli [1], Maristella Maltinti [2], Laura Sabatino [1], Emma Buzzigoli [1], Francesca Mastorci [1], Francesco Sbrana [2], Amalia Gastaldelli [1] and Alessandro Pingitore [1]

1. Institute of Clinical Physiology, CNR, 56100 Pisa, Italy; mgaggini@ifc.cnr.it (M.G.); fabrizia.carli@ifc.cnr.ir (F.C.); laura.sabatino@ifc.cnr.it (L.S.); emma@ifc.cnr.it (E.B.); mastorcif@ifc.cnr.it (F.M.); amalia@ifc.cnr.it (A.G.); pingi@ifc.cnr.it (A.P.)
2. Fondazione CNR-Toscana Gabriele Monasterio per la Ricerca Medica e di Sanità Pubblica, 56100 Pisa, Italy; maristella@ftgm.it (M.M.); francesco.sbrana@ftgm.it (F.S.)
* Correspondence: cristina.vassalle@ftgm.it

Abstract: Background: Exercise may affect lipid profile which in turn is related to inflammation, although changes of ceramides, diacylglycerols-DAG and sphingomyelin-SM and their relationship with inflammatory parameters following a half-marathon have never been examined. Methods: Ceramides, DAG and SM, and markers of inflammation (soluble fractalkine-CX3CL1, vascular endothelial growth factor-VEGF, interleukin6-IL-6 and tumor necrosis factorα-TNFα) were evaluated in trained half-marathoners before, post-race (withdrawal within 20 min after the race end) and 24 h after. Results: IL-6 and CX3CL1 increased immediately after the race, returning to baseline after 24 h. Total ceramides and total DAG significantly decreased post-race. Several ceramide classes decreased after exercise, while only one of the DAG (36:3) changed significantly. Total SM and specific species did not significantly change. Conclusion: Some inflammatory parameters (IL-6 and CX3CL1) transiently increased after the race, and, being reversible, these changes might represent a physiological response to acute exercise rather than a damage-related response. The decrease of specific lipid classes, i.e., DAGs and ceramides, and the lack of their relationship with inflammatory parameters, suggest their involvement in beneficial training effects, opening promising research perspectives to identify additional mechanisms of aerobic exercise adaptation.

Keywords: exercise; ceramides; cytokines; diacylglycerol; biomarkers

1. Introduction

Half-marathon (21.0975 km) is an increasingly popular recreational activity. Its diffusion is in part related to the fact that half-marathon requires less powerful training than the marathon [1]. Nonetheless, one reason for its importance in terms of clinical risk is that half-marathon is performed by a growing number of people in the world, although it still remains a powerful training, which might potentially retain adverse health repercussions. In fact, studies focusing on the role of exercise and inflammatory response have underlined that several cytokines increased after a competitive marathon [2]. In this context, it is interesting to assess the role of sphingolipids, bioactive lipids that regulate diverse cell functions, since the activity of sphingomyelinases (sphingolipid metabolizing enzymes) is increased under inflammation and oxidative stress [3]. Thus, ceramides have been associated with oxidative stress status and inflammatory processes [3]. However, changes of ceramide concentration after a half-marathon race have never been examined. Moreover, to the best of our knowledge, the relationship that may exist between bioactive lipids and markers of inflammation/immune response has never been studied in trained subjects following acute physical exertion such as a half-marathon. In this context, how changes in the balance between inflammatory mediators, immune response or lipid may contribute to the response in the post-race phase and affect the health status of subjects participating in such events also remains unclear. Thus, we aimed to evaluate levels of bioactive lipids related to inflammation signaling pathways, and to this purpose, we studied plasma ceramides, diacylglycerol and SM. These lipids can modulate the activity of intracellular enzymes (e.g., those involved in insulin signaling). In detail:

- Ceramides exert their influence in cellular stress response, inflammatory processes, apoptosis and signaling pathways. They are also accumulated in skeletal muscle, promoting insulin resistance and oxidative stress, contributing to the onset and development of cardiometabolic diseases and renal dysfunction [4]. Several inflammatory cytokines may generate ROS and also induce ceramide formation in several cell types [5].
- Diacylglycerols (DAG) act as second messengers affecting signal transduction from many immune cell receptors and can be produced and metabolized through multiple mechanisms. Moreover, DAG induces the hydrolysis of SM to ceramides.
- Sphingomyelins (SM) are reservoirs for other sphingolipids, influencing cell signaling through their structural role in lipid rafts or through the effects of their catabolic mediators (e.g., ceramides) [6]. Changes in SM concentration directly impact cell membrane physiology by modifying its transmission signal.

Thus, we aimed to evaluate the changes in plasma levels of these bioactive lipids in healthy runners performing a half-marathon, at the end of the race and after 24 h recovery, and their associations with new recently proposed and common biomarkers of immune activation, which are:

- The soluble fractalkine CX3CL1, a potent chemoattractant of T cells and monocytes, which has a recognized role in both immune cell migration and adhesion and is involved in many inflammatory processes and diseases [7].
- Vascular endothelial growth factor (VEGF) is a multifactorial cytokine that derives from endothelial cells and pericytes in response to hypoxia, and is implicated in angiogenesis and microvascular hyperpermeability events [8]
- Interleukin-6 (IL-6), which is generated by different cell types (e.g., macrophages, endothelial cells and T cells). The contraction of skeletal muscle may induce the release of IL-6 into the interstitium as well as into blood in response to an exercise burst. Moreover, IL-6 may modulate the immunological and metabolic reactions to exercise [9].
- Tumor necrosis factor alpha (TNFα), an inflammatory cytokine produced by macrophages/monocytes during acute inflammation, which affects different ranges of signaling pathways, including those leading to necrosis or apoptosis [10].

2. Materials and Methods

2.1. Characteristics of the Participants

The studied population included 13 healthy Caucasian trained runners belonging to the "Gruppo Podistico Rossini" enrolled during the 2018 edition of the Pisa half-marathon. Inclusion criteria of athletes were regular training and absence of cardiovascular disease or any other systemic disorder. Preliminarily to the race, each participant was submitted to a questionnaire to obtain demographic and clinical data and training history. Body mass index (BMI) was calculated by height and weight, measured in each subject. Body fat composition (fat-free mass (FFM); fat% and fat mass) was evaluated by TANITA. The study was conducted according to the guidelines of the Declaration of Helsinki, and was approved by the Pisa Ethics Committee, Italy (protocol number for study acceptance 2805). Informed consent was obtained from all subjects enrolled in the study.

2.2. Sample Collection, Preparation and Evaluation of Lipids and Inflammatory Markers

Three blood samples were collected from the peripheral vein of the athletes (in fasting conditions): (1) the day before the race (baseline), (2) within 20 min after the end of the half-marathon (post) and (3) 24 h after the run (24 h, recovery period). Blood samples were immediately centrifuged at 2500 g for 10 min and stored at $-80\,°C$ until assayed.

Ceramides, SM and DAG were evaluated from 20 µL of plasma (upon being deproteinized using 200 µL of cold methanol) in 13 healthy Caucasian trained runners.

An aliquot of 20 µL of a mix of internal standards SM (d18:1/17:0), ceramide (d18:1/17:0), (Avanti Polar Lipids, Alabaster, AL, USA); DAG (17:0/17:0) (Larodan Solna SE) was added to the sample before deproteinization. The extract was injected in high performance liquid chromatography (Agilent UHPLC 1290, Santa Clara, CA, USA), coupled with a quadrupole time-of-flight mass spectrometry QTOF (QTOF-MS, Agilent 6540, Santa Clara, CA, USA), equipped with electrospray ionization source (ESI). For liquid chromatography analysis, we used ZORBAX Eclipse Plus C18 2.1 × 100 mm 1.8-micron column at 50 °C (Agilent, Santa Clara, CA, USA). The mobile phase A was made by water with 0.1% formic acid and the mobile phase B was made by isopropanol/acetonitrile (1:1, v:v) with 0.1% formic acid. Injection volume was 1 µL. Lipids were measured in positive electrospray ionization and identified using an internal spectral library. The data were normalized by internal standard representative lipids present in the sample and the analysis of the peaks was performed with Agilent MassHunter software program [11]. DAG species founded in plasma were 32:0, 32:1, 34:1, 34:2, 36:3 and 36:4, while ceramide species evaluated in plasma sample were 18:1/16:0, 18:1/18:0, 18:1/25:0, 18:1/26:0, 18:1/22:0, 18:1/24:1, 18:1/24:0, 18:0/24:0. The metabocard for ceramide species was reported as supplementary material (supplemental data). Fractalkine CX3CL1, VEGF, IL6 and TNFα were analyzed in 25 µL of plasma by a specific assay (MILLIPLEX MAP Millipore corporation, Billerica, MA, USA) using an integrated multi-analyte detection platform (high-throughput technology MagPix system, Luminex xMAP technology) with combined analyst software (MILLIPLEX®) for the biomarkers quantification developing new curve fitting algorithms and optimizing mathematical methods to minimize fitting errors.

2.3. Statistical Analysis

Data were expressed as mean ± SD. **Repeated-measures ANOVA** was used for compared data from the same subjects measured more than once (baseline, post, 24 h). Correlation analysis was performed by Spearman parametric test to assess the relationship between continuous variables. Post Δ and 24 h Δ values from baseline (differences) and % change at different successive time periods with respect to values observed at baseline were calculated for fractalkine (pg/mL), IL-6 (pg/mL), TNFα (pg/mL) and VEGF-α (pg/mL). Owing to skewness, log transformation of fractalkine and TNFα was used for statistical analyses. Log-transformed values were then back-transformed for data presentation.

Data statistical analyses were performed with the Statview statistical package, version 5.0.1 (SAS Institute, Abacus Concept, Berkeley, CA, USA). A p value of <0.05 was considered statistically significant. Heatmapping was performed using MetaboAnalyst R 1.0.3 (XiaLab at McGill University, Montreal, QC, Canada). The data in heatmaps were analyzed by t test, the algorithm used was the average method and the measure of distance was Euclidean.

3. Results

3.1. Demographic and Training Characteristics

The characteristics of the runners are summarized in Table 1. Each athlete was regularly engaged in marathon training for more than 3 years, 3–7 times/week in 1–2 h/session. Athletes performed a running race over the distance of 21.0975 km. Race time ranged between 1.33 and 1.46 h. No correlation of inflammatory parameters or sphingolipids with demographic and training characteristics was observed. No gender-related differences were observed for all the biomarkers evaluated.

Table 1. Anthropometric measurement of runners and physical activity.

Anthropometric Measurement	Runners N (13)
Age (years)	47 ± 6
Gender (M/F)	7/6
Height (cm)	171.6 ± 2
Weight (kg)	67.5 ± 2.2
BMI (kg/m^2)	21.6 ± 0.7
WAIST (cm)	78.2 ± 3.1
PAS (mmHg)	128.3 ± 5.2
PAD (mmHg)	72.16 ± 2.3
FFM (kg)	55.6 ± 3.6
FAT% (kg)	11.54 ± 1.5
Physical activity	
Day/week of training	4 ± 0.3
Km/week	50.1 ± 4.7
Years of training	6 ± 1
Half-marathon race finish time (min)	105.2 ± 3.7

Abbreviations: BMI: body mass index, PAS: systolic arterial pressure, PAD: diastolic arterial pressure, FFM: free fat mass.

3.2. Lipids Levels and Race-Related Trends

3.2.1. Total Ceramides, DAG and SM

Total ceramides, total DAG and SM at baseline, post and 24 h after the race are reported in Figure 1 (panel A, B and C, respectively). When plasma levels of total ceramides were considered, a significant decrease was observed after the race and after 24 h compared to baseline (12.25 ± 3.0, 8.68 ± 0.62, $p = 0.011$ vs. baseline; 9.70 ± 0.51, µmol/L, $p = 0.059$ vs. baseline; baseline, post-race, 24 h, respectively), Figure 1A. DAG total analysis evidenced a significant decrease post-race compared to baseline (53.26 ± 21.83 vs. 36.07 ± 18.75 µmol/L, post-race vs. baseline, $p = 0.04$; and 51.56 ± 34.25 24 h µmol/L, not significant), Figure 1B. Instead, SM tended to decrease after the race and at 24 h, although not significantly (145.66 ± 44.83; 100.2 ± 8.9; 105 ± 7.31 µmol/L), Figure 1C.

3.2.2. Ceramides, DAG and SM Species

The specific DAG and SM ceramide species at baseline, post and 24 h after the race are shown by heatmaps that provide intuitive visualization of the data table. Each colored cell on the map corresponds to a concentration value in the data file, with samples in rows and compound in columns (supplemental data).

Trends of DAG classes at baseline and after the race are reported in Figure 2. The greatest changes were attributed to the DAG 36:3 that decreased significantly post-race (25.56 ± 10.6 basal vs. 14.89 ± 8.14 post-race $p = 0.01$; 22.44 ± 8.14 24 h µmol/L). The other DAG species followed the same pattern but did not significantly change: DAG 32:0 (1.06 ± 0.26; 2.32 ± 4.6; 1.21 ± 0.71 µmol/L, baseline, post-race, 24 h, respectively); 32:1 (2.07 ± 0.71; 1.64 ± 0.94; 2.24 ± 1.62 µmol/L); 34:1 (8.22 ± 2.68; 5.85 ± 3.32; 8.66 ± 4.54 µmol/L); 34:2 (12.1 ± 4.85; 8.45 ± 4.76; 12.76 ± 9.39 µmol/L) and 36:4 (4.24 ± 4.13; 2.92 ± 2.04; 4.24 ± 3.95 µmol/L) (Figure 2).

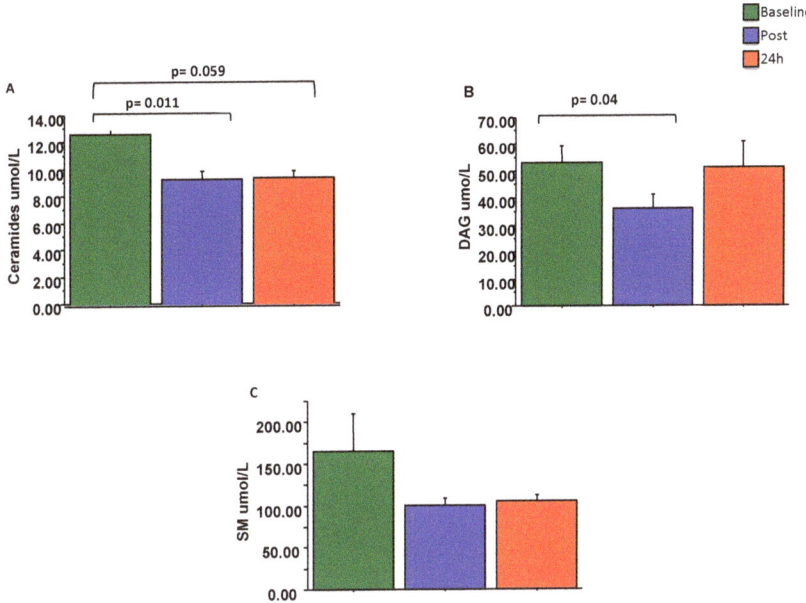

Figure 1. Bar chart reporting mean and SD of total ceramides, total DAG and SM (panel **A**, **B** and **C**, respectively) at baseline, post and 24 h after the race.

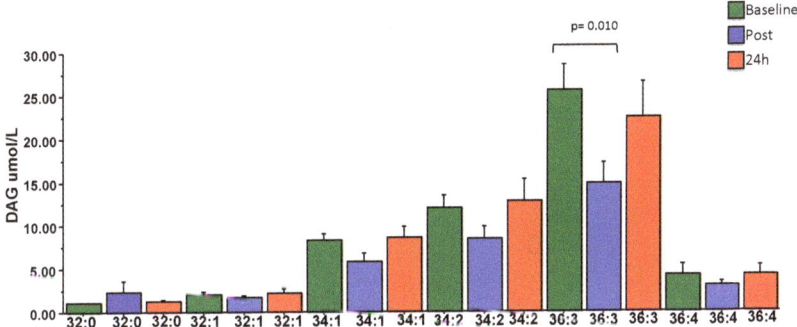

Figure 2. Bar chart reporting the trend of DAG classes as mean and SD at baseline, post and 24 h after the race.

Trends of ceramide species at baseline and after the race are reported in Figure 3. Ceramide species containing long chain fatty acids (18:1/16:0; 18:1/18:0) transiently increased after the race, to significantly decrease at 24 h (0.16 ± 0.06; 0.20 ± 0.05; 0.18 ± 0.04 µmol/L, baseline, post-race, 24 h, respectively); (0.18 ± 0.07; 0.18 ± 0.03; 0.16 ± 0.03 µmol/L) (Figure 3). Instead, ceramides containing very long chain fatty acids, i.e., 18:1/25:0; 18:1/26:0; 18:1/22:0; 18:1/24:1; 18:1/24:0; 18:0/24:0 significantly decreased after the race and at 24 h when compared to baseline (0.82 ± 0.21; 0.55 ± 0.13; 0.62 ± 0.15 µmol/L, baseline, post-race and 24 h, respectively); (0.16 ± 0.05; 0.11 ± 0.03; 0.13 ± 0.03 µmol/L); (1.52 ± 0.35; 1.91 ± 0.50; 1.46 ± 0.43 µmol/L); (3.29 ± 0.91; 2.36 ± 0.60; 2.61 ± 0.38 µmol/L); (5.56 ± 1.4; 1.46 ± 0.43; 4.35 ± 0.95 µmol/L) and (0.17 ± 0.05; 0.12 ± 0.04; 0.13 ± 0.38 µmol/L), Figure 3. SM did not significantly change.

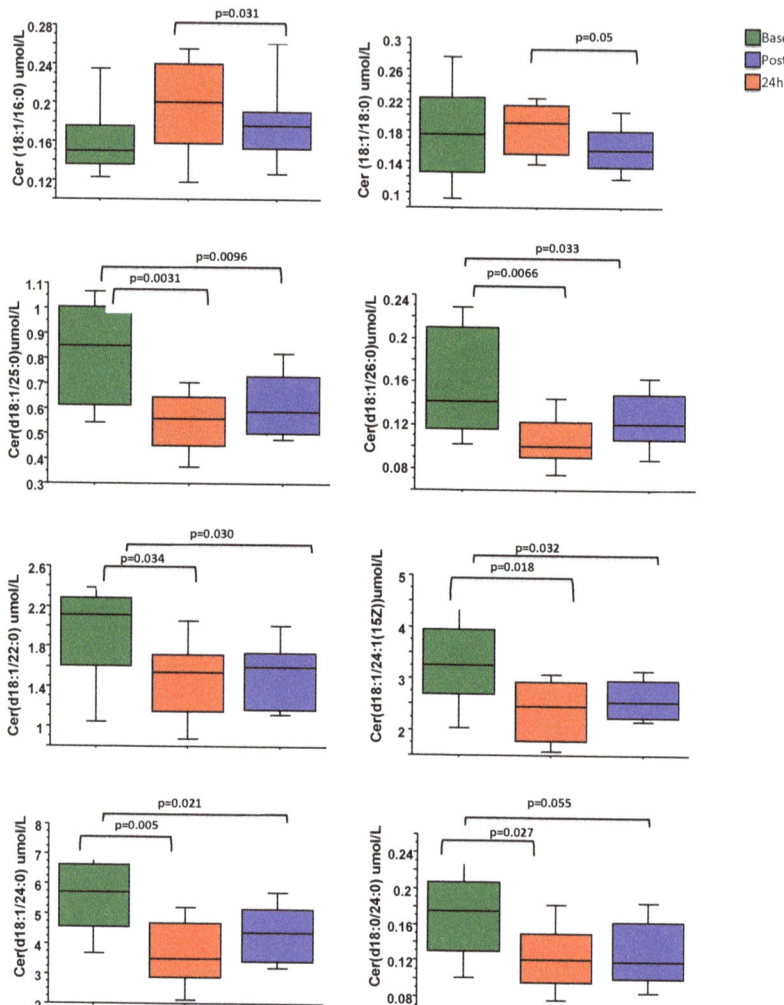

Figure 3. Boxplots with indication of the median, interquartiles and error bars reporting the temporal profile of ceramides are given.

3.3. Inflammatory Levels and Race-Related Trends

Basal plasma levels, post and after 24 h of TNFα, IL-6, fractalkine CX3CL1 and VEGF-A in all runners are reported in Table 2.

Table 2. Plasma values of chemokine and cytokines in runners.

Variables	Mean ± SD		
	Baseline	Post	24 h
Fractalkine (pg/mL)	143.4 ± 124.9	219.6 ± 126.9	107.7 ± 149.4
IL-6 (pg/mL)	0.7 ± 0.6	9.1 ± 6.9	0.64 ± 0.49
TNFα (pg/mL)	32.4 ± 27.8	35.8 ± 29.1	20.5 ± 24.1
VEGF-A (pg/mL)	186.1 ± 128.4	178.5 ± 161.3	147.6 ± 142.8

Cytokines and chemokines at baseline and after the race are reported in Figure 4. IL-6 and fractalkine CX3CL1 significantly changed soon after the race, decreasing towards baseline values after 24 h (Figure 4A,B). TNFα had the same trend but the increment after the race was not significant (Figure 4C). VEGF-A tended to decrease after the race (Figure 4D), but these changes were not significant when compared to baseline. Table 3 shows the exercise-induced change from baseline, as Δ values (% change) for each variable.

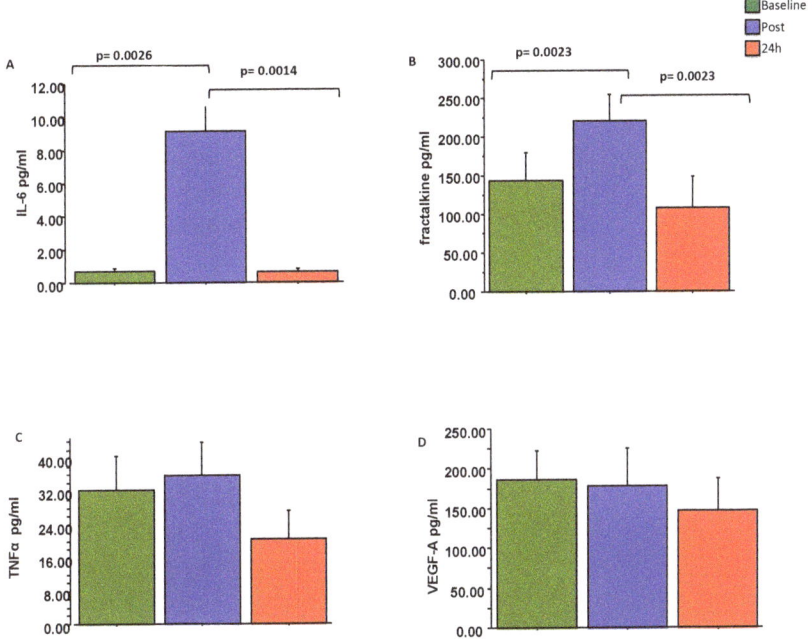

Figure 4. Bar chart reporting mean and SD of cytokines and chemokines at baseline, (**A**) IL-6 (pg/mL), (**B**) Fractalkine (pg/mL), (**C**) TNFα (pg/mL), (**D**) VEGF-A (pg/mL), post and 24 h after the race.

Table 3. Exercise-induced change from baseline, Δ values (% change) in fractalkine, IL-6, TNFα and VEGF-A.

	Pre-Exercise	Post Δ Values from Baseline (% Change)	24 h Δ Values from Baseline (% Change)
Fractalkine (pg/mL)	143.4 ± 124.99	76.2 (53.3%)	−35.7 (−24.9%)
IL-6 (pg/mL)	0.7 ± 0.649	−0.1 (−7.6%)	8.4 (+1208.6%)
TNFα (pg/mL)	32.4 ± 27.844	−11.9 (−36.8%)	3.4 (+10.5%)
VEGF-A (pg/mL)	186.2 ± 128.379	−38.5 (−20.7%)	−7.6 (−4.1%)

Post Δ and 24 h Δ are differences from baseline. % change at different successive time periods with respect to values observed at baseline is reported in brackets.

Interestingly, a strong correlation between basal fractalkine CX3CL1 and TNFα was found at baseline and during recovery (Rho = 0.91 p = 0.0017), Figure 5.

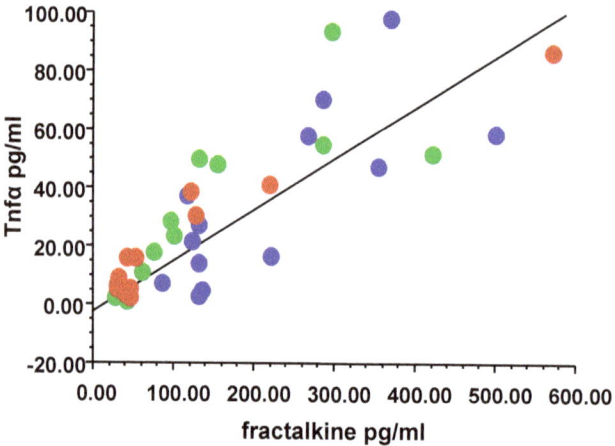

Figure 5. Regression of fractalkine and TNFα in runners (Rho = 0.91 p = 0.0017 24 h). Green dots—baseline, blue dots—post-race, red dots—24 h post-race.

4. Discussion

This is the first study which assessed levels of DAGs and ceramides, and evaluated their relationship with inflammatory parameters in athletes before and after a half-marathon race. Data evidenced the decrease of specific lipid classes, and the lack of relationship between lipids with inflammatory biomarkers, suggesting their possible contribution to exercise-related beneficial effects.

4.1. Demographic and Training Characteristics

The population was similar in demographic and training characteristics; likely, for this reason, we did not observe any correlation concerning inflammatory parameters and sphingolipids. Regarding gender-related differences, it is not clear in literature if ceramides are different in males and females, and neither wheter there is a differential effect of exercise on ceramides in the two sexes. In our population, we did not observe gender-related differences for any of the biomarkers evaluated. Moreover, there is still a lack of a shared consensus on the optimal cutoffs and reference ranges of ceramides to be used. In this context, our data might suggest a lack of need to establish gender-specific reference ranges. However, considering the low number of subjects enrolled in the study, this issue merits further investigation.

Notably, values of inflammatory biomarkers of athletes at baseline did not differ from those observed in a group of 15 sedentary subjects (corresponding to 0.6 ± 3.1 pg/mL for IL-6, 164 ± 145 pg/mL for fractalkine CX3CL1, 23 ± 38 pg/mL for TNFα), except for VEGF-A, which was significantly lower in sedentary subjects (28 ± 61 pg/mL, $p < 0.001$) (unpublished data).

4.2. Lipids Levels and Race-Related Trends

To the best of our knowledge, this is the first report describing half-marathon consequences on circulating sphingolipid metabolism. It is known that exercise may induce modification in plasma levels of numerous circulating biomarkers, inflammatory parameters and lipid metabolites in humans [12] Thus, these changes may affect sphingolipid metabolites as well. In recent years, plasma sphingolipids have attracted attention for their role in pathophysiology of cardiometabolic diseases. In fact, high plasma ceramides may induce endothelial dysfunction, which is closely correlated with aerobic capacity [13], and promote cell growth arrest, cytoskeleton rearrangements, senescence and death (e.g., activation of caspases), impairment of nitric oxide synthase (eNOS) activity and insulin signaling, increasing vascular permeability, oxidative stress and inflammation [14], thus contributing to onset and development of atherosclerosis [15,16]. Accordingly, sphingolipids may represent an independent risk determinant for ischemic disease [17]. In particular, Cer(d18:1/16:0) appears to be independently correlated with the presence of more vulnerable coronary plaques in CAD patients [18]. Conversely, the Mediterranean diet shows the potential to reduce the adverse effects of high ceramide levels in the PREDIMED trial (Prevención con Dieta Mediterranea, a prospective case-cohort study), which is a study including nearly 1000 elderly subjects at high cardiovascular risk [19].

Ceramide metabolism also appears responsive to the exercise stimulus. Better cardiopulmonary fitness correlated with low ceramide concentration in elderly coronary artery disease patients has been observed [20], whereas muscle ceramide levels decreased after chronic aerobic exercise [21]. Moreover, experimental data suggests that total content of ceramides decreased in the muscle in trained rats, contributing to the elevation of the glucose uptake observed in skeletal muscles after training [22]. Previous data suggested that 12 weeks of aerobic exercise training in obese or diabetic subjects [23] and 16 weeks of exercise in overweight/obese subjects may reduce sphingolipids (e.g., C18:0, C20:0 and C24:1) [24].

A decrease in ceramide concentrations hints at increased insulin sensitivity, which contributes, at least in part, to the beneficial exercise effects [25]. According to these previous results, we also observed a decrease in total ceramides after the race in trained subjects. Thus, all together these data suggest that sphingolipid species can represent valuable mediators of cardiovascular risk. Studies related to cardiac lipotoxicity showed that the lipotoxic species were primarily driven by ceramides and DAG and not triacylglycerol [26]. Regarding DAG species, Luukkonen et al. showed that DAG (32:1, 34:1, 36:2, 36:3) were significantly increased in subjects with high peripheral insulin resistance versus low peripheral insulin resistance subjects [27] In our study, DAG 36:3 decreased significantly after the race, indicating an improvement of lipotoxicity, attributable to that species after the acute exercise. Experimental data suggest that total content of ceramides decreases in the muscle of trained rats, contributing to the elevation of the glucose uptake observed in skeletal muscles after training [22]. In overweight, obese subjects or type 2 diabetes (T2D), there is a decrease in total ceramides, indicating that endurance training reduces total content of ceramides, likely improving glucose tolerance [22,25,27–29]. However, ceramide metabolism in patients and obese subjects could be dissimilar to that in lean, trained individuals. In fact, the increased lipid metabolism following the physical exercise reduces the substrate availability required for ceramide synthesis (e.g., palmitate, myristate). Moreover, the analysis of the lipid classes in its total assessment may be unsatisfactory, as the specific and complex relationship of different chains of fatty acids in ceramides with chronic and acute exercise demonstrates the complexity of these biological pathways, which require the assessment of increased, decreased or unchanged specific species. Accordingly, our data, for the first time, associate specific molecular species of lipids to exercise. In particular, Cer18:1/16:0 and Cer18:1/18:0 were very low at baseline in athletes and, after the race, the same ceramides increased, indicating a lower consumption of fatty acids contained in these species (palmitic and stearic acid), making these ceramides a non-preferential species for energy purposes. Mardare, Kruger et al. suggest that endurance training in mice is able to reduce long-chain fatty acids ceramides [28]. In particular, this experimental study suggests that the exercise-induced decrease of very long chain fatty acids ceramides (C24:0 and C24:1) may account, almost in part, for the reduced expression of blood inflammatory markers, as well as the increased glucose tolerance. An elevation in long chain fatty acids (C24:0, C24:1, C26:0, C25:0, C22:0) was associated with mitochondrial damage, apoptosis and cell necrosis [29]. It is not completely clear which are the mechanisms able to prevent the elevation in plasma ceramide level correlated with aerobic exercise. In addition to the possibility that lipid utilization during exercise reduces ceramide production by decreasing the availability of substrates required for ceramide synthesis, there are a number of hypothesis-generating ideas [25]; for example, aerobic exercise may accelerate ceramide degradation and clearance by increasing the expression of genes responsible for ceramide clearance (e.g., acidic and alkaline ceramidase 1 and 3, glucosylceramide synthase and sphingosine kinase 1) [30].

4.3. Inflammatory Levels and Race-Related Trends

IL-6, a pro-inflammatory cytokine, is known to increase after endurance exercise [31]. However, in this setting, IL-6 may have a role as a myokine, and as such, with anti-inflammatory properties, rather than as an inflammatory facilitator [32]. In fact, the observed post-exercise elevations may be in line with exercise-related metabolic IL-6 effects (regulation of glucose homeostasis and fat oxidation) and adaptation to training [33]. Moreover, the release of IL-6 during exercise induces an increase in circulating anti-inflammatory cytokines (e.g., IL-10 and IL-1 receptor antagonist) and decrease of TNFα, or the release of cortisol from the adrenal glands, suggesting that the beneficial effects of exercise (IL-6-mediated) can be expressed, almost in part, through protection against TNFα-induced insulin resistance [34]. These responses, which probably mediate autocrine and paracrine benefits of training, are likely related to training levels, intensity and type of exercise and individual characteristics (e.g., sex and age), and thus may be different in different categories of subjects. Instead, relatively low information is known on the balance between IL-6 and other cytokines and inflammatory biomarkers under such conditions. TNFα did not increase significantly in our population, and this may be the effect of the anti-inflammatory cytokine cascade, which may oppose TNFα increase, giving protection against TNFα-induced damage, as previously observed [35].

CX3CL1 exists in two forms; one form anchors to the membrane, acting as an adhesion molecule, whereas the other form acts as a soluble chemoattractant. CX3CL1 A acts in acute skeletal muscle damage and regeneration through recruitment of macrophages and other immune cells involved in repair and growth of skeletal muscle, influencing the adaptive response to exercise [36,37]. As in our population, previous data suggested an increase of CX3CL1 related to exercise (e.g., cycling) [38]. The variation of circulating CX3CL1 is closely related to changes in muscle gene expression, and as such, might have significance in the adaptive response to exercise [38,39]. Moreover, local CX3CL1 synthesis and expression depend on many factors, including inflammatory cytokines (e.g., TNFα), giving evidence of the relationship that we observed between these two biomarkers [40]. Experimental data suggested that CX3CL1 stimulation of monocytes is associated with a marked increase of TNFα, which is known to stimulate satellite cell proliferation [41,42]. Accordingly, we observed a strong correlation between fractalkine and TNFα, suggesting that this effect could represent an indirect mechanism by which CX3CL1 acts as a mitogen for muscle cells. Moreover, CX3CL1 seems to have beneficial effects in muscle regeneration through a direct effect on myogenic cells [43]. Thus, CX3CL1 likely induces the monocytic and myogenic expression of different factors known to increase in human skeletal muscle after exercise, with a role in the adaptive response following an exercise burst.

Interestingly, in our population, inflammatory biomarkers did not influence the relationships between sphingolipids and exercise, not supporting the existence of a link between inflammation and sphingolipids in half-marathon response, although further studies are needed to verify this possibility. In this context, we also did not observe any relationship between total and species of SM, ceramides and DAG and reactive oxygen species (ROM, a biomarker of oxidative stress) (unshown data) [44].

4.4. Strengths and Limitations

This study has limitations. First, the number of athletes enrolled is not high. However, a strength is that studied athletes were very similar according to training characteristics (day/week of training, Km/week, years of training). Moreover, each subject served as a control for him/herself, increasing the statistical power, and reducing the effects of confounding factors.

Second, insulin was not directly assessed in these subjects. This important issue merits further investigation in future studies to understand the link between species of lipids, inflammatory markers and insulin resistance (IR) during exercise. However, all our subjects had no history of IR and type 2 diabetes (T2D) and they showed normal body mass index; therefore, this relationship could be negligible. Nonetheless, it will be interesting to assess exercise effects on lipid-related biomarkers in IR, T2D or obese subjects in future studies.

5. Conclusions

IL-6 and CX3CL1 transiently increased soon after the half-marathon. As they are promptly reversible, these changes might represent a physiological response to acute exercise rather than a damage-related response. The decrease in plasma ceramide concentration observed after the race and the lack of their relationship with inflammatory mediators suggested the involvement of lipids in exercise adaptation, as well as their possible role in mechanisms underlying beneficial effects of regular physical activity on disease prevention, especially regarding cardiometabolic disease. This opens up a new area of investigation for future research to establish whether the measurement of specific plasma ceramides could provide new biomarkers useful to assess exercise adaptation and to evaluate specific exercise interventions in different categories of healthy subjects and patients.

Supplementary Materials: The following are available online at https://www.mdpi.com/article/10.3390/app11104622/s1.

Author Contributions: All authors discussed the results and contributed to the final manuscript. M.G., C.V. and A.P.: study concept; L.S.: certified English revision; F.S., F.C., M.M., E.B., F.M. and L.S.: acquisition, measurement and analysis of data; M.G., C.V., A.P. and A.G.: interpretation of data; M.G. and C.V.: drafting of the manuscript. All authors contributed to the manuscript's intellectual content and gave approval for the final version. All authors have read and agreed to the published version of the manuscript.

Funding: This research received no external funding.

Institutional Review Board Statement: The study was conducted according to the guidelines of the Declaration of Helsinki and was approved by the Pisa Ethics Committee, Italy, (protocol number for study acceptance 2805).

Informed Consent Statement: Informed consent was obtained from all subjects involved in the study.

Data Availability Statement: Data are available from authors upon reasonable request.

Acknowledgments: The authors acknowledge the athletes of "Gruppo Podistico Rossini (www.podisticarossini.it accessed on 15 May 2021)" for the fundamental contribution.

Conflicts of Interest: The authors declare no conflict of interest.

References

1. Knechtle, B.; Nikolaidis, P.T.; Zingg, M.A.; Rosemann, T.; Rüst, C.A. Half-marathoners are younger and slower than marathoners. *SpringerPlus* **2016**, *5*, 1–16. [CrossRef]
2. Nieman, D.C.; Henson, D.A.; Smith, L.L.; Utter, A.C.; Vinci, D.M.; Davis, J.M.; Kaminsky, D.E.; Shute, M. Cytokine changes after a marathon race. *J. Appl. Physiol.* **2001**, *91*, 109–114. [CrossRef]
3. Nikolova-Karakashian, M.N.; Reid, M.B. Sphingolipid Metabolism, Oxidant Signaling, and Contractile Function of Skeletal Muscle. *Antioxidants Redox Signal.* **2011**, *15*, 2501–2517. [CrossRef] [PubMed]
4. Nishi, H.; Higashihara, T.; Inagi, R. Lipotoxicity in Kidney, Heart, and Skeletal Muscle Dysfunction. *Nutrients* **2019**, *11*, 1664. [CrossRef]
5. Portt, L.; Norman, G.; Clapp, C.; Greenwood, M.; Greenwood, M.T. Anti-apoptosis and cell survival: A review. *Biochim. Biophys. Acta (BBA) Bioenerg.* **2011**, *1813*, 238–259. [CrossRef]
6. Chakraborty, M.; Jiang, X.-C. Sphingomyelin and Its Role in Cellular Signaling. *Chem. Biol. Pteridines Folates* **2013**, *991*, 1–14. [CrossRef]
7. Conroy, M.J.; Maher, S.G.; Melo, A.M.; Doyle, S.L.; Foley, E.; Reynolds, J.V.; Long, A.; Lysaght, J. Identifying a Novel Role for Fractalkine (CX3CL1) in Memory CD8+ T Cell Accumulation in the Omentum of Obesity-Associated Cancer Patients. *Front. Immunol.* **2018**, *9*, 1867. [CrossRef] [PubMed]
8. Gunga, H.-C.; Kirsch, K.; Behn, C.; Koralewski, E.; Davila, E.H.; Estrada, M.I.; Johannes, B.; Wittels, P.; Jelkmann, W. Vascular endothelial growth factor in exercising humans under different environmental conditions. *Graefe's Arch. Clin. Exp. Ophthalmol.* **1999**, *79*, 484–490. [CrossRef] [PubMed]

9. Fischer, C.P. Interleukin-6 in acute exercise and training: What is the biological relevance? *Exerc. Immunol. Rev.* **2006**, *12*, 41.
10. Idriss, H.T.; Naismith, J.H. TNFα and the TNF receptor superfamily: Structure-function relationship(s). *Microsc. Res. Tech.* **2000**, *50*, 184–195. [CrossRef]
11. Hackl, M.T.; Fürnsinn, C.; Schuh, C.M.; Krssak, M.; Carli, F.; Guerra, S.; Freudenthaler, A.; Baumgartner-Parzer, S.; Helbich, T.H.; Luger, A.; et al. Brain leptin reduces liver lipids by increasing hepatic triglyceride secretion and lowering lipogenesis. *Nat. Commun.* **2019**, *10*, 1–13. [CrossRef]
12. Lewis, G.D.; Farrell, L.; Wood, M.J.; Martinovic, M.; Arany, Z.; Rowe, G.C.; Souza, A.; Cheng, S.; McCabe, E.L.; Yang, E.; et al. Metabolic Signatures of Exercise in Human Plasma. *Sci. Transl. Med.* **2010**, *2*, 33–37. [CrossRef] [PubMed]
13. Montero, D. The association of cardiorespiratory fitness with endothelial or smooth muscle vasodilator function. *Eur. J. Prev. Cardiol.* **2015**, *22*, 1200–1211. [CrossRef] [PubMed]
14. Haus, J.M.; Kashyap, S.R.; Kasumov, T.; Zhang, R.; Kelly, K.R.; DeFronzo, R.A.; Kirwan, J.P. Plasma Ceramides Are Elevated in Obese Subjects With Type 2 Diabetes and Correlate With the Severity of Insulin Resistance. *Diabetes* **2008**, *58*, 337–343. [CrossRef]
15. Ichi, I.; Nakahara, K.; Miyashita, Y.; Hidaka, A.; Kutsukake, S.; Inoue, K.; Maruyama, T.; Miwa, Y.; Harada-Shiba, M.; Tsushima, M.; et al. Association of ceramides in human plasma with risk factors of atherosclerosis. *Lipids* **2006**, *41*, 859–863. [CrossRef]
16. Bismuth, J.; Lin, P.; Yao, Q.; Chen, C. Ceramide: A common pathway for atherosclerosis? *Atherosclerosis* **2008**, *196*, 497–504. [CrossRef]
17. Jiang, X.-C.; Paultre, F.; Pearson, T.A.; Reed, R.G.; Francis, C.K.; Lin, M.; Berglund, L.; Tall, A.R. Plasma Sphingomyelin Level as a Risk Factor for Coronary Artery Disease. *Arter. Thromb. Vasc. Biol.* **2000**, *20*, 2614–2618. [CrossRef]
18. Anroedh, S.S.; Hilvo, M.; Akkerhuis, K.M.; Kauhanen, D.; Koistinen, K.; Oemrawsingh, R.; Serruys, P.; van Geuns, R.-J.; Boersma, E.; Laaksonen, R.; et al. Plasma concentrations of molecular lipid species predict long-term clinical outcome in coronary artery disease patients. *J. Lipid Res.* **2018**, *59*, 1729–1737. [CrossRef]
19. Wang, D.D.; Toledo, E.; Hruby, A.; Rosner, B.A.; Willett, W.C.; Sun, Q.; Razquin, C.; Zheng, Y.; Ruiz-Canela, M.; Guasch-Ferré, M.; et al. Plasma Ceramides, Mediterranean Diet, and Incident Cardiovascular Disease in the PREDIMED Trial (Prevención con Dieta Mediterránea). *Circulation* **2017**, *135*, 2028–2040. [CrossRef]
20. Saleem, M.; Herrmann, N.; Dinoff, A.; Marzolini, S.; Mielke, M.M.; Andreazza, A.; I Oh, P.; Venkata, S.L.V.; Haughey, N.J.; Lanctôt, K.L. Association Between Sphingolipids and Cardiopulmonary Fitness in Coronary Artery Disease Patients Undertaking Cardiac Rehabilitation. *J. Gerontol. Ser. A Biol. Sci. Med. Sci.* **2020**, *75*, 671–679. [CrossRef]
21. Bruce, C.R.; Thrush, A.B.; Mertz, V.A.; Bezaire, V.; Chabowski, A.; Heigenhauser, G.J.F.; Dyck, D.J. Endurance training in obese humans improves glucose tolerance and mitochondrial fatty acid oxidation and alters muscle lipid content. *Am. J. Physiol. Metab.* **2006**, *291*, E99–E107. [CrossRef]
22. Dobrzyń, A.; Zendzian-Piotrowska, M.; Górski, J. Effect of endurance training on the sphingomyelin-signalling pathway activity in the skeletal muscles of the rat. *J. Physiol. Pharmacol. Off. J. Pol. Physiol. Soc.* **2004**, *55*, 305–313.
23. Kasumov, T.; Solomon, T.P.; Hwang, C.; Huang, H.; Haus, J.M.; Zhang, R.; Kirwan, J.P. Improved insulin sensitivity after exercise training is linked to reduced plasma C14:0 ceramide in obesity and type 2 diabetes. *Obesity* **2015**, *23*, 1414–1421. [CrossRef] [PubMed]
24. Dubé, J.J.; Amati, F.; Toledo, F.G.S.; Stefanovic-Racic, M.; Rossi, A.; Coen, P.; Goodpaster, B.H. Effects of weight loss and exercise on insulin resistance, and intramyocellular triacylglycerol, diacylglycerol and ceramide. *Diabetologia* **2011**, *54*, 1147–1156. [CrossRef]
25. Scherer, P.E.; Hill, J.A. Obesity, Diabetes, and Cardiovascular Diseases. *Circ. Res.* **2016**, *118*, 1703–1705. [CrossRef] [PubMed]
26. Luukkonen, P.K.; Zhou, Y.; Sädevirta, S.; Leivonen, M.; Arola, J.; Orešič, M.; Hyötyläinen, T.; Yki-Järvinen, H. Hepatic ceramides dissociate steatosis and insulin resistance in patients with non-alcoholic fatty liver disease. *J. Hepatol.* **2016**, *64*, 1167–1175. [CrossRef] [PubMed]
27. Dubé, J.J.; Amati, F.; Stefanovic-Racic, M.; Toledo, F.G.S.; Sauers, S.E.; Goodpaster, B.H. Exercise-induced alterations in intramyocellular lipids and insulin resistance: The athlete's paradox revisited. *Am. J. Physiol. Metab.* **2008**, *294*, E882–E888. [CrossRef] [PubMed]
28. Bergman, B.C.; Brozinick, J.T.; Strauss, A.; Bacon, S.; Kerege, A.; Bui, H.H.; Sanders, P.; Siddall, P.; Kuo, M.S.; Perreault, L. Serum sphingolipids: Relationships to insulin sensitivity and changes with exercise in humans. *Am. J. Physiol. Metab.* **2015**, *309*, E398–E408. [CrossRef] [PubMed]
29. Mardare, C.; Krüger, K.; Liebisch, G.; Seimetz, M.; Couturier, A.; Ringseis, R.; Wilhelm, J.; Weissmann, N.; Eder, K.; Mooren, F.-C. Endurance and Resistance Training Affect High Fat Diet-Induced Increase of Ceramides, Inflammasome Expression, and Systemic Inflammation in Mice. *J. Diabetes Res.* **2015**, *2016*, 1–13. [CrossRef] [PubMed]
30. Hartmann, D.; Lucks, J.; Fuchs, S.; Schiffmann, S.; Schreiber, Y.; Ferreirós, N.; Merkens, J.; Marschalek, R.; Geisslinger, G.; Grösch, S. Long chain ceramides and very long chain ceramides have opposite effects on human breast and colon cancer cell growth. *Int. J. Biochem. Cell Biol.* **2012**, *44*, 620–628. [CrossRef]
31. Cappuccilli, M.; Mosconi, G.; Roi, G.; De Fabritiis, M.; Totti, V.; Merni, F.; Trerotola, M.; Marchetti, A.; La Manna, G.; Costa, A.N. Inflammatory and Adipose Response in Solid Organ Transplant Recipients After a Marathon Cycling Race. *Transplant. Proc.* **2016**, *48*, 408–414. [CrossRef] [PubMed]

32. Gill, S.K.; Teixeira, A.; Rama, L.; Prestes, J.; Rosado, F.; Hankey, J.; Scheer, V.; Hemmings, K.; Ansley-Robson, P.; Costa, R.J.S. Circulatory endotoxin concentration and cytokine profile in response to exertional-heat stress during a multi-stage ultra-marathon competition. *Exerc. Immunol. Rev.* **2015**, *21*, 114–128.
33. Pedersen, B.K.; Åkerström, T.C.A.; Nielsen, A.R.; Fischer, C.P. Role of myokines in exercise and metabolism. *J. Appl. Physiol.* **2007**, *103*, 1093–1098. [CrossRef]
34. Ostrowski, K.; Rohde, T.; Asp, S.; Schjerling, P.; Pedersen, B.K. Pro- and anti-inflammatory cytokine balance in strenuous exercise in humans. *J. Physiol.* **1999**, *515*, 287–291. [CrossRef]
35. Febbraio, M.A.; Pedersen, B.K. Muscle-derived interleukin-6: Mechanisms for activation and possible biological roles. *FASEB J.* **2002**, *16*, 1335–1347. [CrossRef]
36. Chapman, G.A.; Moores, K.E.; Gohil, J.; Berkhout, T.A.; Patel, L.; Green, P.; Macphee, C.H.; Stewart, B.R. The role of fractalkine in the recruitment of monocytes to the endothelium. *Eur. J. Pharmacol.* **2000**, *392*, 189–195. [CrossRef]
37. Goda, S.; Imai, T.; Yoshie, O.; Yoneda, O.; Inoue, H.; Nagano, Y.; Okazaki, T.; Imai, H.; Bloom, E.T.; Domae, N.; et al. CX3C-Chemokine, Fractalkine-Enhanced Adhesion of THP-1 Cells to Endothelial Cells Through Integrin-Dependent and -Independent Mechanisms. *J. Immunol.* **2000**, *164*, 4313–4320. [CrossRef]
38. Catoire, M.; Mensink, M.; Kalkhoven, E.; Schrauwen, P.; Kersten, S. Identification of human exercise-induced myokines using secretome analysis. *Physiol. Genom.* **2014**, *46*, 256–267. [CrossRef] [PubMed]
39. Pillon, N.J.; Bilan, P.J.; Fink, L.N.; Klip, A. Cross-talk between skeletal muscle and immune cells: Muscle-derived mediators and metabolic implications. *Am. J. Physiol. Metab.* **2013**, *304*, E453–E465. [CrossRef] [PubMed]
40. Wojdasiewicz, P.; Turczyn, P.; Dobies-Krzesniak, B.; Frasunska, J.; Tarnacka, B. Role of CX3CL1/CX3CR1 Signaling Axis Activity in Osteoporosis. *Mediat. Inflamm.* **2019**, *2019*, 1–9. [CrossRef]
41. Strömberg, A.; Olsson, K.; Dijksterhuis, J.P.; Rullman, E.; Schulte, G.; Gustafsson, T. CX3CL1—A macrophage chemoattractant induced by a single bout of exercise in human skeletal muscle. *Am. J. Physiol. Integr. Comp. Physiol.* **2016**, *310*, R297–R304. [CrossRef] [PubMed]
42. Li, Y.-P. TNF-α is a mitogen in skeletal muscle. *Am. J. Physiol. Physiol.* **2003**, *285*, C370–C376. [CrossRef] [PubMed]
43. Sonnet, C.; Lafuste, P.; Arnold, L.; Brigitte, M.; Poron, F.; Authier, F.J.; Chrétien, F.; Gherardi, R.K.; Chazaud, B. Human macrophages rescue myoblasts and myotubes from apoptosis through a set of adhesion molecular systems. *J. Cell Sci.* **2006**, *119*, 2497–2507. [CrossRef]
44. Vassalle, C.; Del Turco, S.; Sabatino, L.; Basta, G.; Maltinti, M.; Sbrana, F.; Ndreu, R.; Mastorci, F.; Pingitore, A. New inflammatory and oxidative stress-based biomarker changes in response to a half-marathon in recreational athletes. *J. Sports Med. Phys. Fit.* **2020**, *60*. [CrossRef]

MDPI
St. Alban-Anlage 66
4052 Basel
Switzerland
Tel. +41 61 683 77 34
Fax +41 61 302 89 18
www.mdpi.com

Applied Sciences Editorial Office
E-mail: applsci@mdpi.com
www.mdpi.com/journal/applsci

www.ingramcontent.com/pod-product-compliance
Lightning Source LLC
LaVergne TN
LVHW070439100526
838202LV00014B/1626